SERVICING MEDICAL & BIOELECTRONIC EQUIPMENT

No. 930
$10.95

SERVICING MEDICAL & BIOELECTRONIC EQUIPMENT

by Joseph J. Carr, Senior Bioelectronics Technician—
The George Washington University Medical Center

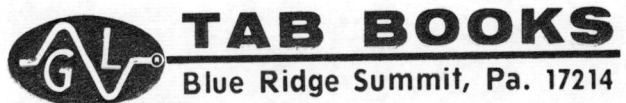

TAB BOOKS
Blue Ridge Summit, Pa. 17214

FIRST EDITION

FIRST PRINTING—FEBRUARY 1977

Copyright © 1977 by TAB BOOKS

Printed in the United States
of America

Reproduction or publication of the content in any manner, without express permission of the publisher, is prohibited. No liability is assumed with respect to the use of the information herein.

Library of Congress Cataloging in Publication Data

Carr, Joseph J
  Servicing medical & bioelectronic equipment.

  Bibliography: p.
  Includes index.
  1. Medical instruments and apparatus--Maintenance and repair. 2. Medical electronics--Equipment and supplies--Maintenance and repair. I. Title.
R856.5.C37   681'.761   77-73
ISBN 0-8306-7930-8
ISBN 0-8306-6930-2 pbk.

Preface

Medical instrumentation is one of the fastest growing areas of electronic technology and promises to continue its growth for some time to come. This has created a rather substantial employment market for electronic personnel at all but the most elementary levels.

In this book we introduce you to medical instrumentation from the point of view of the service technician, who may have to repair, install, calibrate, or even operate such equipment. We are pretty much forced to limit the discussion to coverage of the more common *clinical* instruments such as might be found in almost any well-equipped, modern hospital. Highly specialized research instruments—which are themselves the subject of research—and some of the more sophisticated and esoteric instruments found in the laboratory and nuclear medicine cannot be treated here.

It is assumed that you have some minor knowledge of human anatomy and physiology. This is necessary so that you can understand the medical personnel who use the equipment. For this knowledge you can go to almost any nursing-level anatomy and physiology textbook or to *Introduction to Medical Electronics* by Burton Klein (TAB book No. 830). I consider Klein's book something of a prerequisite to this work and well worth reading because you will gain an introduction to descriptive physiology.

You will find that some employers of electronic technicians in the medical area—especially hospitals—either require or give preference to technicians who are certified. Many other employers will either offer premium pay or career advancement to the certified technician. You will soon note that fully half the people who wander about hospitals have name tags boasting some sort of initials after their names, such as John Doe, C.E.T.

For electronics people there are several options open. If qualified as an engineer, there is the professional engineer (P.E.) registration. P.E. licensure is a function of the individual states and those interested should contact the proper authorities. Incidentally, considering the malpractice climate, it might be wise to have a P.E. on the staff.

Another alternative for the engineer is certification as a clinical engineer. There are two groups offering such certification. One is the American Board of Clinical Engineering Examiners, the other is the Association for the Advancement of Medical Instrumentation (AAMI). This latter group also arranges certification for Biomedical Equipment Technicians (BMET). Its address as of this writing is:

> A.A.M.I.
> Suite 602
> 1901 Fort Myer Drive
> Arlington, Va., 22209

Also offering certification for medical electronics technicians is the International Society of Certified Electronics Technicians (ISCET), which now offers a biomedical option to the well known Certified Electronic Technician (C.E.T.) program. Their address is:

> I.S.C.E.T
> 1715 Expo Lane
> Indianapolis, Ind., 46224

A study guide is available for the C.E.T. medical option, which was written by the author of this book: *C.E.T. License Handbook, 2nd Edition* (TAB book No. 901).

In some places throughout this book, I have departed from standard practice in the medical sciences in the use of *mm Hg* for the pressure unit. Instead, I have used *torr* as the unit of pressure, in keeping with standard practice in the physical sciences of chemistry and physics. But do not be confused, 1 torr = 1 mmHg.

The preparation of any book requires assistance from many people and organizations. It is fitting that these be publicly thanked for their services, advice, forbearance, or whatever contribution they were able to make. First of all, I would like to thank my co-workers, Mr. Milton Shockley and Mr. Chuck McCullough of the Bioelectronics Laboratory at The George Washington University Medical Center, and Mr. Michael Shaffer, director of the laboratory. Also of the university medical center, and due great appreciation, are the chief monitoring technician in the Department of Anesthesiology, Miss Jeanette Kuhn, R.N. and her crew of monitoring technicians. I would like to express thanks to Mr. Gene Banasiak and Mr. Norman McElroy (radiologic engineer and radiation physicist, respectively) for assistance with the chapter on X-rays and parts of the scientific instruments chapter. Technical advice was generously given by Professor Marvin F. Eisenberg, Director of the Medical Engineering Program at the School of Engineering and Applied Science of The George Washington University.

Special thanks go to Mr. Ron Hatch of Hewlett-Packard Service and Mr. Al Magnusen of American Optical. Technical information and illustrations were supplied by Hewlett-Packard and by Mr Al Norment and Mr. George Lambert of American Optical. Also supplying photos and other assistance were Electronics-for-Medicine, Parke-Davis, Neurodyne-Dempsey, General Medical Industries, The Ritter Company, Park Electronics Laboratories, Tektronix, Roche Medical Electronics, Bio-Design, and Honeywell Metrology (a servicer of medical electronics).

I would also like to extend special thanks to the nursing staffs of CCU and PCCU at The George Washington University Hospital for waking me up by telephone in the middle of the night often enough for me to find out what medical electronics is *really* all about. Extra, super-special appreciation is due one particular (*very* particular) CCU nurse, Bonita L. Carr, R.N., mostly because she is married to and adored by the author!

Joseph J. Carr
Bioelectronics Laboratory
The George Washington University
Medical Center

Contents

1 Electrocardiograph Machines — 11
ECG Leads—ECG Machine Operation—Evaluating ECG Machine Performance—ECG Electronics

2 Medical Electrodes and Transducers — 34
Medical Electrodes—Temperature Transducers—Plethysmographic Transducers—Blood Pressure Transducers—Crystal Transducers—Extending Transducer Usefullness

3 Blood Pressure Amplifiers — 48
Direct Measurement—Blood Pressure Amplifier Circuitry—Pressure Processors

4 Medical Oscilloscopes — 67
Oscilloscope Sweep Circuits—Sweep Triggering—Vertical Amplifiers—Non-Fade Displays—Testing Oscilloscopes

5 Bedside and Portable Monitors — 90
General Features—Typical Bedside Monitor Systems—ECG Preamplifiers—Cardiotachometers—Monitor Alarms—Portable Monitors

6 ICU/CCU Multibed Monitoring Systems — 115
Typical System Configuration—System Connections—Recording Instruments—Alarm Modules—Selecting and Displaying Information—Computerized Systems—Servicing Considerations in Central Systems

7 Strip Chart Recorders — 128
Writing Techniques—PMMC Galvanometer—Recorder Electronics—Adjustments and Typical Faults—Servorecorders

8 Defibrillators and Cardioverters 148
Basic Configurations—Cardioverters—Quantitative Testing—Spares and Repairs

9 Electrosurgical Generators 165
How They Work—Cut Oscillator—Spark Gap Coagulator—Modern Designs—Maintenance

10 Cardiographic and Catheterization Lab Equipment 180
Cath Lab Instrumentation—Phonocardiographs—Exercise ECG Laboratories—Computer-Based Systems—Holter Monitors—Cardiac Output Computers

11 Cardiac Radio Telemetry 196
FM Terms and Techniques—Typical ECG Telemetry Transmitters—Frequency Modulation Receivers—Servicing FM Telemetry

12 Scientific Instruments in Clinical Use 210
pH Meters—A Typical pH Meter—Blood Gas Analyzers—Radiation Detectors—Scintillation Counters—Semiconductor Radiation Detectors—Typical Geiger Counter Circuits—Densitometers—Filter and Flame Photometers

13 Ultrasonic Instruments 228
Ultrasonic Transducers—Properites of Sound Waves—Ultrasonic Doppler Flow Detector—Fetal Heart Detectors—Servicing Doppler Equipment—Echoencephalographs

14 Balloon Pumps, Pneumotachometers, and Cardiomemories 245
Intra-Aortic Balloon Pumps—Pneumotachometers—ECG Memory Recorders

15 Test Instruments and Repair Facilities 266
Facilities—Special Test Equipment—Medical Instrumentation Calibration System

16 Electrical Safety 282
Electrical Shock—Mechanics of Microshock—Potentially Dangerous Situations—Equipotential Ground Systems—Isolated Electrical Systems—Points Insuring Safe Systems

17 X-Ray Apparatus 294
Properties of X-Ray—Photoelectric Effect—Compton Effect—Bremsstrahlung—X-Ray Tubes—High-Voltage Power Sources—Typical X-Ray Machines—Design Variations—Scatter Reduction—Image Intensifiers—Some X-Ray Terms

18 Lung, Blood Gas, and Dialysis Machines 314
Respiratory Measurements—Spirometers—Gas measurements—Kidney Dialysis Machines—Some Final Advice

Appendices 325

1 Bibliography 327

2 Medical Prefixes, Suffixes, and Roots 330

3 Medical Glossary 336

Index 342

Chapter 1
Electrocardiograph Machines

Electrocardiographs (abbreviated ECG, or EKG after the German spelling) are probably the oldest class of electronic medical instruments. Their long clinical history and almost universal distribution to even the smallest doctor's office and clinic attest to their importance. The basic ECG machine picks up minute voltages on the surface of the patient's skin that are generated by the heart. The function of the ECG machine is to draw an amplitude-vs-time graph of the waveform on a special graph paper. Figures 1-1 and 1-2 show typical roll-around and portable versions of this useful machine.

The weak bioelectric potentials picked up and displayed by the ECG machine are generated by the cells of the heart. These cells, as well as many other types of cells in the body, can be viewed as a form of miniature, biological battery. Under normal circumstances, both sodium and potassium are found on each side of the cell wall, or *membrane*. In illustration Fig. 1-3, only one element on each side of the wall is shown because the relative concentrations are so different. Inside the cell, for example, the fluid has a concentration of potassium that is approximately thirty times that of sodium. On the outside, the concentration of sodium is approximately ten times that of potassium. These concentration gradients produce an electrical potential difference across the cell wall of about 90 millivolts (mV), with the inside being negative with

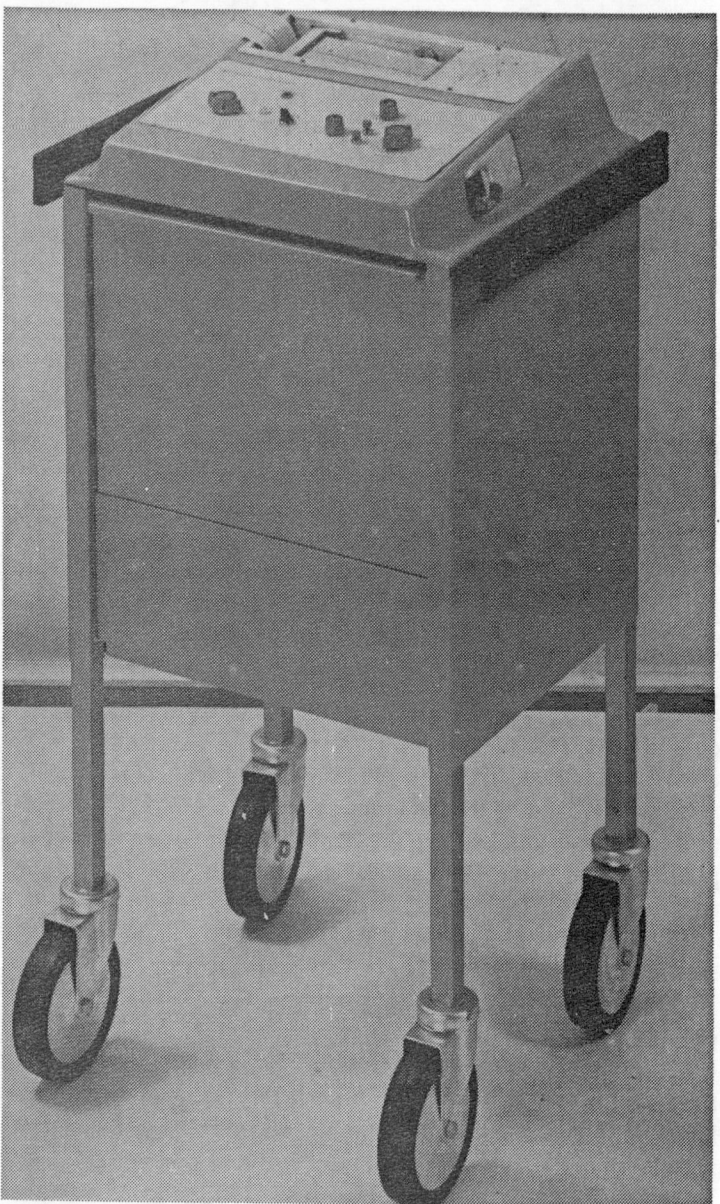

Fig. 1-1. A bedside electrocardiograph on wheels. (Courtesy Hewlett-Packard)

respect to the outside. Not exactly a powerhouse, but a battery of rather substantial voltage nonetheless.

When the heart cell is stimulated, the nature of its membrane wall changes so that it becomes more permeable to sodium ions. This allows sodium ions to rush into the cell in an attempt to reduce or neutralize the imbalance in concentration. The voltage drop across the cell wall during this period (Fig. 1-4) switches rapidly from approximately −90 mV, the *resting* potential, to an *action* potential of approximately +20 mV. At this point the cell is said to be *depolarized*. The characteristics of the cell wall then change back to the prestimulus condition. During this period, called the *repolarization period*, the membrane potential gradient drops back to its −90 mV resting level. Once the cell is triggered by a stimulus, it will go through this cycle completely and cannot be retriggered until after it is repolarized. In this sense, the cell is anologous to the familiar electronic circuit called the monostable multivibrator or one shot.

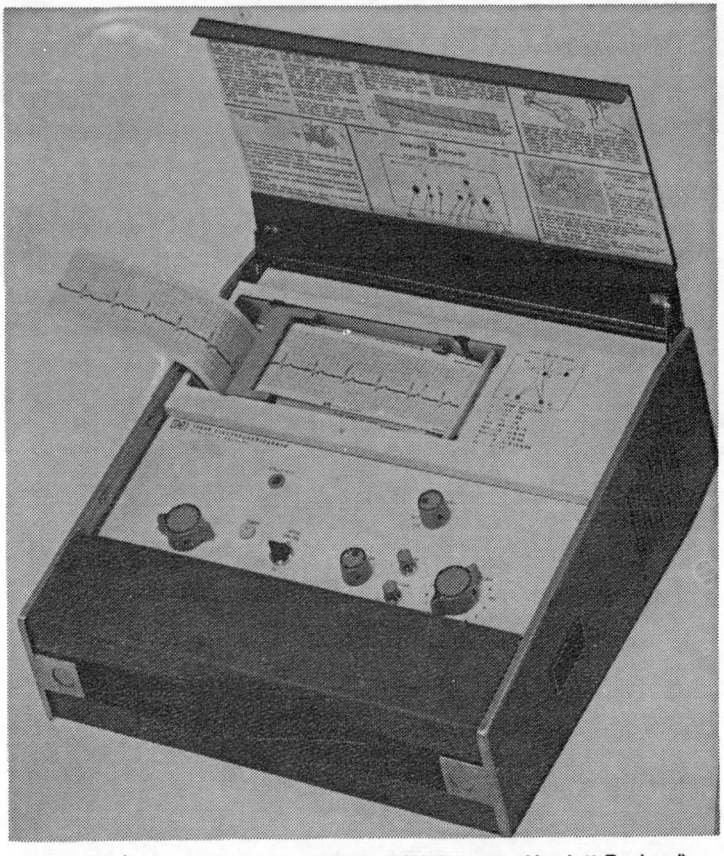

Fig. 1-2. A portable electrocardiograph. (Courtesy Hewlett-Packard)

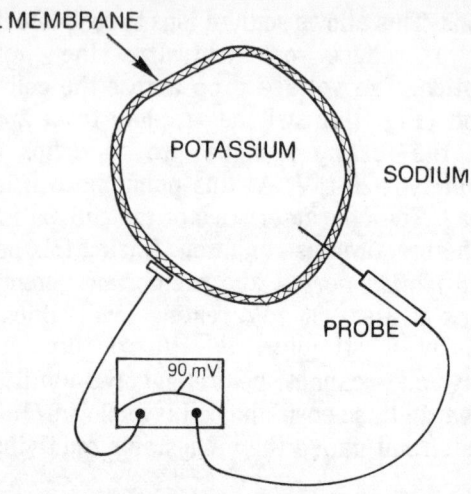

Fig. 1-3. Sodium and potassium concentrations inside and outside of the cell membrane generate small voltages as the heart beats.

The cells of the heart generate a current from the cell depolarizations as it beats. The vector sum of these currents can be picked up as voltage drops across various points on the surface of the skin (Fig. 1-5). Different views of the heart's electrical activity result in different waveforms, and these are obtained from different points on the patient's body. Each of these views is called a *lead* in ECG terminology. (Since you can expect your medical customers or colleagues to use this

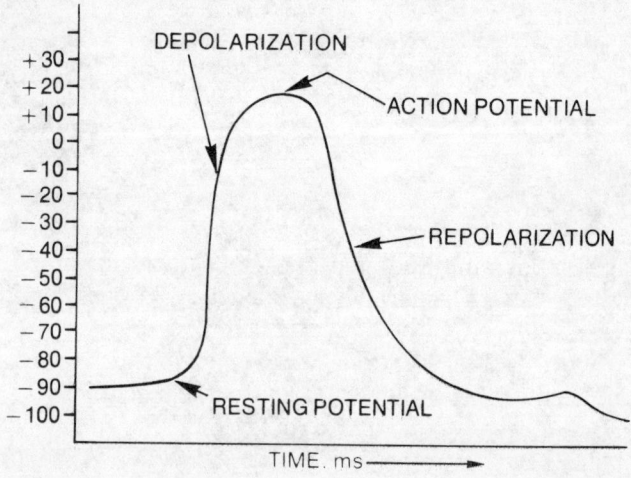

Fig. 1-4. Voltage drop across the cell membrane shown in Fig. 1-3.

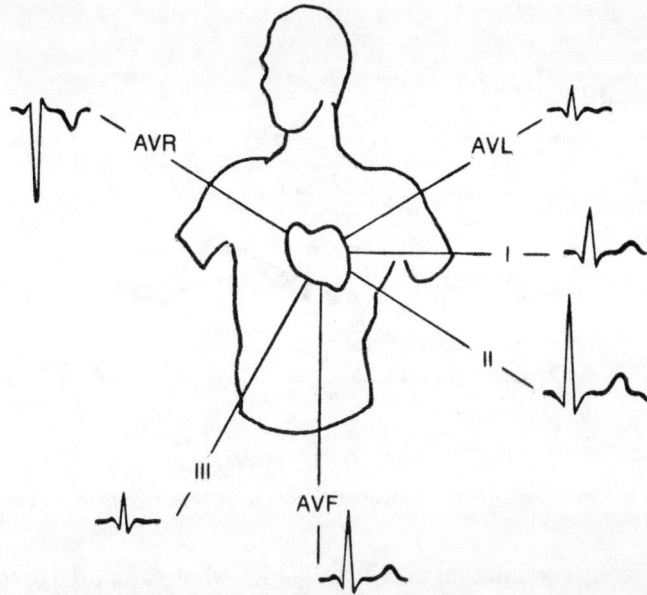

Fig. 1-5. More than one lead is used for ECG measurements since we want voltages from different areas of the heart. Each lead gives information from a particular portion of the heart muscle and is therefore useful in diagnosing troubles particular heart ailments.

word in that context, don't make the mistake of thinking that they are talking about a short length of hookup wire with alligator clips on either end.) The reason why so many different views of the heart's electrical activity are desired by medical people is that it helps them diagnose disease conditions more accurately. A multiplicity of views assists them in localizing and analyzing the areas that are diseased.

ECG LEADS

Figure 1-6 shows the major features of one of the classic ECG waveforms, called *lead I* in proper terminology. Here we see the major amplitude features of the waveform and the alphabetic letters generally used to identify those features. The first feature, on the left, is called the *p wave*. Following the p wave is the *QRS complex*, which is easily the most predominent feature of the entire waveform. The QRS complex generally has the highest amplitude in the lead-I display. Its major property, however, is its fast rise and fall times and rapid slope reversal. This, incidentally, indicates a

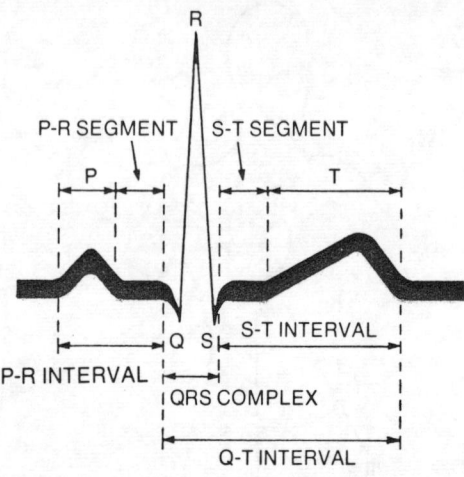

Fig. 1-6. Time measurements locate the position of each event in the pulse cycle of the heart.

frequency content that is relatively high when compared to the approximately 0.5 to 1.0 Hz fundamental rate. Generally, a frequency response of 0.5 to 100 Hz is required from instruments that are expected to faithfully reproduce this waveform. The relative amplitudes compared with a standard 1 mV calibration pulse are shown in Fig. 1-7.

The basic waveform acquisition system from a typical ECG machine is shown in Fig. 1-8. Wires from a patient cable are connected through a lead selector switch to the inputs of a differential amplifier. This amplifier usually has push-pull output that is then used to drive a permanent-magnet moving

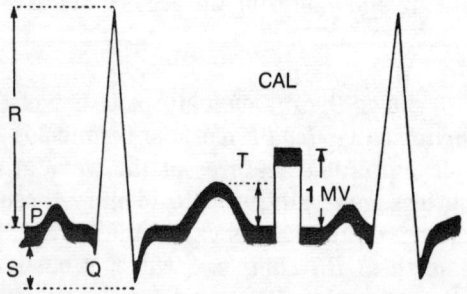

Fig. 1-7. Voltage measurements show the amplitudes of the ECG signals received by the patient electrodes. Note the 1 mV calibration signal used to measure relative amplitudes. A good ECG should be sharp, have a stable baseline, be clear, and be exact.

coil (PMMC) galvanometer pen assembly. The pen draws the vertical component of the waveform on a special graph paper passed under its tip at a fixed rate, in most cases 25 mm/sec. Figures 1-9, 1-10, and 1-11 show the common ECG leads. In all cases, the common (or *reference ground* if you prefer) is connected to the patient's right leg.

The three simplest leads are the *bipolar limb* leads, designated leads I, II, and III. These are known collectively as the *Einthoven Triangle* leads because of the triangle formed by the right arm, left arm, and left leg.

Three more leads are called either the *augmented* or *unipolar limb* leads, which are designated by the letters *aVR*, *aVL*, and *aVF*. These are created by simply summing currents

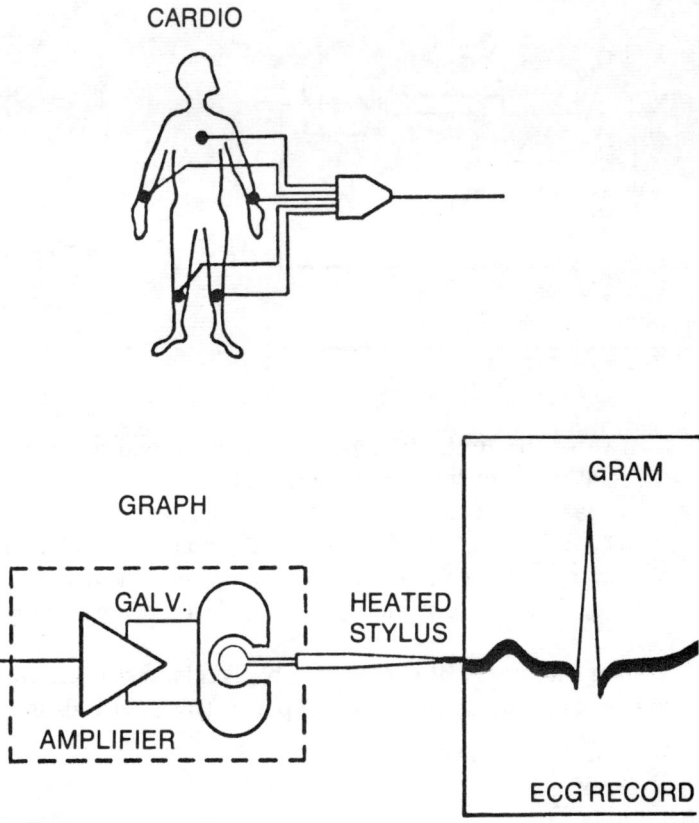

Fig. 1-8. Basic ECG hookup. The heart (cardio) signals are received by the electrocardiograph machine to produce a record, or electrocardiogram.

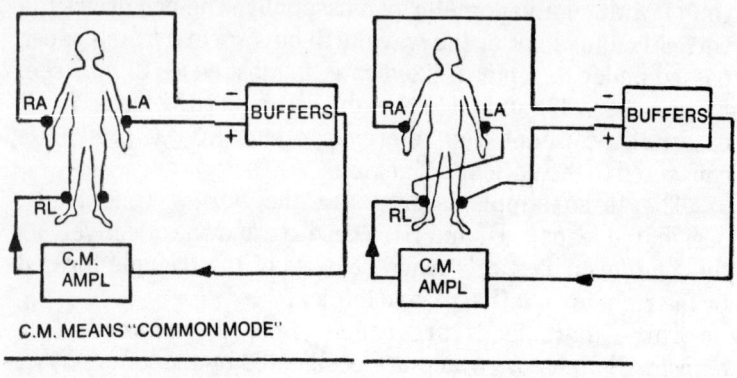

C.M. MEANS "COMMON MODE"

LEAD I

LEAD II

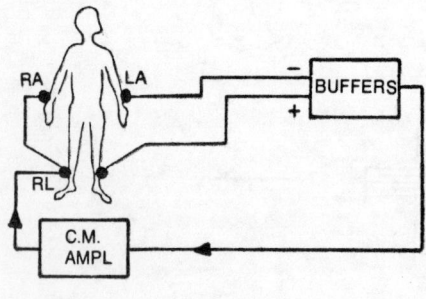

Fig. 1-9. Bipolar limb leads.

LEAD III

from two of the limbs in a resistor network and measuring them relative to the third remaining limb.

The last set of common standard leads are the *V leads* (V1–V6). These are taken by summing currents from all three limbs in a resistor network and measuring them against signals picked up from one of six standard positions on the chest.

Each wire on an ECG patient cable is color coded so that it won't be connected to the incorrect place. This color code is:

RA—white
LA—black
RL—green
LL—red
Chest—brown

ECG MACHINE OPERATION

Figure 1-12 shows a simplified drawing of a typical ECG machine drive mechanism. Such devices are actually part of a larger family of scientific instruments known collectively as strip chart recorders, and these are dealt with in more detail in Chapter 7. The most common single-channel, one-trace paper used in ECG recording is 50 mm wide and is divided into 1 and 5 mm squares to form a kind of graph paper. The paper is normally stored in a special compartment on a roll or in a Z-fold stack.

The working edge of the paper is stretched across a writing bar or a knife edge, a table, and through a set of drive rollers. One roller is actually a driver while the other an idler roller. The driven roller is coupled through a gear train or drive chain and sometimes a speed governor clutch to the drive motor. The idler roller is almost universally made of

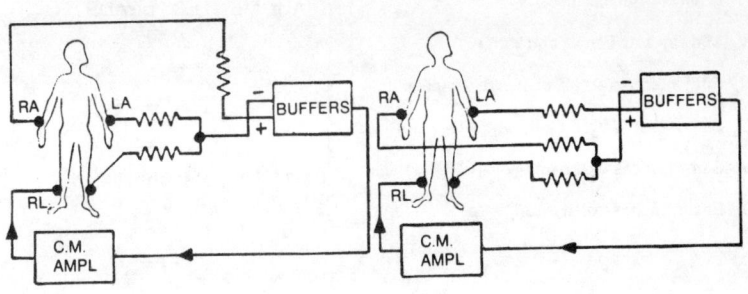

LEAD AVR**   LEAD AVL**

**ALSO KNOWN AS "AUGMENTED" LEADS

LEAD AVF**

Fig. 1-10. Unipolar limb leads.

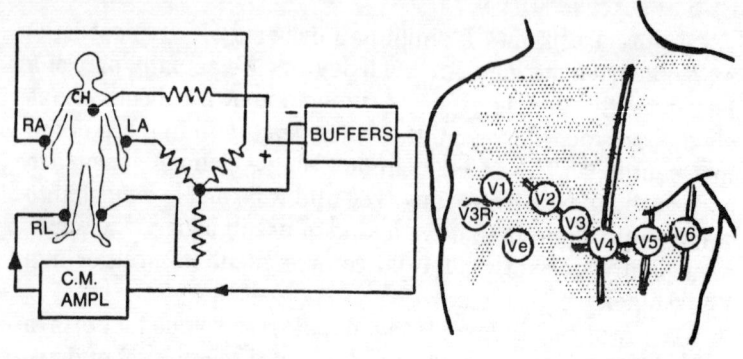

LEAD V**

V_1 Fourth intercostal space, at right sternal margin.

V_2 Fourth intercostal space, at left sternal margin.

V_3 Midway between V_2 and V_4.

V_4 Fifth intercostal space, at mid-clavicular line.

V_5 Same level as V_4, on anterior axillary line.

V_6 Same level as V_4, on midaxillary line.

V_E Ensiform, base of sternum.

CH POSITIONS

**ALSO KNOWN AS "AUGMENTED" LEADS

Fig. 1-11. Unipolar chest leads.

CH POSITIONS

hard rubber, but the drive roller may be manufactured of either rubber or aluminum. The pen, or *writing stylus* as it is often called, will lay against the paper at the knife edge or writing bar, as the case may be.

In repairing ECG machines you will soon note that few drive motors ever go bad (I have not seen one in several years). However, a large number of idler rollers and somewhat fewer but still substantial numbers of drive rollers will be needed. Machines used in high traffic areas, such as the emergency room or heart station, can be expected to wear out rollers in a short time. The usual symptoms are a drive roller that seems to turn normally, yet the paper moves either not at all or only haltingly.

Another common problem area is the write stylus. There are actually two types encountered in ECG machines: ink and thermal. It is the thermal, by far, which is most frequently seen in ECG machines. Both, however, are subject to a variety of assorted faults. You can expect pens to clog with dried ink (especially if not used for several days) and thermal types to burn out. Both types of stylus are very delicate and will easily bend if allowed to slam against the high- or low-end mechanical stops or travel limits. This may occur if too high an amplitude signal is applied to the input, which is often the result of pulling the cable electrodes off the patient before turning the machine off or to an inactive condition. Expect to replace a lot of styluses.

Still another mechanical defect is poor paper tension. Normal functioning ECG machines will produce a nice clean trace such as Fig. 1-13. When paper tension across the knife edge is reduced, either by a machine mechanical defect or improper paper loading by the operator, the paper strip chart will be allowed to skew under the tip of the stylus and a smeared trace is produced. In fact, it is the drag of the pen on the paper surface that tends to aggravate the skew effect. This type of trace is shown in Fig. 1-14. Although the fault may be either mechanical or human failure, it is very common for the nurse, doctor, or technician using the machine to complain of a worn out or bad stylus. For the sake of doing a good job, let me hasten to admonish the new technician to examine each machine before automatically replacing an expensive stylus!

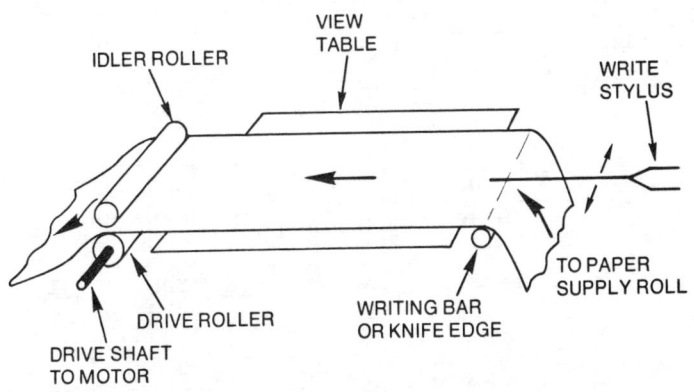

Fig. 1-12. Simplified drive scheme of ECG machine.

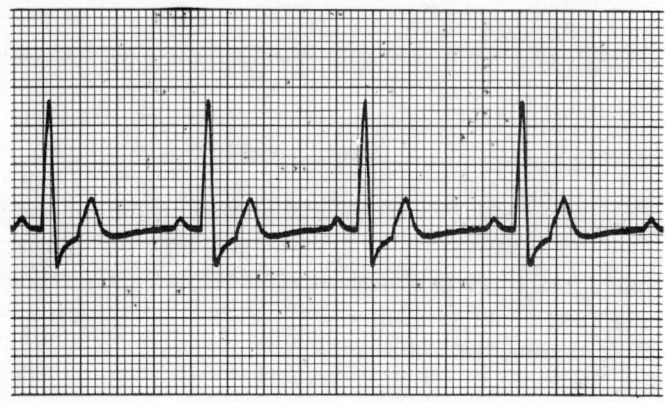

Fig. 1-13. Normal ECG trace.

Interfering voltages applied to the input of the ECG machine may tend to obscure the real waveform and render it unreadable. Anomalies on the tracing that represent either machine errors or voltages present but not generated by the patient's heart, are called *artifacts*. Most of the time, artifacts can be easily diagnosed and corrected by the nurse, ECG technician, or other medical person making the ECG recording. In some cases, though, artifacts will be referred to an electronics person for correction. You will therefore see both machine defects and user errors causing various artifacts. Thus, learn to recognize and correct some of the more common ECG recording artifacts.

Figure 1-15A shows a reasonably clean ECG tracing with few, if any, artifacts. In Fig. 1-15B and C, however, we see

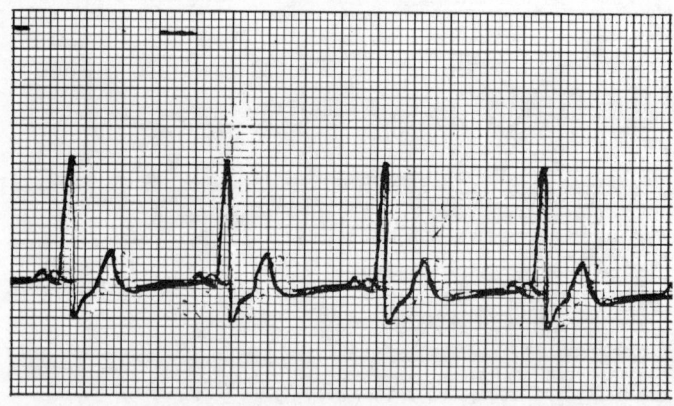

Fig. 1-14. Defective ECG trace caused by inadequate paper tension.

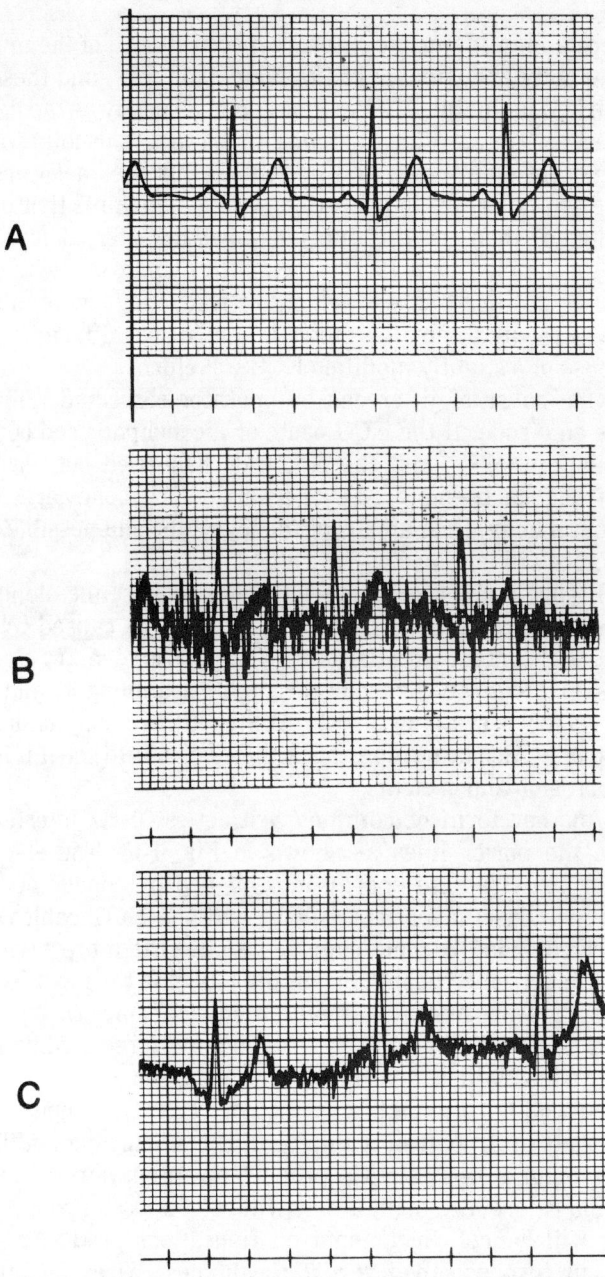

Fig. 1-15. Artifacts are extraneous signals appearing on the ECG. (A) is a normal ECG. (B) shows severe muscle jitter resulting in an erratic waveform that obliterates significant details of the ECG pattern. (C) is mild muscle jitter causing reduced and slower-changing interference.

severe and mild muscle jitter, respectively. All of the muscles in the body are capable of producing voltages, and these will be picked up by the ECG machine just as easily as the desired voltages. The cure for this class of artifact is usually to have the patient calm down and lie still. If this does not work and there are no errors in operation or machine faults that can be corrected, then try the internal machine filter, if any. This may be labeled as a *filter* or *monitor-diagnostic* switch. The monitor position has a lower cutoff frequency low-pass filter, and this will attenuate much of the noise although at the expense of a slightly modified ECG waveform.

One cause of jitter can be operator corrected. This is a loose electrode. If the ECG paste or alcohol pad used between the patient's skin and the electrode has dried out, or if the electrode has been placed over a particularly boney area of the patient's body, then apparent muscle jitter and possible other artifacts will increase.

Figure 1-15C also shows a wandering baseline along with the muscle artifact. This defect can also be caused by poor electrical contact with the skin. When this is seen, try cleaning the skin under the electrode (or slightly abrading it) and use a new alcohol swab or fresh dab of ECG paste under the electrode. Also be sure to check the electrode to see if it is free of corrosion and is clean.

Another form of common aritfact is 60 Hz interference from the power lines as shown in Fig. 1-16. The electrical power lines radiate energy into all nearby conductors—and that includes the patient's body and the ECG cables. This effect can also be demonstrated somewhat more vividly to many electronics people by simply touching the input leads to an oscilloscope or audio amplifier. In the former case you will see a sine-wave trace on the oscilloscope screen, while in the latter a buzz will be heard from the loudspeaker.

An ECG preamplifier, though, has two input leads, balanced to ground in a differential configuration. Although each input of this pair will produce an output in response to a ground referenced signal, they will be of opposite polarity and thus will cancel. Such input configurations produce outputs only in response to *differential* voltages. Wires feeding the ECG inputs should pick up roughly equal amounts of 60 Hz energy, provided they are of equal length. If the input circuits remain balanced, the preamplifier sees these as *common*

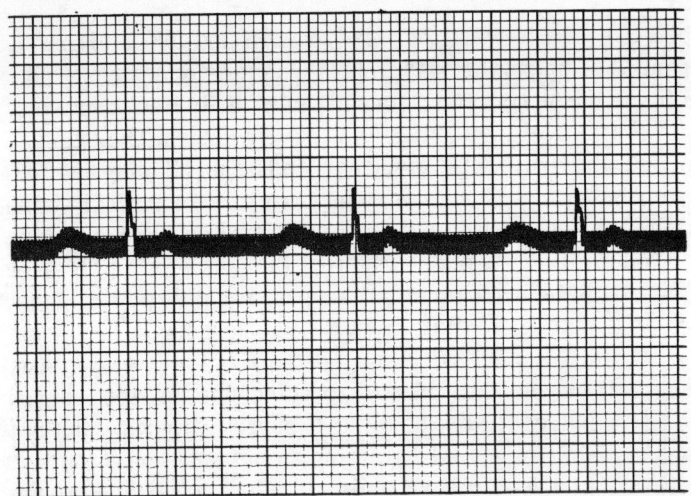

Fig. 1-16. Power-line interference results in this steady 60 Hz pattern appearing on the ECG trace. Severe amounts of 60 Hz pickup can completely destroy the ECG pattern.

mode (equal voltages at each input) signals and no output can be produced.

Several common defects tend to upset the input balance and allow the 60 Hz signal voltage to become differential. If an electrode is in poor contact with the skin, or if the skin itself is in such a condition to produce a poor contact, 60 Hz interference will result. Another frequently found cause of 60 Hz interference is a broken wire in the patient cable. In a few cases the trouble is in the ECG machine electronics. Look for broken input wires or a faulty or dirty lead selector switch—clean with a good contact cleaner or electronic switch degreaser solvent. A bad input socket is often found because of the torque placed on the socket by the heavy patient cable and the abuse usual to such equipment—TLC is for patients, not equipment.

Diagnosing the cause of 60 Hz interference is usually pretty simple, straightforward, and can be performed rapidly. First, short together all of the electrodes. If this causes the interference to disappear altogether, then suspect the connection to the patient. If it persists, then look to the cable. One means of testing the cable is to replace it with one that is known to be good; another way is to measure continuity using an ohmmeter. Keep in mind, though, that some ECG patient cables use a series resistor of between 1K and 10K, and so may appear to be open if an inappropriate ohmmeter scale is used.

Some hospitals keep a special lamp-and-battery continuity tester that is designed to test ECG patient cables. The machine end and the individual electrode ends are all plugged into appropriate jacks. A switch is then turned to connect first one and then the other end to the test lamp circuitry. You can also keep a dummy ECG plug with all of the pins shorted together so that it can be inserted into the input jack; this puts all input lines at ground potential. If 60 Hz interference still is seen, then you may suspect a defect inside the machine. In that case, incidentally, you can almost predict one of the causes discussed above will be the fault. It is relatively rare, but not unheard of, for the actual electronic amplifiers to be at fault.

Do not overlook the possibility of a bad power line ground as the cause of the 60 Hz interference. All ECG machines use a three-wire power cord that has the third wire connected to chassis ground. If the ground is broken or is not as good as it should be, then interference will result. If an ohmmeter check reveals an open or high resistance ground to the chassis of the ECG machine, replace the power cord or plug. In most cases the break will be at the plug end of the cord immediately behind the connector, which is the major point of stress in most power cords. Also replace the plug if the blades or the ground lug appear to be worn, or even if they appear to be simply ratty.

If the power cord and plug seem to be alright, suspect a bad duplex outlet in the wall. It is often the case that a soon-to-be-bad outlet on the wall will give itself away by causing interference on ECG machines or bedside monitors. Loss of tension on the ground lug can cause this problem, as well as presenting additional problems with regard to patient safety. This condition can be easily tested by plugging the machine into another outlet that is known to be good. Another means of testing the outlet is with a special tension guage. Have the house electrician replace the ac outlet if it is found to be defective.

EVALUATING ECG MACHINE PERFORMANCE

There are several parameters that we use to examine and evaluate the typical ECG machine. Although the actual specifications may vary somewhat from one manufacturer to another, the commonality of purpose for which they are designed makes some tests common to all instruments of the class.

Every ECG machine has a voltage calibration button used to place a 1.0 mV pulse across the differential inputs of the preamplifier. This is usually labelled *standardize, STD,* or 1 *mV*. The calibration pulse is used by the operator to adjust the amplifier gain till the 1 mV signal produces a stylus deflection of 10 mm (2 large squares on standard ECG paper). This button is located at a point in the circuit that will allow you to make a quick and cheap evaluation of machine performance without any additional test equipment. Simply press the calibration button and hold it for 2 seconds (Fig. 1-17). The amplitude should drop about 5 to 7 mm in this time period. Next, make a few 1 mV pulses in quick succession by pressing and releasing the button several times. Make sure the amplifier has sufficient gain to give more than the required minimum amplitude.

A somewhat more comprehensive analysis of overall ECG machine performance can be realized by using some of the more sophisticated test equipment in the electronics laboratory. Do not make the mistake, however, of assuming that all that high-cost test equipment is the *be all* and *end all* of ECG testing. You may well—in fact you will—find defects that only show up when a real, live (hopefully) human test subject is used as the ECG "signal generator." ECG repair technicians tend to see their own ECG a great deal, since they make a handy portable signal source that can walk to the job site unassisted and uncarried!

Seriously, though, there are some tests that are important. You will need a square-wave generator that is capable of producing a 1 Hz signal with an amplitude of several volts. These specifications, incidentally, are well within the range of most of the low-cost function generators on the market today. With older generators that only go down to 10 or 20 Hz, you can use digital IC logic dividers, such as the *7490* series in the TTL family (its cheap!), to build an adapter that will frequency-divide the output of the generator.

Since few generators come with a balanced output, it may prove wise to construct a balancing attenuator pad such as in Fig. 1-18. This circuit takes the single-ended input and delivers a balanced, although greatly attenuated, output. Resistors R1

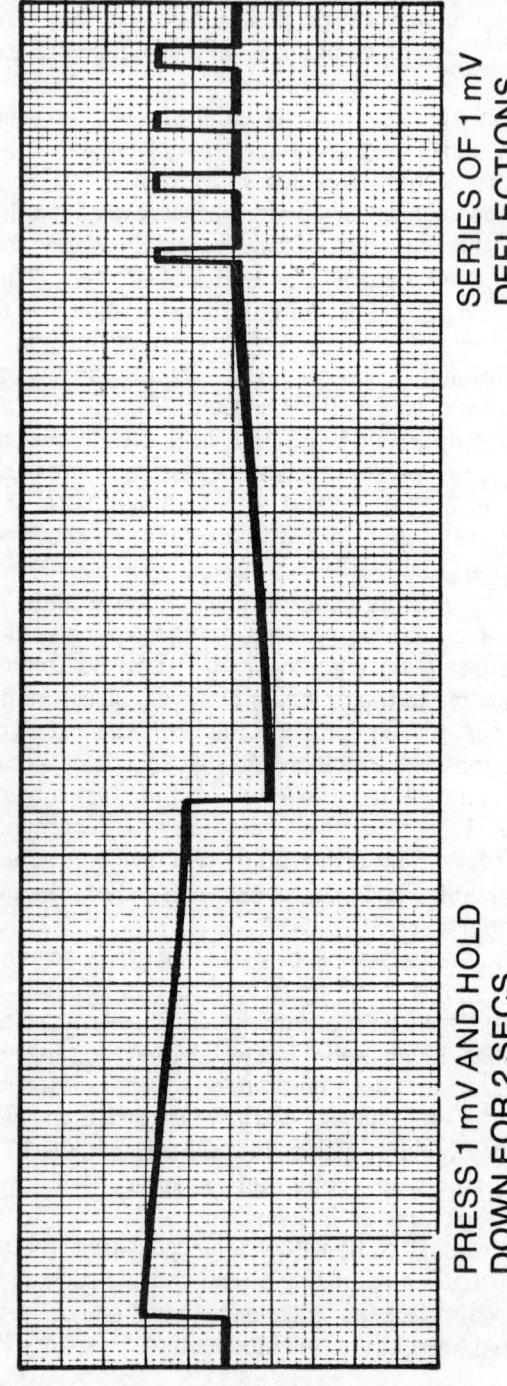

Fig. 1-17. ECG test procedure illustrating decay curve due to normal low-frequency response, followed by short square deflections resulting from normal high-frequency response.

through R3 in the circuit form a voltage divider in which output E1 will be approximately one-third of the input. This output voltage is impressed across a balanced voltage divider consisting of resistors R4 through R6. This is the voltage actually delivered to the ECG machine and it has a value of

$$\frac{E_1 \; R_6}{R_4 + R_5 + R_6}$$

The values listed for the resistors in Fig. 1-18 will attenuate voltage E1 approximately 60 dB (1/1000), so in order to yield an output voltage of 1.0 mV, you will require an input of about 3V peak from the function generator. Connector J1 can be a BNC type or whatever is compatible with your signal source. (It is a good idea to have a collection of test equipment patch cords.) Connector P2, on the other hand, must be compatible with the ECG input jack on your machine. In most cases this means a 5-pin, size 14 AN (also called MS by some manufacturers) connector wired in the now standard Sanborn ECG configuration:

        RA—pin A   C—pin D
        LA—pin B   RL—pin E
        LL—pin C

(The pins selected in Fig. 1-18 are for lead I.)

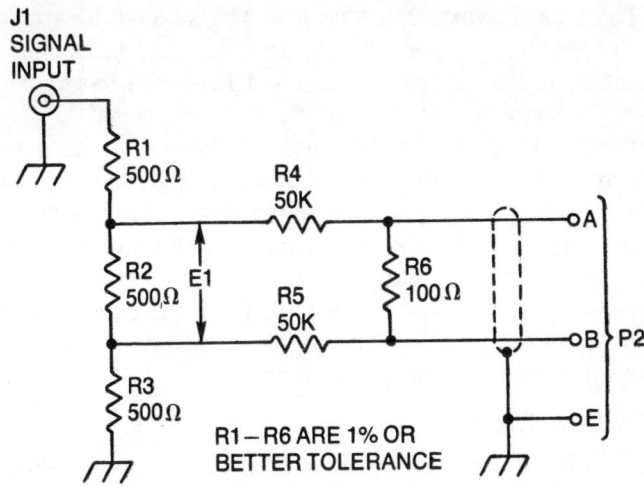

Fig. 1-18. ECG test circuit for converting high-level oscillator square-wave signals into balanced output of 1 mV amplitude.

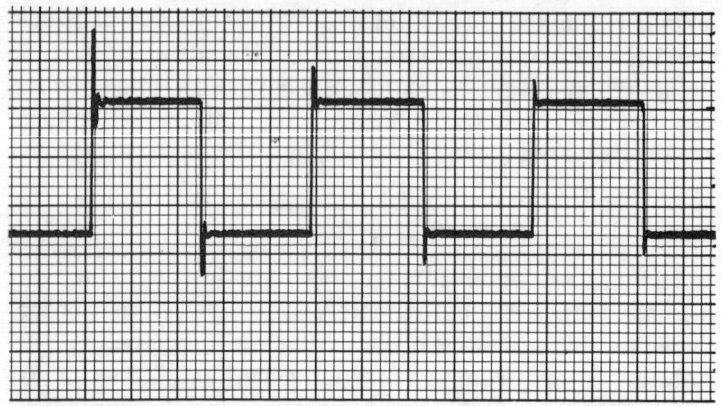

Fig. 1-19. Overshoot and ringing results from misadjusted instrument compensation. The damping adjustment should be corrected to yield an almost perfect square wave.

The ECG machine can be tested in several ways using this adapter and a 1 Hz square wave. Figure 1-19 shows a pattern of square waves taken from an ECG machine tracing. Note that the pulses to the left overshoot and ring a little bit. This fault is characteristic of misadjusted damping. In a few models this is caused by adjustment of stylus pressure while in most an electrical adjustment is required. In the latter case you will find a damping control somewhere on the machine; adjust it for the best possible square shape.

The square wave can also give you a rough idea of the proper frequency response in the amplifiers and galvanometer assembly. If the waveshape of the 1 Hz signal has rounded corners, suspect poor high-frequency response. Low-frequency attenuation is indicated if the top of the square wave appears to tilt. Be aware that some ECG machines have their high-frequency response intentionally limited so that muscle jitter and 60 Hz artifacts are reduced naturally. These instruments are normally used for long-term monitoring purposes rather than diagnostic ECG strips. On those machines the square wave response will always be poor, and no repair is either possible or feasible.

ECG ELECTRONICS

Figure 1-20 shows a block diagram of a common type of ECG preamplifier. The overall gain provided by stages A1 and A2 must be several thousand. Their frequency response should be of 0.5–100 Hz. Amplifier A1 has differential inputs, for reasons already discussed, and a push-pull output so that it can drive the differential input of amplifier A2. In machines typically found in hospitals, you can expect to see all of the well known amplifier technologies of the past 20 years—vacuum tubes, transistors, and integrated circuits.

The frequency response at the lower end of the range is limited by capacitors C5 and C6. These will normally have a value in the 10 to 100 μF range in solid-state equipment, and 0.1–0.5 μF in vacuum-tube designs.

One further requirement is that amplifier A1 have a high input impedance. Since these circuits are actually no more than voltage amplifiers, you would ideally want a low source impedance (the patient) and a high input impedance. With the patient's impedance at the electrodes on the order of 10K to 50K, you would thus require a very high input impedance. The usual rule is 10 to 100 times the source impedance! In actual design practice, this is a little hard to accomplish, but it is approached through techniques discussed in the chapter on bedside monitors.

Since we shall return to this same topic when discussing bedside monitors, we shall not belabor the point here. But it is appropriate and instructive to mention some details of typical ECG input preamplifier circuitry shown in Fig. 1-20. We show everything following the input lead selector switch. The 1 mV calibration section is the circuit that places the 1 mV dc potential in series with one input line. Such circuits consist of a couple of resistors, a pushbutton switch, and some sort of power source. In many machines a single mercury battery such as the No. 1 instrument battery (RM1, hg1, etc) is used, while in others a voltage divider from a regulated dc power supply is used Capacitors C1 and C2 are used to bypass rf signals from outside the machine (see Chapter 9), which may be picked up by the patient cables.

Amplifier A3 serves both to increase patient safety and to improve the common-mode rejection ratio (CMRR) of differential input amplifier A1. Amplifier A3 is usually called the *common-mode* amplifier in scientific strip chart recorders and the *right leg* amplifier in ECG machines. Common-mode signals such as 60 Hz interference are summed in two RC networks: R3-C3 and R4-C4. These are connected to the input of amplifier A3, which incidentally is an inverting follower. Since the output of such an amplifier is 180° out of phase with

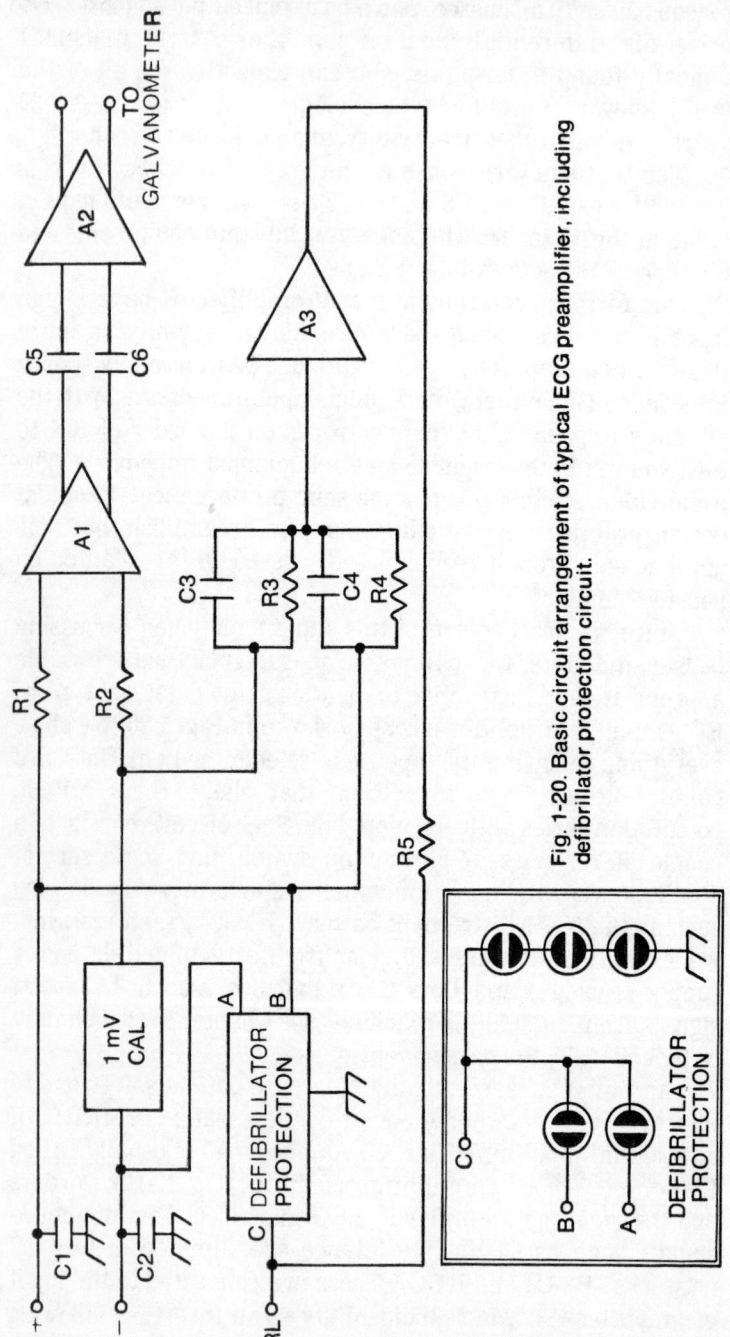

Fig. 1-20. Basic circuit arrangement of typical ECG preamplifier, including defibrillator protection circuit.

32

the input, the summed common-mode signals add destructively with the original common-mode signals. This causes an effective cancellation, which results in a substantially reduced level of interference and a much improved CMRR. Resistor R5 is needed to protect the patient by limiting the maximum current that can be applied to the patient, in case of a radical or catastrophic electrical component failure within the ECG machine.

Although the input section of most instrumentation amplifiers may resemble that of the ECG preamplifier, there is one feature that is unique to those differential amplifiers designed and used for ECG work—defibrillator protection. Defibrillators are devices used to electrically shock the patient's heart to correct certain types of heart attack. Unfortunately for the poor ECG machine, most defibrillators can place several hundred to several thousand volts across the ECG input! If there was no protection, this would surely blow the ECG input circuitry.

The defibrillator protection circuitry consists of resistors R1 and R2, plus a collection of strategically placed neon glow lamps. The resistors attenuate any voltage applied to the input, affording some degree of protection by themselves. Some manufacturers also place voltage dependent resistors (VDR) or JFET constant-current diodes in series with the two input lines.

The first line of defense and the protectors used to take the main blow from the defibrillator is the neon glow lamps. Normally, voltages presented across the ECG input are several orders of magnitude too low to fire these lamps, so they will remain extinquished. But if an excessive voltage appears across the input, they will fire and allow current to flow to ground. In machines using several lamps connected in series, the firing potential is approximately 250−300V. After the voltage deminishes (a couple dozen milliseconds in the machines using the Lown circuit), the lamps extinguish and return to their previous state.

These neon lamps should be changed not less than once a year—more often on machines used frequently in conjunction with defibrillators (e.g., those in ER, CCU, or ICU). It seems that the repeated firing of the lamps tends to deteriorate their firing point. When the firing voltage rises to a certain level, the amount of protection afforded the preamplifier input circuitry becomes negligible.

Chapter 2

Medical Electrodes and Transducers

Before any electronic medical monitoring can be performed, there must be some means for acquiring a significant signal or an electrical analog of some nonelectrical parameter from the patient. In some forms of monitoring, we are interested in displaying a time-varying bioelectric potential, so only a simple electrode connection is required. In other cases, however, the desired parameter might not be electrical, so a form of transducer device is required. In this context, a *transducer* is a device that generates an electrical analog signal in response to some physical parameter such as pressure, position, velocity, and temperature.

MEDICAL ELECTRODES

Electrocardiography (ECG), electroencephalography (EEG), and electromyography (EMG) use simple electrodes to acquire bioelectric potentials from the patient. The sources of these voltages were discussed briefly in Chapter 1. The most common of these is the ECG. It would be ludicrous to attempt to fully cover the subject of medical electrodes. You might be tempted to ask just what is so complicated, but let me assure you that whole books have been written on the sole subject of medical electrodes!

Reusable flat electrodes made of a brass-like material are used in many instances for ECG. These are connected to the patient's limbs at the wrists and ankles by sets of rubber straps that hold them in place. Chest electrodes made of the same material are fashioned in the form of suction cups, so that attachement can be made to acquire the precordial ECG leads. The electrodes themselves will not make good electrical connection, so either an alchohol swab or a special ECG paste is used between the electrode surface and the patient's skin. There are two forms of paste used: one is a conductive mixture while the other is an abrasive jelly that conditions the top layer of skin to make better connection.

Reusable electrodes have not proven too viable on ICU and CCU patients requiring long-term monitoring of the ECG. This is partially due to the fact that such electrodes tend to work loose and have to be constantly readjusted. You can easily see this is an aggravation that the nursing staff can do without.

Disposable electrodes have been developed, and they help eliminate or at least greatly reduce this particular problem. Disposable electrodes have a metallic electrical contact surface, immersed in jelly or paste, and affixed to the sticky side of a circular adhesive patch. The back side of the electrical contact piece has a snap fitting for connection to the patient cable. The actual electrical contact in the typical disposable electrode patch measures about 1 cm in diameter.

EEG electrodes are somewhat smaller than ECG types. They are often made of gold- or silver-plated construction. EEG electrodes require the use of a special electrode paste to insure a decent electrical contact with the patient's scalp. In both EEG and ECG recording, needle electrodes are sometimes used. But in most cases these are small-diameter needles using a length of wire (and often a male connector) to make connection to the patient cable from the instrument. This construction facilitates gas sterilization of the needles between uses. Sterilization is not required of noninvasive surface electrodes such as those described previously.

Electrodes can be a major source of trouble in medical monitoring systems, and they are a primary source of artifacts. They must be kept clean, and any paste used must be fresh. Before taking an instrument to the lab for troubleshooting, make sure the problem is not in the patient cable or electrodes. If the alchohol pad or paste has dried out, it may be necessary to clean the patient's skin at the point of contact and install a fresh pad or apply fresh jelly.

A surprising number of "equipment defects" turn out to be little more than operator defects. I recall one case where an ICU nurse reported large amounts of 60 Hz interference. The monitoring technician found that she improvised a way to keep the electrode patch (a disposable) in place. It seems that she smeared a little betadine solution on the patient's skin. This dries tacky and can act as an adhesive. However, it also acts as an insulator, and this made the ECG preamplifier see an open electrode. That unbalanced the differential input and created the interference problem.

TEMPERATURE TRANSDUCERS

Probably the most common form of temperature transducer is the *thermistor*—a temperature-sensitive resistor. These devices change their electrical resistance a certain amount for every degree of temperature change. Most thermistors are specified with a certain resistance at room temperature, usually taken to be 25°C. In most medical thermistors, this is the bottom edge of the range of interest—normal human temperature is around 37°C. But because of certain medical considerations, it is desirable for electronic thermometers to read down to at least 28°C. In most clinically used temperature monitors, the thermistor is in one leg of a Wheatstone bridge.

Transistor and diode PN junctions also exhibit properties similar to those of the thermistor and can respond much faster. Several medical, scientific, and industrial temperature transducers are known that actually have a transistor in the probe tip. Heat is coupled from the outside world to the metal case of the transistor, which in turn is thermally connected to the transistor collector.

Thermocouples represent still another form of temperature transducer. Traditional thermocouples, known and used for many decades, have been bimetallic junctions. Strips made from different but carefully chosen metals are connected together at one end, forming a junction. A voltage will appear across the unconnected ends when this junction is heated. Modern thermocouples are often made from semiconductor materials and are generally considered to be superior in terms of both sensitivity and linearity. The thermocouple finds application in certain scientific and control-system instruments (an example is the pyrometer).

Medical equipment generally uses the thermistor, though, because of lower cost and the fact that an acceptable linearity is availible despite the low cost and slow reaction time.

The actual mechanical form taken by medical temperature transducers depends entirely upon their intended use. Some types appear to be small blobs on the end of a wire and are intended for use in the nostrils or ear canal. Those intended for oral use are generally used to take the temperature of an awake patient, but not for long-term continuous monitoring of temperature. Oral transducers can thus be fashioned into a plastic housing similar to some of the more recent probes used on voltmeters and oscilloscopes. Most oral temperature probes are permanently attached to an electronic thermometer (such as the ubiquitous IVAC). These have plastic sterile covers so the instrument can be used on several patients in succession without having to sterilize the thing every time (an economic impossibility). Such electronic thermometers, incidentally, are in common use in almost all U.S. hospitals.

Long-term ICU or CCU monitoring of patient's temperature is usually done with a rectal temperature probe, in which the thermistor is constructed inside of an 8- to 10-inch plastic or rubberized tube. This type of transducer can be left in place for a length of time but must be gas sterilized between patients.

Thermistors find other uses in medical instrumentation, but these are relatively minor compared with thermometry. Some respiratory instruments, for example, use the temperature variation in exhaled breath gases to yield a respiratory waveform. At least one respiratory alarm has been constructed using a thermistor thermometer.

PLETHYSMOGRAPHIC TRANSDUCERS

Plethysmographs are devices that measure change in volume. Blood volume measurements are used for detection of vessel obstructions and for determination of the pulse waveform velocity. True plethysmographs are pneumatic devices and are somewhat difficult to operate. Certain electrical devices are available, though, which mimic and approximate the performance of the real plethysmograph—but are a lot easier to use clinically.

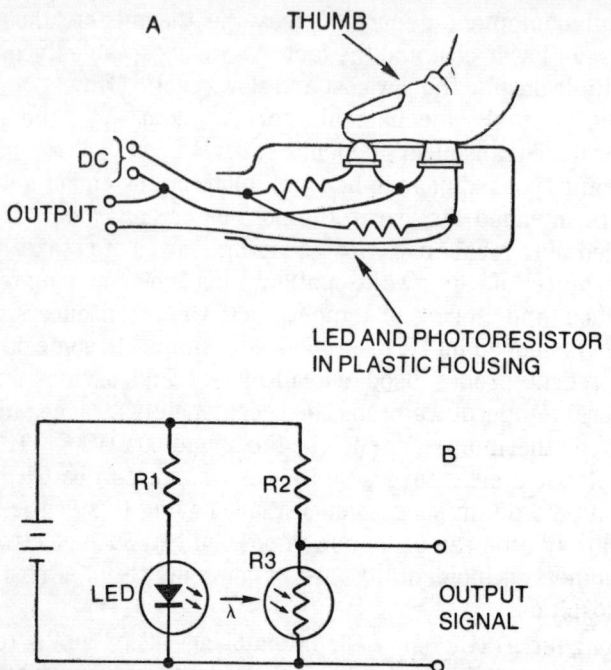

Fig. 2-1. The photoplethysmograph obtains an output that is proportional to variations in light energy passing through patient tissues. (A) shows relative component positions for a thumb sensor. (B) shows the electrical circuit, containing an LED and photoresistor.

One such device is shown in Fig. 2-1. This is called the *photoplethysmograph* because it operates using light. In Fig. 2-1A we see how the device is attached to the patient. In other versions, the components are fashioned into a plastic earclip. The circuit for this type of transducer is shown in Fig. 2-1B and consists of a light source such as a lamp or light emitting diode (LED) and a photoresistor. Light from the source passes through the tissue of the finger or ear lobe to the photoresistor. Pulsating blood flow causes the optical density of the tiny vessels in the tissue to change as the heart beats. This causes a varying light to fall on the photoresistor, which changes its resistance in step with the tissue density changes. The output waveform is a voltage that resembles the human blood pressure waveform.

The photoplethysmograph cannot be easily calibrated in units of blood pressure, but it can be used to determine the existence of blood flow or the velocity of the waveform. It can also be used to drive a cardiotachometer, which reads out the heart rate in beats per minute.

BLOOD PRESSURE TRANSDUCERS

Figure 2-2 shows a transducer typical of those used in medical monitoring of blood pressure. This particular model is from the Hewlett-Packard *1280* series, and it is an example of the inductive Wheatstone bridge. Fluid from an arterial line enters the clear plastic dome, where it distends a diaphram an amount proportional to the applied pressure. A threaded screw-on collar allows these domes to be removed for cleaning and occasional replacement. The use of clear plastic also allows inspection for air bubbles and any other anomaly that could affect the actual reading or produce artifacts in the waveform. Be careful when handling such transducers because they are fragile—in fact, very fragile. Any handling of the diaphram, which is exposed when the dome is removed, could conceivably result in damage.

One common form of blood pressure transducer is the resistive Wheatstone bridge strain gauge of Fig. 2-3. An excitation voltage is applied between pins B and D. Under normal circumstances of zero pressure above atmosphere (0 torr, where 1 torr equals 1 mmHg), the strain gauge is in its unstrained or rest condition, and all four resistors have approximately the same value. Applying pressure causes one, two, or all four resistive elements (depending upon design) to change value, and this unbalances the bridge to produce a voltage proportional to the applied pressure. A potentiometer scales the output to compensate for individual differences in sensitivity.

Resistive strain-gauge transducers come in two general catagories: bonded and unbonded. In the bonded variety, resistance wires are cemented to, or semiconductor material deposited upon, a thin metallic diaphragm that can be deformed by the applied pressure. Most bonded strain-gauge transducers have all four resistance arms attached to the diaphram in such a way that two will be stretched (resistance increased) while the other two are compressed (resistance decreased) by the applied pressure.

Typical unbonded strain gauges have resistance wires stretched between supports that can be deformed by applying pressure to the diaphram. This arrangement will stretch one pair of wires and compress the others.

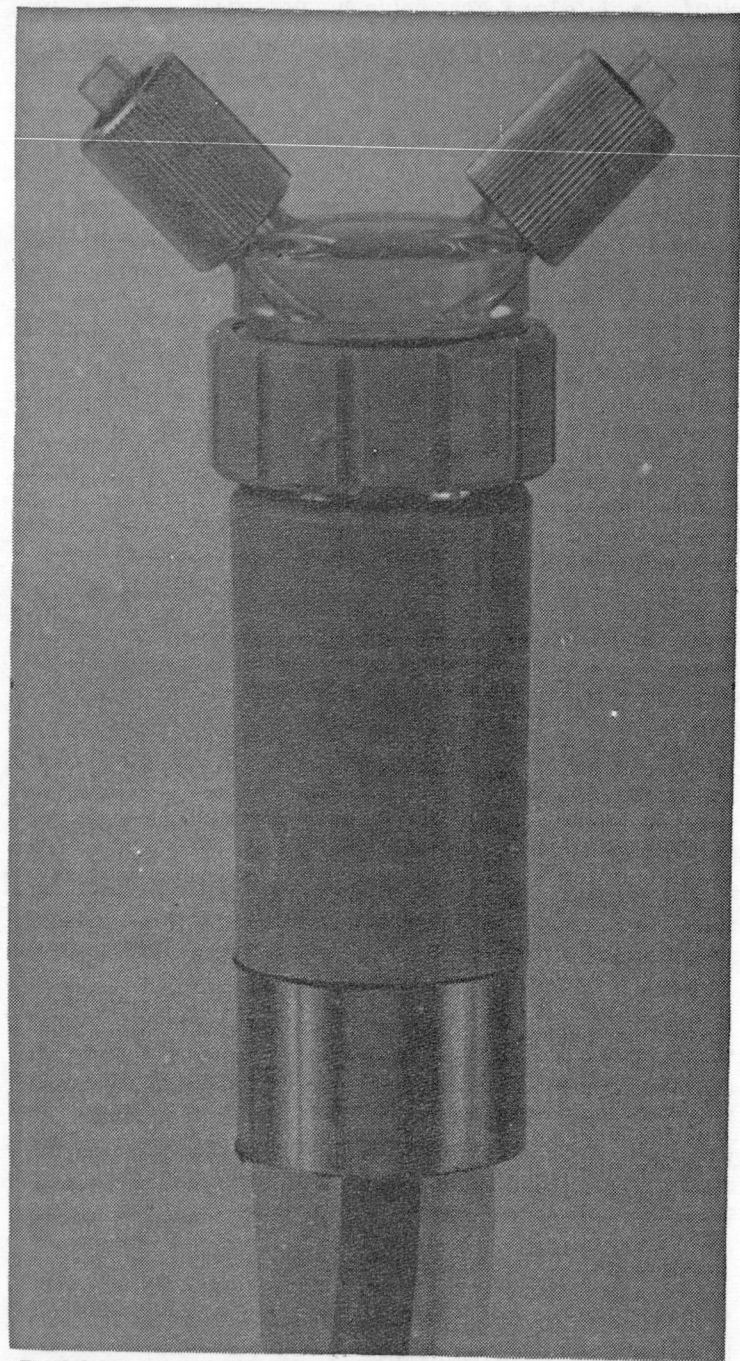

Fig. 2-2. Inductive blood pressure transducer. (Courtesy Hewlett-Packard)

Transducers are rated by *gauge factor* and by *sensitivity* as well as by range and measured parameters. The gauge factor is defined as the percentage change in resistance per unit change in length of the resistance elements. In other words,

$$\text{gauge factor} = \frac{\frac{\Delta R}{R}}{\frac{\Delta L}{L}}$$

Metallic strain gauges have gauge factors from about 2 up to about 4. Modern semiconductor strain gauges, however, have guage factors over 100.

Another parameter used to specify strain gauges is the sensitivity. Each transducer will have a rating expressed in microvolts per volt of excitation per unit of pressure:

$$\text{sensitivity} = \mu\text{V/V-torr}$$

For example, let us assume a certain transducer has a sensitivity of 50 μV/V-torr. Let us also assume a 5V excitation

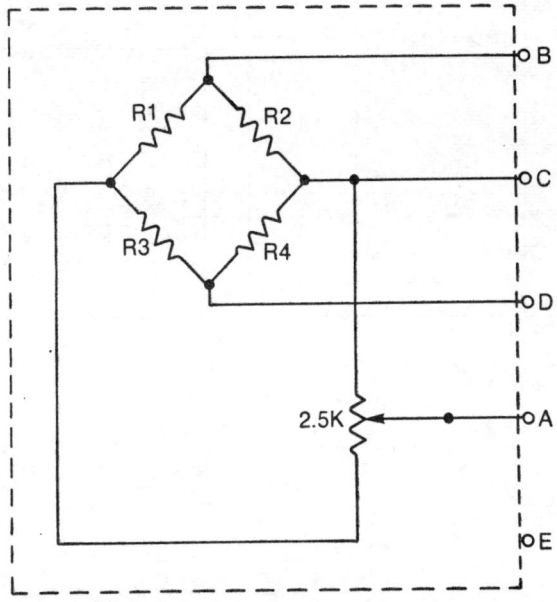

Fig. 2-3. A resistive strain gauge is based upon the familiar Wheatstone bridge circuit. Circuit resistances are such that the bridge is balanced when no pressure is applied.

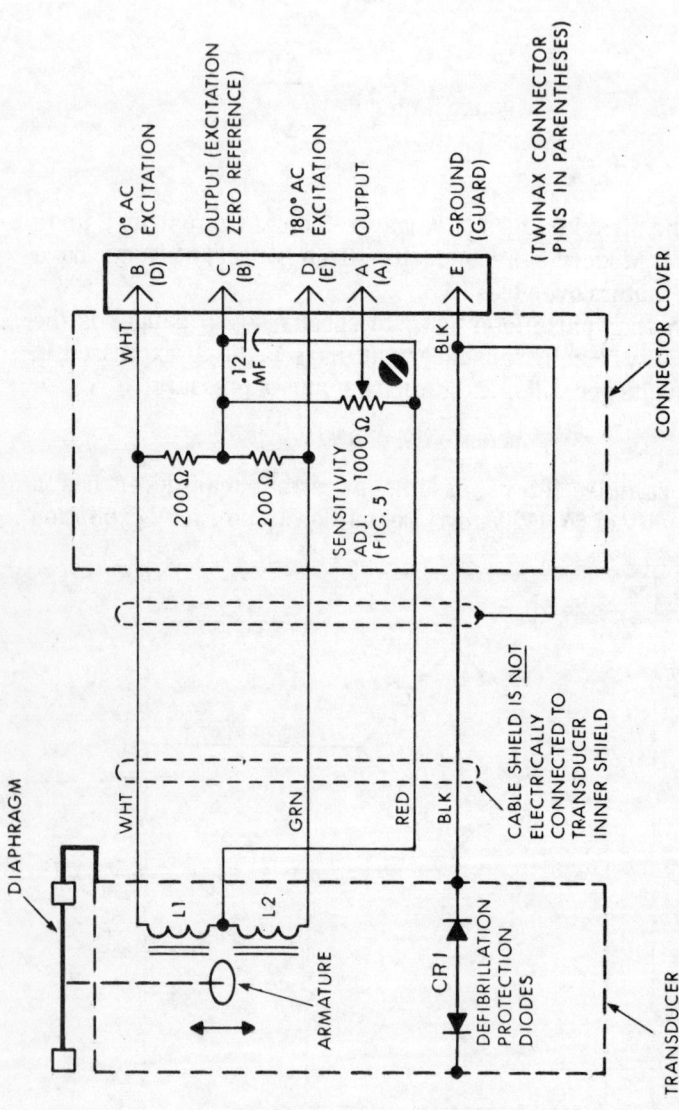

Fig. 2-4. The inductive strain gauge is also a bridge circuit, but it relies upon pressure exerted against a diaphragm connected to a moving armature. As the armature moves, it varies the inductance of the two coils relative to each other, and this unbalances the bridge circuit to produce an output voltage proportional to pressure.

signal (which is typical) and an applied pressure of 100 torr. What is the output voltage produced by the Wheatstone bridge?

$$E_{OUT} = \text{sensitivity} \times \text{excitation} \times \text{pressure}$$
$$= (50 \; \mu\text{V/V-torr}) \, (5\text{V}) \, (100 \, \text{torr})$$
$$= 25{,}000 \; \mu\text{V}$$
$$= 0.025\text{V}$$

Once the sensitivity and excitation voltage are known or determined, the gain of an amplifier can be scaled to read out values of pressure.

An inductive Wheatstone bridge circuit is shown in Fig. 2-4. This is the internal circuitry of the Hewlett-Packard *1280* series transducers. Two arms of the bridge are fixed resistors while the other two are variable inductors. The cores of these coils are connected to the pressure deformable diaphram. At atmospheric pressure (0 torr gauge pressure), the cores will be positioned equally in both coils. This will cause the coils to have equal inductances and, therefore, equal inductive reactances. When a pressure is applied, the cores are shifted so that more is in L2 than in L1. This changes the relative inductances and upsets the bridge's balance.

The sensitivity of an inductive bridge is generally much greater than the resistance types. A disadvantage of this type of transducer, though, is that the excitation voltage must be ac, while resistance types seem equally happy with either ac or dc excitation. This disadvantage often diminishes because many pressure amplifiers are designed for ac operation because drift is easier to control through use of feedback. Figure 2-5 shows the graph of transducer output voltage as a function of applied pressure.

One last type of pressure transducer is the *linear voltage differential transformer* (LVDT) of Fig. 2-6. The transducer is excited by an ac carrier. Note that the secondaries are connected in series opposing. When zero gauge pressure is applied to the diaphram, the core is equally divided between both secondaries, so their respective flux linkages with the primary are equal. Because of the opposing connection, the currents in these secondary windings are equal in amplitude, but of opposite polarity, and therefore cancel. When a pressure is applied, the core moves into one of the coils more than it is in the other. This causes the first coil to have a greater flux

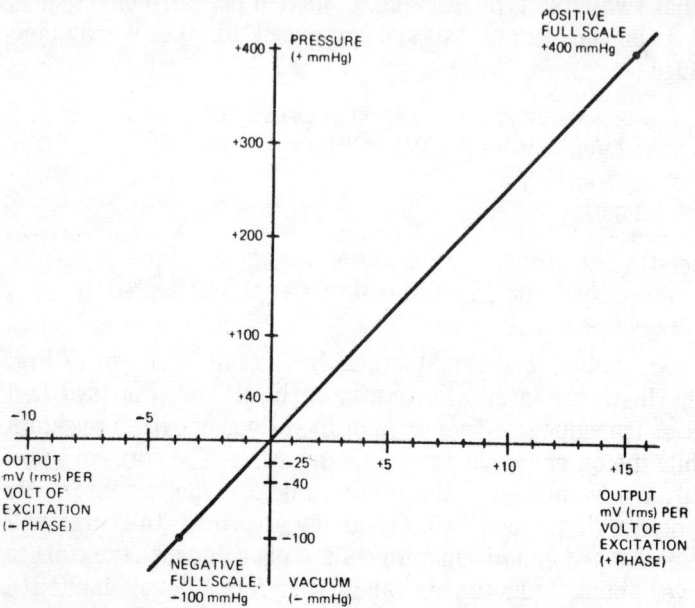

Fig. 2-5. Typical transfer characteristic of an inductive pressure transducer using ac excitation. Note the good linearity of the response, indicated by the straight line of the transfer curve.

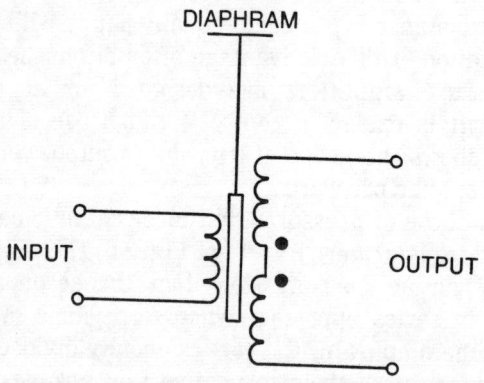

Fig. 2-6. Linear voltage differential transformer. The input ac excitation voltage induces voltages in each secondary output winding. However, the windings are connected in opposite phases (note position of dots) so that the balanced output is zero. As pressure is applied to the diaphragm, the position of the core is altered, permitting different amounts of magnetic flux to pass through each secondary, which yields an output voltage proportional to applied pressure.

linkage with the primary and greater induced current. Since the induced currents are no longer equal, complete cancellation does not take place, and this generates an output voltage that is proportional to the applied pressure. The output voltage can be amplified and displayed as the voltage analog of blood pressure. Generally speaking the LVDT is more sensitive and has superior linearity compared with other transducer types. On the minus side, though, they also tend to be more expensive.

Figure 2-7 shows a method for calibrating and testing pressure transducers. The piece of test equipment shown in this figure can be homebrewed from a discarded or purloined sphygmomanometer used for manual measurement of patient blood pressures. A *tee* or Y fitting and several convenient lengths of surgical tubing connect the gauge, squeeze-ball/valve assembly, and the transducer together. At the transducer end of the tubing, there must be a male Luer-lock fitting so that it can connect to standard transducer fittings. The other transducer port must be dead-ended into either a Luer dead plug or a turned-off Luer-lock stopcock. If a pressure amplifier is available, it can be used to assist in the calibration or examination of the transducer. If none is available, you can still test the transducer by connecting it to a suitable source of excitation, such as a signal generator or dc power supply, and a voltmeter or oscilloscope. Check to see if

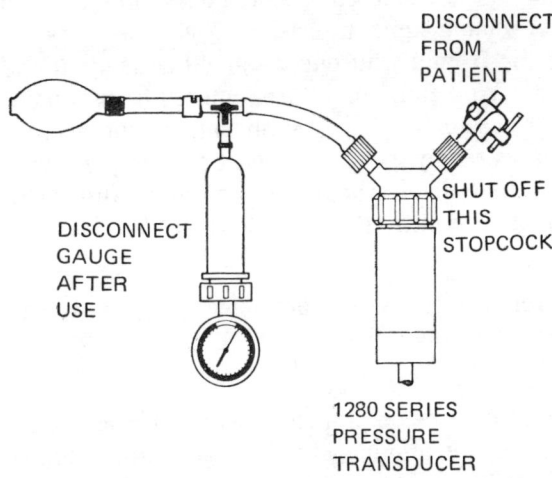

Fig. 2-7. Test apparatus for calibrating pressure transducers.

the output level is consistent with the applied excitation and pressure level read from the manometer. Alternatively, a mercury column or water column can be used. Water manometer columns are easily obtained, but the reading must be divided by a factor of 13.6 if it reads in mmH$_2$O to obtain mmHg or torr.

CRYSTAL TRANSDUCERS

One type of transducer seen occassionally is the crystal transducer. Some crystalline structures exhibit a phenomenon called *piezoelectricity*—meaning pressure electricity. If a slab of piezoelectric material is mechanically deformed, a voltage is generated that can be picked up by surface electrodes. When the crystal is allowed to regain its shape and then deformed in the opposite direction, a similar voltage of opposite polarity is generated. Interestingly enough, most crystal piezoelectric elements are *bimodal*—a voltage can also be applied to the electrodes to generate a mechanical flexure.

These phenomena are important in certain areas of medical ultrasonics, which is covered in a later chapter. Crystals can oscillate at a rate determined by their size and other factors, and these rates can exceed 10 MHz.

EXTANDING TRANSDUCER USEFULNESS

Through the use of electronic integrators, differentiators, and other analog signal processing tricks, we can gain a lot of information from a transducer signal that is not immediately apparent. We can, therefore, measure parameters not originally possible with only simple amplification of the signal output delivered by the transducer. For example, from physics we know that velocity can be derived by differentiating a position function of time. In calculus notation

$$v = dx/dt$$

By differentiating the resultant velocity signal, we can derive the acceleration signal,

$$a = dv/dt = d^2 x/dt^2$$

In some cases, a simple linear potentiometer can be ganged to some moving object to generate a time-varying voltage function that is the electrical analog of position. Acceleration and velocity can be derived using electronic (op-amp) differentiators of suitable design. A slide potentiometer is used for rectilinear motion, while rotary potentiometers are used for angular motion. Similarly, you can often acquire an electrical analog of some flow rate, and this can be integrated to derive the flow volume; such instruments are sometimes used in respiratory measurements.

Chapter 3
Blood Pressure Amplifiers

The hydraulic pressure in the aorta is at its minimum value when the heart is relaxed in *diastole*. When *systole* commences, the heart is contracting and aortic pressure climbs to a maximum value, which then falls off toward the diastolic value as the chambers of the heart empty of blood.

Figure 3-1 shows the pressure-vs-time graph of this cycle. Point A in the figure is the pressure existing during the period when the heart is relaxed. This value is called the *diastolic pressure*. *Systolic pressure*, the maximum value in the cycle, is shown at point B. As the left ventricle of the heart empties, pressure in the aorta begins to fall. The smooth falling characteristic that might be expected is interrupted by the closing of the heart's aortic valve. This creates a glitch in the waveform and is the feature at point C in the graph. This feature is called the *dicrotic notch*. Following this feature, the pressure will continue its decline and fall back to the diastolic value untill a new cycle begins.

Medical people generally quote arterial pressure in terms of systolic and diastolic pressures. So the pressure shown in the figure would be given as *120 over 80* or *120/80*. Notice that the actual pressure never falls all the way back to zero.

There are two general techniques for measuring blood pressure: direct and indirect. Direct methods require going into an artery and actually measuring the dynamic pressure.

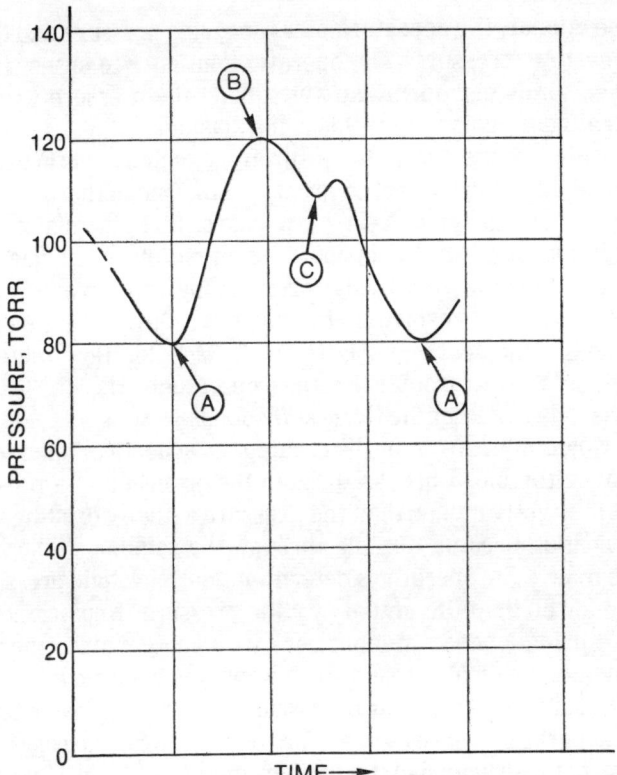

Fig. 3-1. Typical blood-pressure waveform of heart pulse, showing diastole (A), systole (B), and dicrotic notch (C).

The indirect method is, by far, the most common and should be familiar to almost everyone who has been examined by a doctor.

The indirect method actually measures the air pressure in an aneroid chamber called the *blood pressure cuff*. The pressure gauge used to measure aneroid pressure is called a *sphygmomanometer*. The cuff is wrapped around the patient's arm and its pressure is pumped up until the cuff occludes the artery in the arm and shuts off blood flow. The operator listens with a stethoscope placed over the artery in the arm at a point downstream from the cuff location. Air pressure in the cuff is slowly leaked out while the operator listens with the stethoscope. When the pressure in the cuff falls to a level approximately equal to the systolic pressure level in the artery, blood will spurt through the occlusion and generate certain characteristic sounds called *Korotkoff sounds*. When these appear, the operator notes the gauge pressure and this is the systolic pressure. The operator continues to observe until these sounds disappear, at which point the pressure value on the gauge is again noted; this is the diastolic value.

Although the indirect measurement technique is in general clinical use, it is subject to great errors. One authority claims that 5–10% is typical. In most cases, though, this error is negligible in normal decision making, so the technique lives on. But there are methods for reducing this error to a low value without resorting to invasive direct-measurement methods. One technique is to use a Doppler flow meter or electronic (ultrasonic) stethoscope such as the Roche Fetasonde to detect the Korotkoff sounds.

Normally, an error is created in acoustical monitoring because the blood breaks through the occlusion at a pressure that is slightly higher than the pressure actually existing when the sounds become audible through the regular stethoscope. This makes the operator's determination of systolic pressure a little lower than the actual systolic pressure. Replacement of the spring-loaded manometer with a genuine mercury manometer will also result in an improved accuracy. But even with ordinary acoustical monitoring and spring manometers, the accuracy is satisfactory for most medical purposes. If it were not, you can bet that other methods would have been found a long time ago.

The main problem with normal indirect methods is that they are not suitable for long-term continuous monitoring, as might be desirable in an operating room or intensive care unit. There are some instruments that automate the indirect method (an example is the Roche Arteriosonde) and these will be considered in due course. For the time being, however, we are going to restrict our discussion to invasive, direct methods of blood pressures monitoring.

DIRECT MEASUREMENT

In order to perform a direct measurement of human blood pressure, it is necessary to get inside the artery. Although instruments exist that measure pressure directly using a water or mercury column, they are (except in one case) obsolete. So electronic instruments dominate the field. Pressure is a physical parameter, but electronic instruments can only respond to electrical signals. In order to translate pressure values into analogous electrical signals, you need a transducer such as those described in Chapter 2.

Some blood pressure transducers are so tiny that they can be inserted directly into the artery. Others, also very small, are fitted with a single Luer-lock connector so they can be directly attached to a needle inserted into the artery. The most common configuration, however, is to use a relatively large transducer mounted at bedside. The transducer is hydraulically coupled to the artery by a thin, rigid-wall, hollow tube, called a *catheter*. This is inserted into the artery by a doctor using either percutaneous puncture or cut-down techniques. A column of saline solution couples the arterial pressure wave to the transducer diaphram.

Since the laws of physics still apply, we must take certain precautions regarding the transducer. One very important point is to be sure the transducer is mounted at the same height above the floor as the point where pressure is being measured. This, of course, is the site where the catheter enters the patient's body. If this is not done, a certain amount of artifact is introduced into the measurement because gravity induces hydrostatic pressure against the transducer diaphram.

The frequency response of the system can be important, especially if certain features on the arterial waveform are to be examined in detail. At the operator level, this can be accomplished by selecting of a catheter with relatively rigid walls. Of course, there has to be a trade-off between rigidity for the transducer's sake and flexibility for ease of operation and installation.

Air bubbles in the system can cause bad artifacts. They must be purged from the catheter, lines, and dome. Medical transducers typically have a transparent dome made of plastic located over the diaphram, and this makes it easy to spot bubbles and facilitates in their removal. Most modern arterial pressure monitoring systems use a constant flush technique to keep the lines open and free of blood.

Figure 3-2 shows a transducer setup typical of medical pressure monitoring systems. The three-way stopcock can also be used to inject medications and to draw blood. Most transducers cannot stand much vacuum (negative pressure) and will be easily damaged if a vacuum is drawn against the diaphram. One mechanism by which this can occur is through

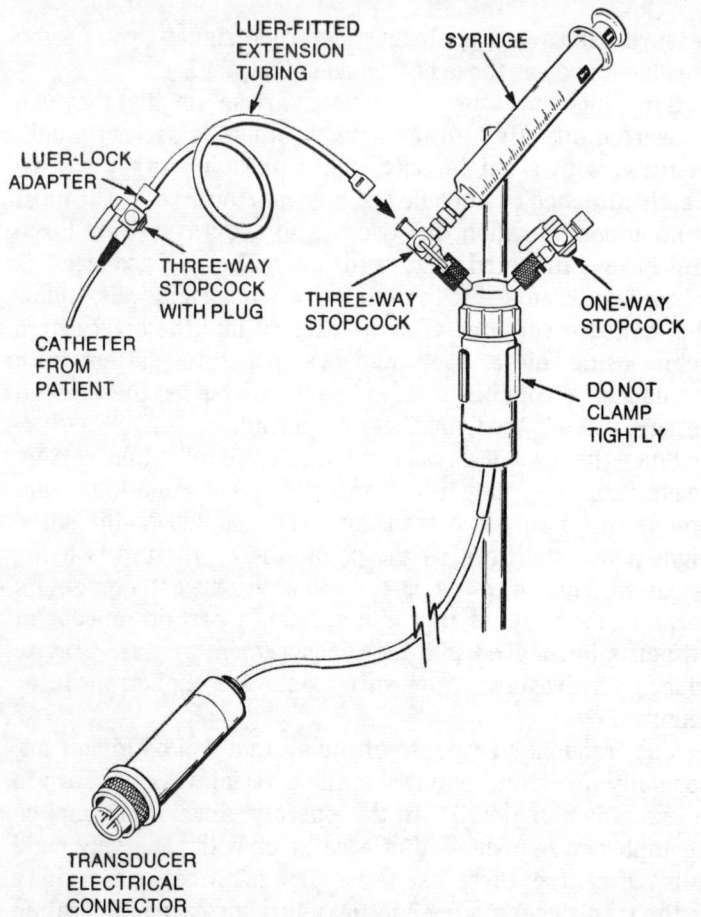

Fig. 3-2. Typical setup for measuring blood pressure by direct means through a catheter. The location of the stopcocks is important to permit bleeding air from the system, enable blood to be withdrawn or medication to be injected, and to protect the pressure transducer from damage.

an incorrect setting of the three-way stopcock. If the stopcock is turned to the wrong position and an attempt is made to withdraw blood, a vacuum is created in the dome and the diaphram is permanently strained in the negative direction. And believe me, a hypodermic syringe makes a very good, small-volume vacuum pump! In one case I watched a nurse as she attempted to draw blood through a one-way stopcock connected to the transducer.

The transducer's electrical connector is attached to the pressure amplifier input. The purpose of the pressure amplifier is to process and present, in a form suitable for display, the signal analogous to blood pressure. This output signal may be required to drive a meter readout, strip chart recorder, or oscilloscope. In order to calibrate this system, you must adjust the zero point and gain (sensitivity) of the amplifier. Transducers are imperfect devices and are rarely exactly nulled when zero pressure (atmosphere) is applied. Wire and semiconductor strain gauges exhibit slightly different values of resistance in each of the arms, while inductive types are often afflicted with different values of stray capacitance between the primary and two secondary windings in the bridge. Both of these conditions result in an unbalanced bridge and a zero-point displacement on the pressure readout device. Adjustment of the *zero* control is done with the transducer open to atmosphere because we are really measuring gauge pressure rather than absolute pressure, which is relative to a vacuum.

Amplifier gain is adjusted with either a standard pressure pumped into the system or by depressing a *calibrate* button on the amplifier's front panel. In this latter case, you are actually supplying an internal signal presenting a standard pressure. The amplifier gain is adjusted so that the pressure indicated on the readout device agrees with the value of the applied pressure or standardized electrical calibrate signal.

Figures 3-3 and 3-4 show three different pressure amplifiers as might be used in medical settings. In Fig. 3-3 we have two models by American Optical. The top unit is a model *261131* and features a digital readout. The lower instrument is very similar but uses the more traditional analog meter for readout. This combination allows simultaneous display of both systolic and diastolic pressures. Most blood pressure amplifiers used for medical monitoring have some form of alarm to detect over- or under-pressure limits that may be exceeded. These alarms are features of these two units as well as the unit in the following figure. One interesting aspect of the A-O models is the use of automatic zeroing. The transducer stopcock is opened to atmosphere and the *zero* button is pressed. Internal circuitry takes over and generates a null by sampling and holding the off-zero condition at the output and creating an input that counteracts this condition, thereby forcing the output to zero.

Figure 3-4 is a Hewlett-Packard pressure system made from two subassemblies (models *78205A* and *78206A*) in a

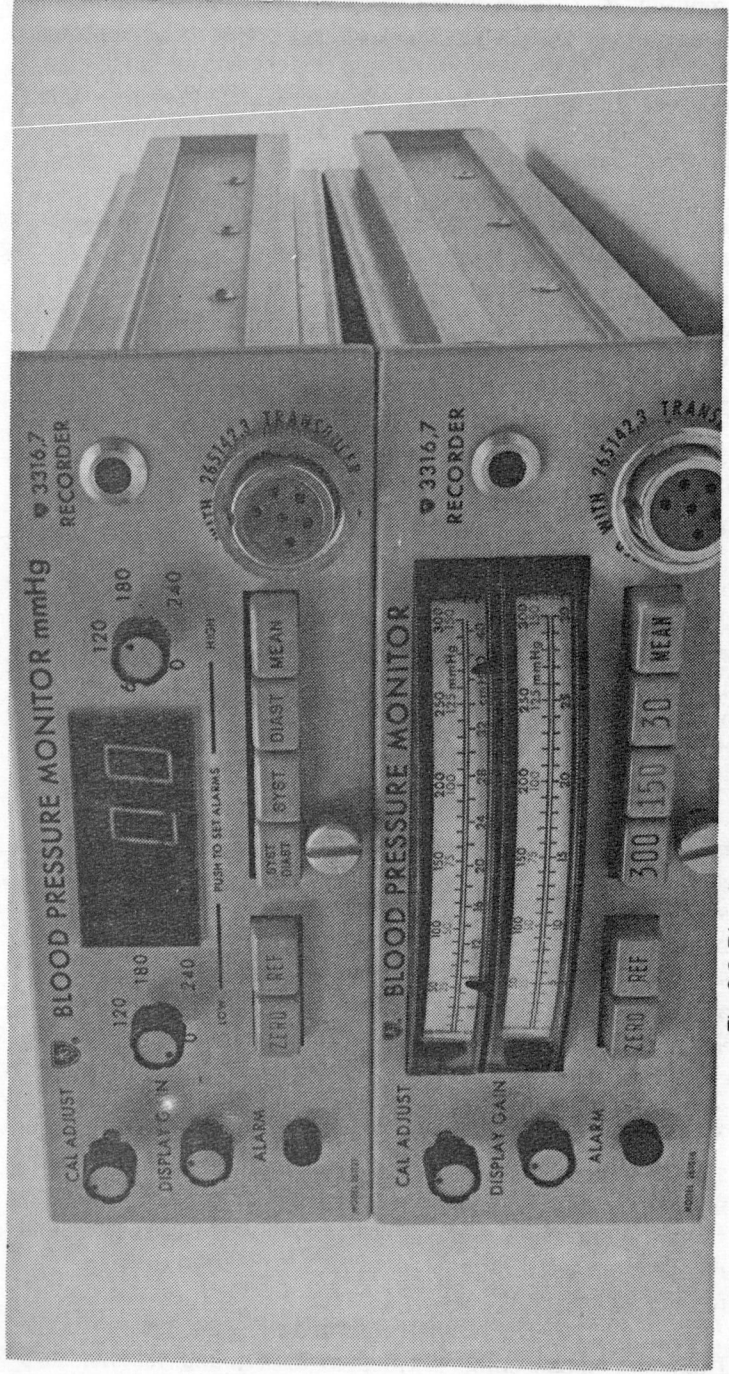

Fig. 3-3. Blood pressure amplifiers. (Courtesy American-Optical)

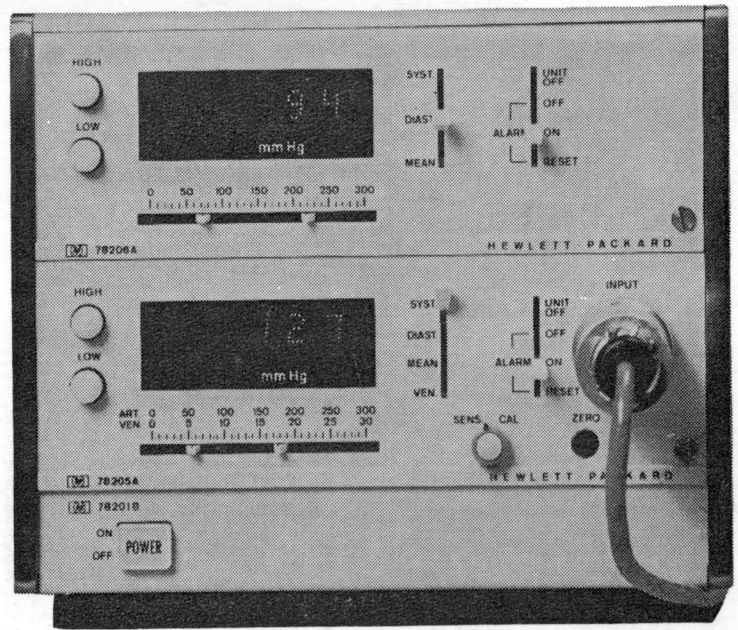

Fig. 3-4. Blood pressure amplifiers. (Courtesy Hewlett-Packard)

standard system mainframe. This instrument package has many features of the A-O instruments. The alarm points are set by slide potentiometers on the front panel. Instruments of this type usually bring signals out to a connector on the rear panel to allow system interconnection with a minimum of mess and trouble.

BLOOD PRESSURE AMPLIFIER CIRCUITRY

The number of different circuits representing any one class of instrument is far too large for any book to cover in detail. There are, fortunately, only two general circuit catagories, and these can be profitably discussed. The feature distinguishing these classes is the method of transducer excitation: ac or dc.

In Fig. 3-5 we see the block diagram of a dc-excited system. Of course, the pressure amplifier must be a dc amplifier and that implies all direct coupling. A highly regulated dc potential is used as the excitation signal and is applied across the Wheatstone bridge. If no pressure is applied, transducer output voltage E_T will be zero, and amplifier output voltage E_O will also be zero.

55

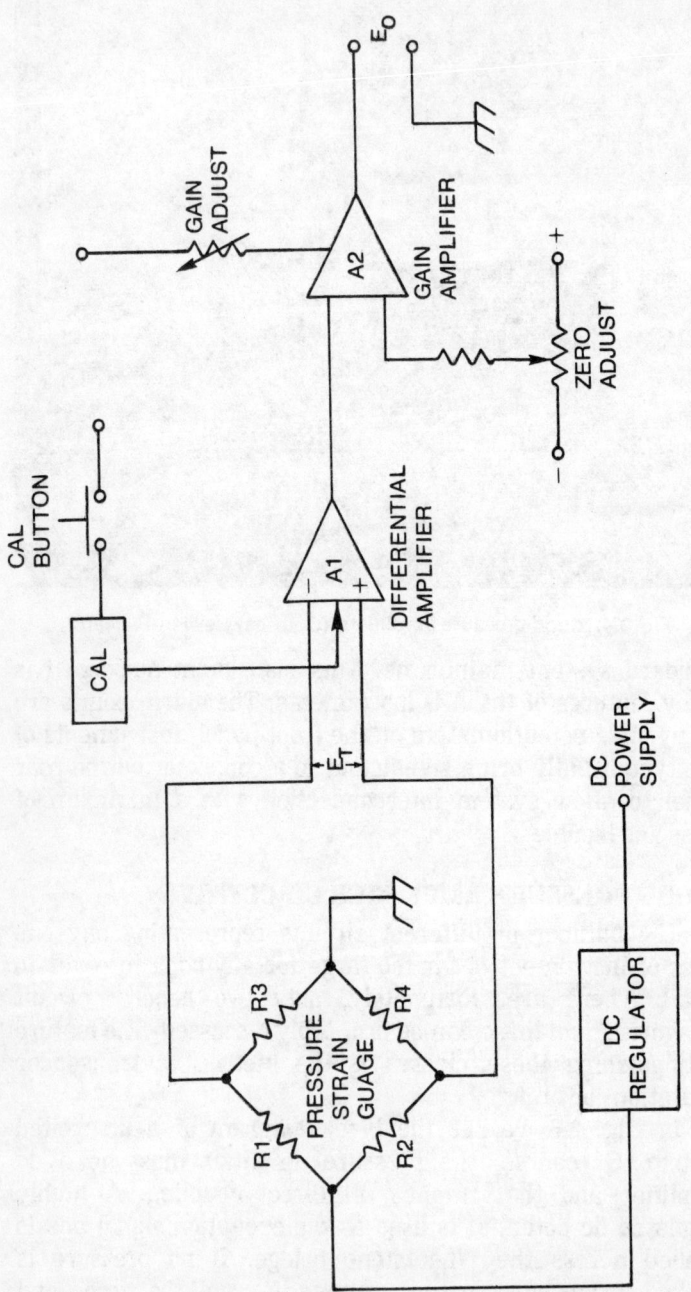

Fig. 3-5. A dc-excited pressure amplifier system.

In this present discussion we are going to assume—at least temporarily—that the transducer is perfectly nulled. This is, in reality, very seldom the true case. Also assumed, is that the amplifier has no offset voltages on the output, or anyplace else.

If a pressure is applied to the diaphram of the transducer, the Wheatstone bridge will become unbalanced and produce a value of E_T proportional to that applied pressure. This is a *differential* voltage, and it is applied to the differential inputs of amplifier A1. The remainder of the needed gain is supplied by amplifier A2. The *zero* control is needed because real equipment is not perfect. This control is used to compensate for errors in transducer balance at zero pressure and for amplifier output offsets existing in the amplifier.

The gain control is used to set the value of E_O to a certain prescribed level when a certain standard pressure is applied to the transducer or when the *cal* button is pressed. For example, if the calibration control applies a simulated 200 torr pressure signal, the gain or sensitivity control is adjusted until the readout meter says *200*. If you know the scale factor, it may be possible to get a better measurement using a 3½- or 4½-digit digital multimeter (DMM). Then the meter calibration can be checked and an adjustment made, if necessary. Hewlett-Packard uses a scale factor of 10 mV/torr, so a 200 torr pressure would generate a potential of 2.00 volts. Not all manufacturers, however, make things so rationally convenient thereby forcing you to use a little arithmetic when using a vol meter on the output.

Direct-current excitation has several severe disadvantages. One is the fact that only a resistive strain gauge may be used—LVDT and inductive bridges are not compatible. Another serious defect is that regulated dc power supplies and dc amplifiers have the nasty habit of drifting which is not too nice in medical and scientific equipment.

Pressure monitors using ac excitation, often called *carrier amplifiers*, form the bulk of medical blood pressure and scientific pressure monitors. These devices produce an excitation signal between 2 and 10 volts rms at frequencies between 500 and 2500 Hz. Carrier amplifiers have several advantages over dc-excited types. For instance, they will operate with all three common types of blood pressure transducers. Also, all of the early stages are ac amplifiers, and this implies the use of capacitor coupling. This latter feature, along with judicious use of feedback, makes ac amplifiers superior to dc amplifiers in the matter of slow baseline drift.

There are at least two different carrier-amplifier configurations used in medical monitoring of pressures. The simplest units are usually set up for bedside or operating-room monitoring with a limited number of transducer types. These are designed for reasonably good accuracy with a minimum number of user-operated controls, and they will usually have a built-in alarm system. Examples of such instruments are shown in Figs. 3-3 and 3-4, already discussed. The reason for this approach is that absolute accuracy can be a trade-off in monitoring systems where less experienced staff are required to learn the equipment quickly.

Where accuracy is needed, or where a large variety of transducer models may be called into use, you will find the more complex configuration. Although basically the same, these units include features that make them more flexible. Most instruments in this class take the form of rack-mountable preamplifiers such as the Hewlett-Packard *8800* series. These can be installed in either a single-channel power-supply housing to make a simple instrument or in the preamplifier rack of a large multichannel oscilloscope or strip chart recorder. Although such systems are occassionally found in ICU bedside, operating room, or other day-to-day clinical use, they are generally confined to catheterization laboratories, research facilities, or centralized OR monitoring. The operators there have a slower personnel turnover and can be trained on more complex equipment.

Among the advantages of the more complex type of pressure amplifiers is the ability to accommodate wider ranges of transducer types, all of which seem to have different sensitivity ratings. They also provide for zero suppression, correction of resistance and capacitance errors, include null controls to balance the transducer, and feature the ability to measure other parameters, such as temperature, if a suitable transducer is supplied.

Figure 3-6 shows in block form a simple carrier amplifier used in pressure monitoring. The excitation signal (or ac carrier, if you prefer) is developed in an oscillator and is fed to the transducer at a relatively high amplitude and power level. Most models seem to use a carrier level around 5V, which is in

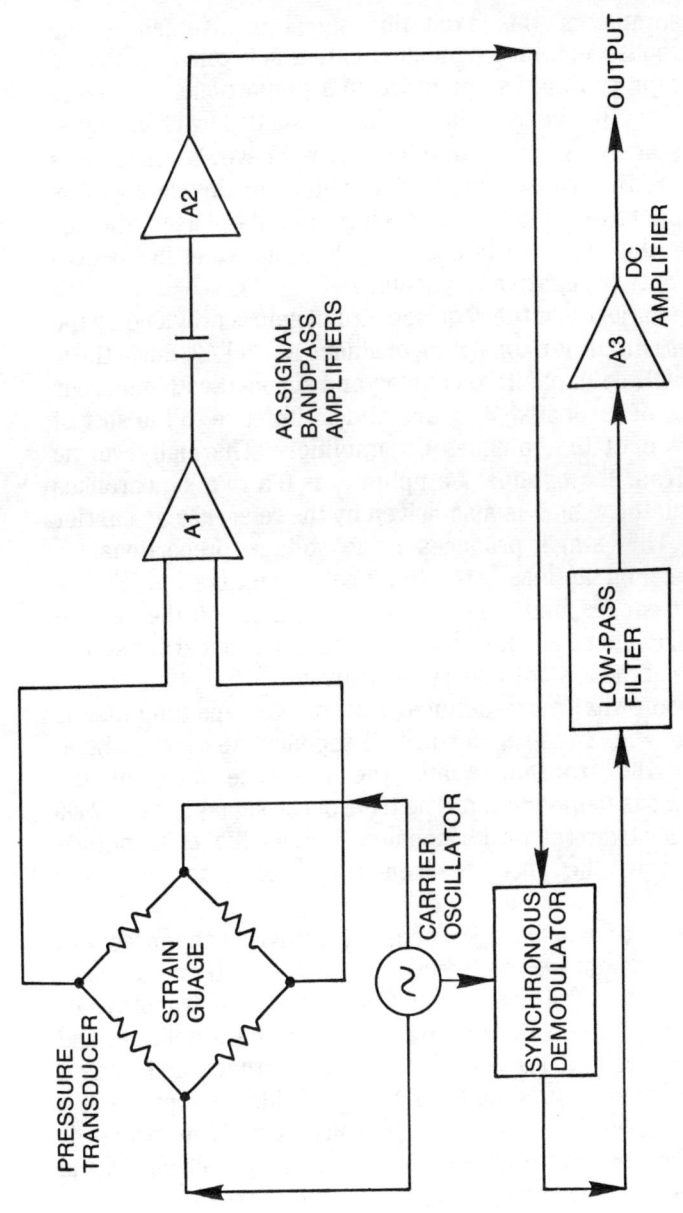

Fig. 3-6. Carrier amplifier block diagram.

keeping with transducer manufacturer's recommendations and requirements.

A sample of this excitation signal is also fed to the synchronous detector (demodulator), which converts the ac signal representing the pressure to a proportional dc signal for delivery to the readout device. A small low-level signal appears at the input of amplifier A1 whenever a pressure is applied to the transducer. The amplitude of this ac signal is proportional to the applied pressure, and its phase indicates whether the pressure is positive (the usual case in medical equipment) or negative (a vacuum).

The majority of the required circuit gain is provided by the bandpass amplifier consisting of stages A1 and A2. Since these stages will be capacitive coupled and supplied with generous amounts of feedback, they are almost immune to the sort of baseline drift that plagues dc amplifiers. The high-level ac signal from the bandpass amplifiers is fed to a synchronous demodulator, which is also driven by the reference ac carrier signal. This stage produces a dc voltage proportional to pressure and applies it to the final amplifiers, which are low-gain stages and serve mostly as buffers to the outside world. Drift here is not so much a problem as in earlier stages because of the low voltage gains involved.

A somewhat more detailed view of this type amplifier is shown in Fig. 3-7. Transformer T1 supplies the carrier signal to both the transducer and the reference input of the synchronous demodulator. The transducer signal is a 5V, 2400 Hz carrier from the first secondary. A much higher amplitude signal from the second secondary is used to drive the demodulator input.

Either resistance differences or stray capacitances will tend to unbalance the transducer and create an artifact voltage at the input to the amplifier. The *zero* control provides a sample of the 2400 Hz carrier, having an amplitude and phase appropriate for cancelling out this artifact, and sums it with the transducer signal in R1. If the bridge is connected, it must be opened to air for zero adjustment. If no bridge is connected, it is merely necessary to short together pins A and C on the amplifier input.

The calibration signal represents a pressure of 20 torr in the venous amplifier and 200 torr in the arterial, even though both machines use the same plug-in printed circuit board in

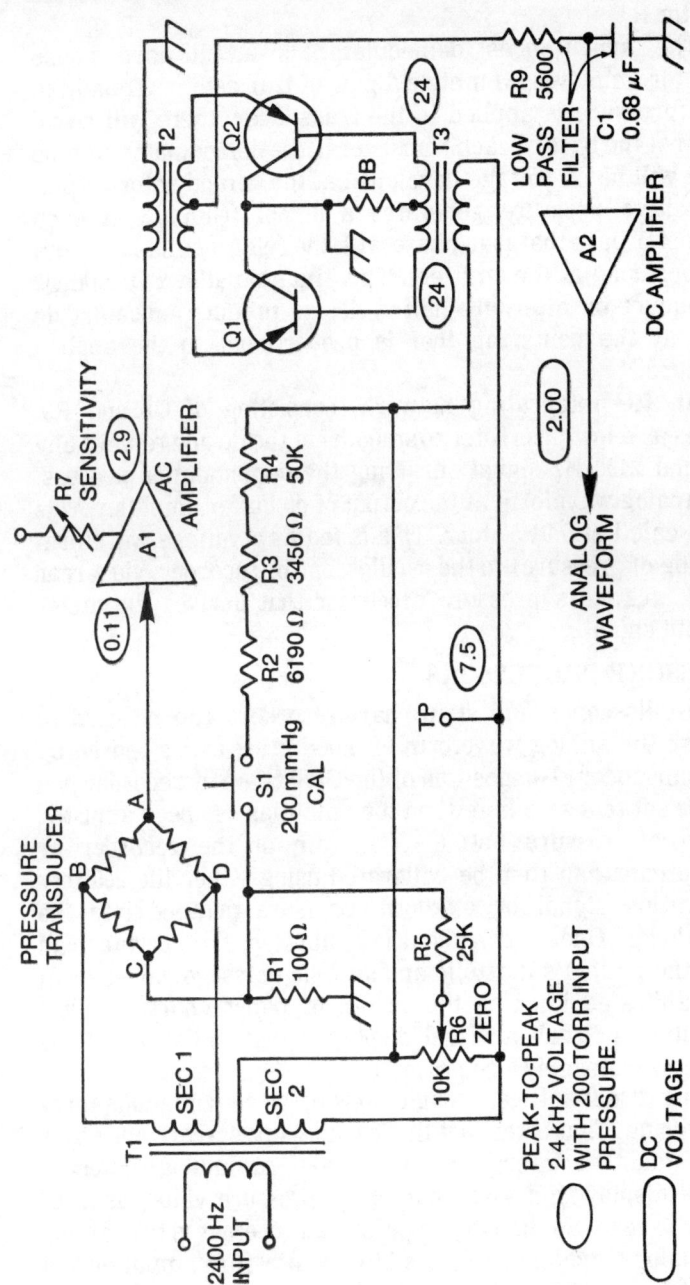

Fig. 3-7. Carrier amplifier circuit.

the carrier section. This signal is also developed across resistor R1.

The synchronous demodulator is a full-wave phase detector employing a matched pair of transistors, Q1 and Q2. If no pressure is applied to the transducer, there will be no signal at the base of each transistor in the demodulator pair, so there will be no voltage developed at the demodulator output. A positive pressure generates a signal from T3 at each transistor base that is in phase with the reference signals from T2 appearing at the emitters. This situation allows Q1 and Q2 to conduct on alternate half-cycles to produce pulsating dc level at the centertap that is proportional to the applied pressure.

An RC integrating network, consisting of C1 and R9, serves as a low-pass filter to smooth out the dc and remove any residual 2400 Hz signal surviving the demodulation process. The analog waveform at the output of dc buffer amplifier A2 is then scaled at 0.01 V/torr. This is fed as a voltage waveform (analog of pressure) to the oscilloscope or recorder, via a rear panel jack, to a pressure processor that derives the meter readout signal.

PRESSURE PROCESSORS

Oscilloscopes and strip chart recorders can be used to display the analog waveform of blood pressure as sensed by the transducer. The position of the CRT beam or recorder pen can be set to a zero line when the amplifier has been adjusted for zero pressure output. The gain of the recorder or oscilloscope can then be calibrated using either the 200 torr calibration signal or a known pressure pumped into the transducer. Once the readout is calibrated, the operator can read the patient's diastolic and systolic pressure values from the calibrated lines on the screen or paper chart. Another advantage of such a visual display is that the shape of the analog waveform is also presented.

One disadvantage, though, pops up when doing long-term monitoring. That is the fact that oscilloscope screens and chart paper must be interperted or "read." An analog meter or digital display that gives numerical pressure values is a lot easier to read. So the job of a pressure processor is to examine the analog waveform delivered by the pressure amplifier and uses it to create a dc voltage level or current that can be read as a steady signal on a panel meter.

Figure 3-8 shows the block diagram of a typical pressure processor used by Hewlett-Packard in its 7809 arterial pressure monitor. The systolic detector is little more than a strobed peak-holding circuit. The diastolic detector is the same sort of thing except that an inverter in the input makes the diastolic or low point on the analog waveform a high point, so that a peak holder will respond to it. The *mean filter* is basically a low-pass filter (integrator) that is used to approximate the mathematical relationship:

mean blood pressure = diastolic + ⅓ (systolic − diastolic)

For example, the mean pressure of a waveform showing an arterial pressure of 120/80 is

mean blood pressure = 80 + ⅓ (120 − 80) = 93.3 torr

Details of the peak-holding circuit are the subject of Fig. 3-9. The analog waveform is applied to the input of amplifier A1 and also to the input of a second, identical amplifier in a parallel peak holder. The output of amplifier A1 is used to charge the 100 μF capacitor, C1. The voltage across C1 is proportional to the peak input, which in this instrument is the systolic pressure. This potential is applied through isolation diode D2 to the amplifier stages and readout meter. This same action simultaneously occurs in the second peak holder, and its voltage is applied through diode D3 in a similar manner.

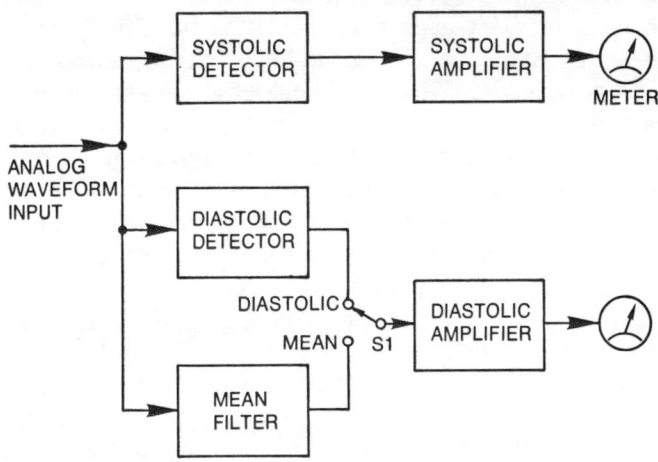

Fig. 3-8. Block diagram of pressure processor for detecting and displaying diastolic and systolic levels.

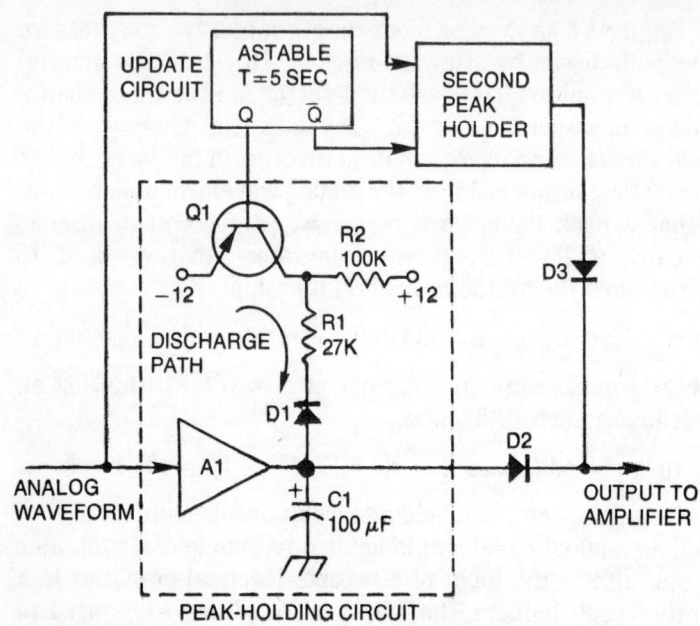

Fig. 3-9. Dual peak-holding system for providing stable systolic pressure readings.

An update circuit strobes the peak holders such that one is being discharged while the other supplies voltage to the systolic amplifier. Strobe action is timed by an astable multivibrator with a period of about 5 seconds. The discharge path used to reset each peak holder is through diode D1, resistor R1, and transistor Q1. A similar circuit is used in the second peak holder. When the Q output of the astable circuit goes high, where it remains for approximately 2.5 seconds, transistor Q1 will turn on and allow C1 to discharge. This will allow the capacitor to recharge to the next systolic value after the Q output of the astable goes low. When that happens, the Q̄ output will be high and cause the discharge of the 100 μF capacitor in the second peak holder.

The reason why a dual peak-holding system is used is to keep the output steady and readable on a panel meter. If only one peak holder was used, the reading would drop as the discharge took place, resulting in an undulating meter pointer that is very difficult to interpret. You may see a similar symptom should one of the systolic peak holders become inoperative.

Checking Pressure Amplifiers

There are several methods used to check pressure amplifiers. The zero point is easy to check, since all that is required is a short across the amplifier inputs. Here we are not now interested in transducer balance but rather the amplifier is output offset. All amplifiers have some amount of offset, but this can be nulled out.

A number of different methods exist for checking the gain of the amplifier. One is to use a calibrated transducer, but since these are so expensive it is simply not feasible to keep one handy just for testing amplifiers. One form transducer simulator that can be used for pressure amplifier analysis is a homebrew Wheatstone bridge. This unit can be made from precision resistors with at least 1% tolerance—0.05% if you can get them. These should be in the 200–300Ω range. The exact value is not too critical so long pseudo-transducer in a small metal box and equip it with a connector or cable at the output. An unbalancing resistor is switched across one arm of the bridge when you want to simulate a standard pressure. Since the resistances selected may vary from case to case, the value of the unbalancing resistor will have to be found experimentally.

One homemade tester—which has proved immensely valuable in testing pressure amplifiers dynamically—uses an optocoupler to switch in the unbalancing resistor. The LED side of the optocoupler is connected to the output of a 1 Hz square-wave generator. Every time the square wave goes high, the LED lights up and this shorts together the output terminals, switching the resistor into the circuit. This will put a 1 Hz square wave on the oscilloscope screen as a measure of the amplifier's performance. There will, however, be some high-frequency rolloff on the corners of the waveform.

Hewlett-Packard recommends the circuit in Fig. 3-10 for testing the pressure amplifiers in its *7800* series instruments. I have also found it useful in testing other pressure amplifiers that depend upon the Wheatstone bridge configuration. Connector J2 mates with your amplifier, although the pin-outs shown are for the male 5-pin AN (MS) connector formerly used by Hewlett-Packard as their standard pressure transducer connector. When the switch is in the *up* position, the amplifier input terminals are shorted together and the *zero* control on the amplifier is adjusted so that there is a 0.00V ±

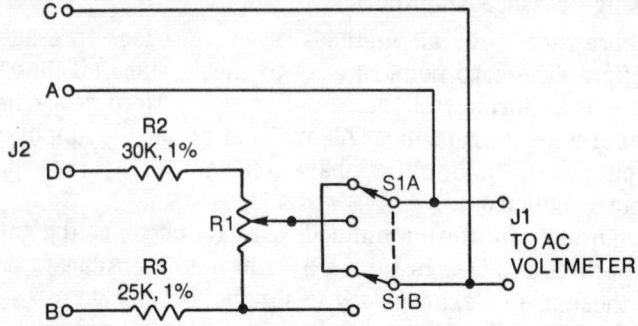

Fig. 3-10. Pseudo-transducer for testing amplifier gain in blood pressure monitors. Resistor R1 should be a 1K, 10-turn potentiometer with a turns-counting dial. Always use high-input-impedance voltmeters for maximum accuracy.

10 mV potential at the output of the amplifier. This is indicated on a dc voltmeter connected to the output jack. For best accuracy, use at least 3½-digit digital multimeter.

In the H-P instrument, the test is made with the internal gain switch set to X1. Adjust R1 in the tester until an ac voltmeter connected to J1 indicates 40 mV rms. Adjust the pressure amplifier sensitivity control for 1.00V ± 10 mV dc on the output meter. The control should have a liberal range to either side of this, and there should be less than 10 mV noise and hum on the output as viewed on an oscilloscope connected in parallel with the voltmeter. Although the voltages and steps may differ, this technique can be extended to other amplifiers made by H-P and to other manufacturers as well.

Chapter 4

Medical Oscilloscopes

Cathode-ray oscilloscopes are used to monitor the output waveforms of ECG preamplifiers, blood pressure amplifiers, and other instruments that produce either an actual waveform or a dc level proportional to some physiological parameter being measured. Medical oscilloscopes differ little from oscilloscopes used in other fields of science and technology, and like their cousins, they come in a seemingly endless and bewildering variety.

Before proceeding with our description of medical oscilloscopes let's review the basic theory underlying the operation of the cathode ray tube (CRT). It is, of course, the CRT that makes oscillography possible. The CRT viewing screen is coated on the inside of the evacuated, glass-tube envelope with a phosphorous material that emits light when struck by a beam of electrons. These electrons are generated by thermionic emission from a cathode and are formed into the required narrow beam by elements of an "electron gun" located in the neck of the CRT. The electrons are accelerated by a high voltage, which can be as low as 1500V dc in small-screen oscilloscopes, to as much as 30,000V dc in some color television receiver CRTs. Light is emitted when the accelerated electrons strike the phosphorous screen. Generally, the intensity of the emitted light is proportional to the accelerating potential, which implies that the kinetic energy of the electrons is a pertinent factor.

Unless the electron beam is deflected to one side or the other, it will travel in a straight line from the electron gun exit aperture to the viewing screen, producing only a small dot in the center of the screen, which is hardly useful. There are two basic methods commonly employed for electron beam deflection: magnetic and electrostatic.

In the magnetic system, coils of wire are wrapped around the neck of the CRT, concentric to the path of the electron beam. This assembly, called a *deflection yoke*, is actually little more than an electromagnet whose field is capable of deflecting the electron beam from its original path according to well-known laws of physics. In the typical yoke assembly there will actually be two sets of mutually perpendicular magnet coils. One set causes deflection of the electron beam from left to right (assuming the mechanical orientation is correct) and this is the *horizontal* winding. The second set of coils, oriented at right angles to the first, supplies *vertical* deflection of the electron beam.

In CRT designs that use the electrostatic deflection system, the beam is deflected by an electric field established between mutually perpendicular sets of deflection plates by a differential voltage.

In most medical oscilloscopes, horizontal deflection is by a sawtooth voltage or current waveform designed to sweep the beam from left to right across the CRT face. When the characteristic sharp drop in the edge of the sawtooth occurs, the electron beam retraces back to the left-hand side of the CRT screen very rapidly. Normally, the CRT electron beam is turned off or *blanked* during this time period. The vertical deflection system will be connected through appropriate amplifiers to an input connector, so that time-varying voltages from other instruments (e.g., the ECG preamplifier) can be traced out on the screen. In some cases, both horizontal and vertical inputs are used to trace out patterns created by two time-varying voltage functions. This method of displaying two related functions in terms of each other creates *vector patterns* and *Lissajous figures*.

Intensity modulation of the CRT screen light can be accomplished by varying the voltage applied to the control grid or cathode (effectively the same thing) in the electron gun assembly. Usually, though, in medical applications only the retrace pulse generated by the sawtooth's falling edge is applied at these points. (We shall discuss at least one exception later on.) A CRT screen, such as found in a television is normally swept both vertically and horizontally, although at different rates, causing a *raster*, which means that the entire viewing area is illuminated.

The simplest forms of medical oscilloscope are the one- or two-channel, recurrent-sweep models used for most bedside monitoring applications. All medical oscilloscopes in this class use long-persistence phosphors, such as the P7, in the CRT screen. This allows most features of slow-moving waveforms, such as the ECG or blood pressure (arterial) signals, to remain visible until the end of the appropriate cycle. They will fade away by the beginning of the next cycle, since the persistence is only on the order of a couple seconds.

More sophisticated medical oscilloscopes use special circuitry to store the waveform pattern on the CRT screen until it is either erased on retrace or is "over-written" by the waveforms of the following sweep. These are the so-called *non-fade* displays that are useful in storing several waveforms of immediate past history at the same time. More about these designs in due course, toward the end of this chapter.

OSCILLOSCOPE SWEEP CIRCUITS

Figure 4-1 is the block diagram of a typical recurrent-sweep, simple medical oscilloscope. Although the model shown in the illustration is a two-channel variety, the discussion and basic theory of operation applies also to single-channel models, provided that the chopper circuit and one vertical amplifier channel are eliminated.

The cathode ray tube will usually be of the long-persistence type and will have a screen measuring 4 to 12 inches diagonally. Either electrostatic or magnetic deflection may be used, depending upon the manufacturer and their choice of CRT type number.

Typical laboratory or service oscilloscopes use electrostatically deflected CRTs because magnetic deflection yokes cannot accommodate the higher sweep speeds and vertical input frequencies required. Even elderly, cheap "audio" oscilloscopes will sweep to at least 150 kHz. Modern, yet moderately priced oscilloscopes might sweep to as much as 10 or 15 MHz. For such oscilloscopes, we find that the vertical channels might be required to accommodate signals

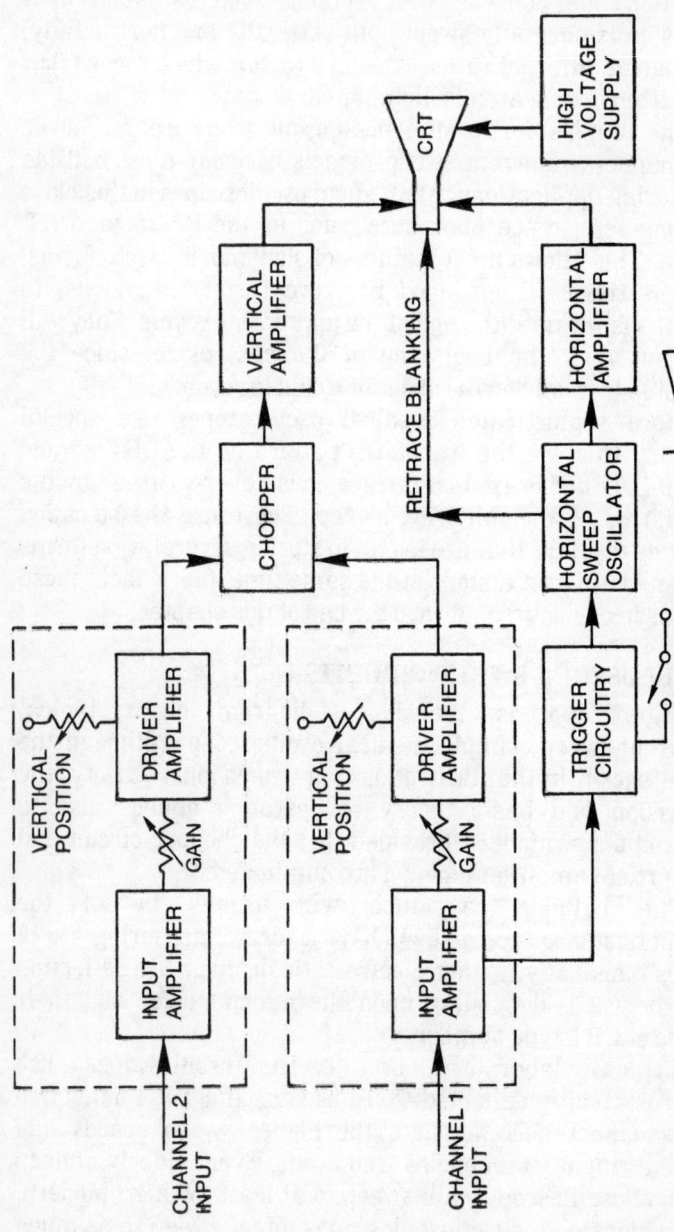

Fig. 4-1. Two-channel medical oscilloscope. In a single-channel design, one vertical amplifier chain and the chopper circuit would not be present. Otherwise, both one- and two-channel scopes work essentially the same.

70

from 500 kHz to well over 100 MHz before showing any appreciable attenuation.

In medical oscilloscopes, on the other hand, we can use either sweep method. The fastest horizontal sweep speed might be only 100 mm/sec on a 10 cm (approximately 4 inch) CRT. This corresponds to only one sweep per second (1 Hz). Typical ECG sweep speeds are 25 mm/sec and 50 mm/sec; the lower of these corresponds to 0.25 Hz on the same size screen. Vertical frequency-response requirements will be no greater than 100 Hz for ECG—and may well be considerably less for oscilloscopes intended only for long-term monitoring purposes. In the strictest requirement, for uses other than ECG, the vertical bandwidth need only go up to about 2000 Hz.

Obviously, then, the medical oscilloscope can use either magnetic or electrostatic deflection since frequency response is not really a limiting factor. It is true that the high-frequency capability of a yoke coil is seriously limited by its own inductance and by the stray capacitance between its windings. But this effect is of little consequence below frequencies of 20 kHz or so. In fact, magnetic deflection for medical oscilloscopes is probably the more common of the two competing methods One reason why this is true may be the fact that magnetic CRT types tend to be a little shorter in length than most electrostatically deflected types, and this allow the manufacturers to offer more attractive packages for their instruments. Also, until fairly recent times, it was generally better to use magnetic deflection in solid-state oscilloscopes because the final amplifier stages driving the deflection circuit could use high-current, low-voltage transistors instead of the less reliable high-voltage types needed to accommodate electrostatic designs. Regardless of certain claims by semiconductor manufacturers and design engineers (who never again see their product), low-voltage transistors have proved to be more reliable from the servicer's point of view.

Besides the usual low-voltage bias, there are four inputs needed to operate the CRT. One is the high-voltage accelerating potential on the second anode. This could be produced by rectifying the secondary of a special low-current, high-voltage 60 Hz transformer, but it is usually derived from a high-frequency oscillator operating a flyback transformer—much in the same manner as in television receivers.

The other signals applied to the CRT are the horizontal sweep, vertical deflection, and retrace blanking.

The horizontal sweep signal is a low-frequency sawtooth waveform generated in a circuit such as in Fig. 4-2, a unijunction transistor (UJT) relaxation oscillator. A UJT will not conduct current across its emitter–base junction until the voltage across that junction rises above a certain critical point. When that voltage is exceeded, the resistance between the base and emitter is greatly reduced and can discharge the timing capacitor.

In the UJT relaxation oscillator (Fig. 4-2), the voltage across the emitter–base junction is controlled by the charge on capacitor C. The emitter voltage will rise as C becomes charged, but only until the critical firing point is reached. At that time, the emitter–base resistance drops sharply and causes the capacitor to discharge rapidly. This produces the classic sawtooth waveform at the emitter.

This waveform has the slowly rising characteristic of the charging capacitor. But in this case, we want a linear (straight line), rather than an exponential characteristic, so that the sweep trace is consistant on all points of the CRT screen. To accomplish this, it is necessary to charge the timing capacitor from some sort of constant current source. Such a circuit might consist of one or more bipolar transistors, a junction

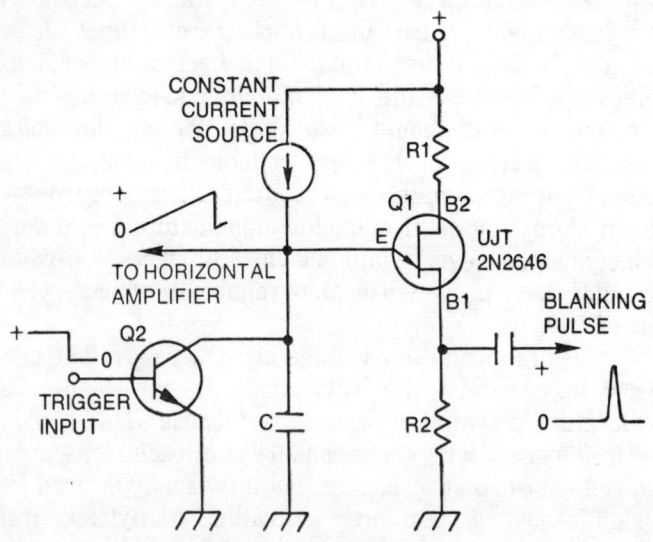

Fig. 4-2. UJT sweep oscillator.

field-effect transistor with gate and source tied together, or a constant current diode. When the constant current source is used to charge capacitor C, we will find a sawtooth output that has a linearly rising ramp.

The UJT relaxation oscillator can also provide the blanking pulse. A capacitor is connected to the grid of the CRT with its other end to the emitter of the UJT. This pulse or spike is generated across resistor R2 by the heavy current flow produced as the charge on the capacitor is discharged through the emitter–base circuitry.

The horizontal circuit of the CRT is designed so that the electron beam will strike the left side of the screen, or even slightly off the screen at the left, when the voltage across capacitor C is zero. As the voltage rises, the CRT beam is swept across the screen at a constant rate toward the right. When the capacitor is discharged, the beam snaps back to its rest position on the left. The blanking pulse generated at this time is used to extinguish the CRT electron beam during this retrace period. This prevents the retracing electron beam from creating a distracting streak of light as it snaps back across the screen.

SWEEP TRIGGERING

If the UJT relaxation oscillator is allowed to free-run, then the oscilloscope is called a *free-running* or *recurrent sweep* model. An alternate model of oscilloscope is called the *triggered sweep* type.

In a triggered-sweep oscilloscope, the sweep oscillator is inhibited until it is unlocked by a special triggering circuit. The electron beam is held to the left-hand side of the screen (either extinguished or so far to the left that it is actually off the screen) until a certain minimum amplitude signal is present in the vertical amplifier channel. Many medical models are also equipped with a trigger timing circuit to create or uninhibit the trace if no signal is received from the trigger within a certain preset period of time, often 1.5 to 4 seconds.

In some laboratory and service oscilloscopes you can often adjust the trigger point to initiate a sweep with some time delay after the required amplitude signal is presented in the vertical amplifier channel. This delayed-sweep feature allows you to examine, on an expanded time scale, almost any feature on the input waveform.

Most medical oscilloscopes, however, are specially designed to trigger only on the ECG's R wave. This constraint allows an easy determination of the patient's heart rate by noting how far from the left-hand side of the screen the first *visible* R wave occurs. In doing this, we are actually using the oscilloscope's internal time base to measure the period of the patient's R-to-R interval, which is simply the reciprocal of frequency of heart rate. Many medical monitors intended mostly for ECG monitoring have a calibrated heart-rate scale printed on the CRT graticule—the higher rates appear to the left (quickly occurring R wave) with the lower rates to the right.

In circuit of Fig. 4-2, trigger switch Q2 is an NPN transistor connected across timing capacitor C. In the *hold* mode, the base of Q2 is kept positive by the trigger input, causing Q2 to be forward biased and therefore conducting heavily from collector to emitter. This condition keeps capacitor C from charging by sinking the current delivered by the constant current source. When a QRS complex waveform is received in the vertical amplifier channel, the minimum threshold is exceeded by the R-wave, and this removes bias from the base of Q2, cutting the transistor off and allowing the capacitor to charge in the normal manner.

The foregoing is a stylization of actual trigger circuit operation and is intended mostly to illustrate the principle of triggered sweep. Although most trigger circuits are actually a bit more complex, it is still fairly typical of simple medical oscilloscope trigger circuits.

VERTICAL AMPLIFIERS

The medical oscilloscope in Fig. 4-1 has two channels and the vertical amplifiers are identical to each other. We shall therefore describe only one of them. Typical input sensitivities for such amplifiers range from 1V/cm to 1V full scale (6–10 cm).

Because of the low-frequency response required in medical monitoring, it is necessary for the medical oscilloscope to easily pass signals down to at least 0.5 Hz; some go all the way down to dc. Since these oscilloscopes usually operate with high-level input signals of 1V or more, we need not worry a lot about baseline drift, which is a common affliction of oscilloscopes boasting millivolt or better sensitivities.

Most medical oscilloscopes come equipped with an external gain control to adjust the display size and a position control to adjust the baseline location on the vertical axis of the CRT screen. The position control merely sets the dc offset of the vertical amplifier.

If this was a single-channel oscilloscope, there would be but one vertical channel and it would feed the vertical power amplifier directly. In this case, however, we have a two-channel design, so a *chopper* is required in addition to a second vertical channel.

A chopper is a high-frequency square-wave generator that drives certain switching circuits so that one vertical channel is connected to the vertical power amplifier on positive square-wave peaks and the other is connected on negative square-wave peaks. The repetition or chopping rates of a typical chopper must be sufficiently high so as to not distort the signal to be displayed on the screen of the oscilloscope.

Typical laboratory and service oscilloscopes often have vertical amplifiers with frequency-response characteristics high enough that the chopping rate becomes too low. When this occurs, the square wave actually appears on the screen. In this condition, which occurs at faster sweep speeds, the vertical input signal appears to be broken up and has what could be called the "sampled" look. In medical designs, fortunately, we use only low-frequency vertical amplifiers, so a chopping rate in the low ultrasonic range is sufficient.

Simple oscilloscopes using but two or four channels work well with the chopper technique, but the method is often found to be wanting when more than four channels are desired. Figure 4-3 shows an old Sanborn (now Hewlett-Packard) multichannel oscilloscope. The lower assembly is the gating amplifier—the unit which actually breaks up the single beam into the eight separate beams seen on the screen of the CRT. Actually, this series of oscilloscope models may be found in any of several configurations, depending upon which of several devices is installed in the gating amplifier slot. The space occupied by the gating amplifier in this version is actually a standard preamplifier rack assembly, which can accommodate up to six preamplifiers (ECG, EEG, pressures carrier, PPG, etc.) and a small four-channel gating amplifier. In other versions, the oscilloscope is fitted with up to eight single-channel gating amplifiers. In this current discussion,

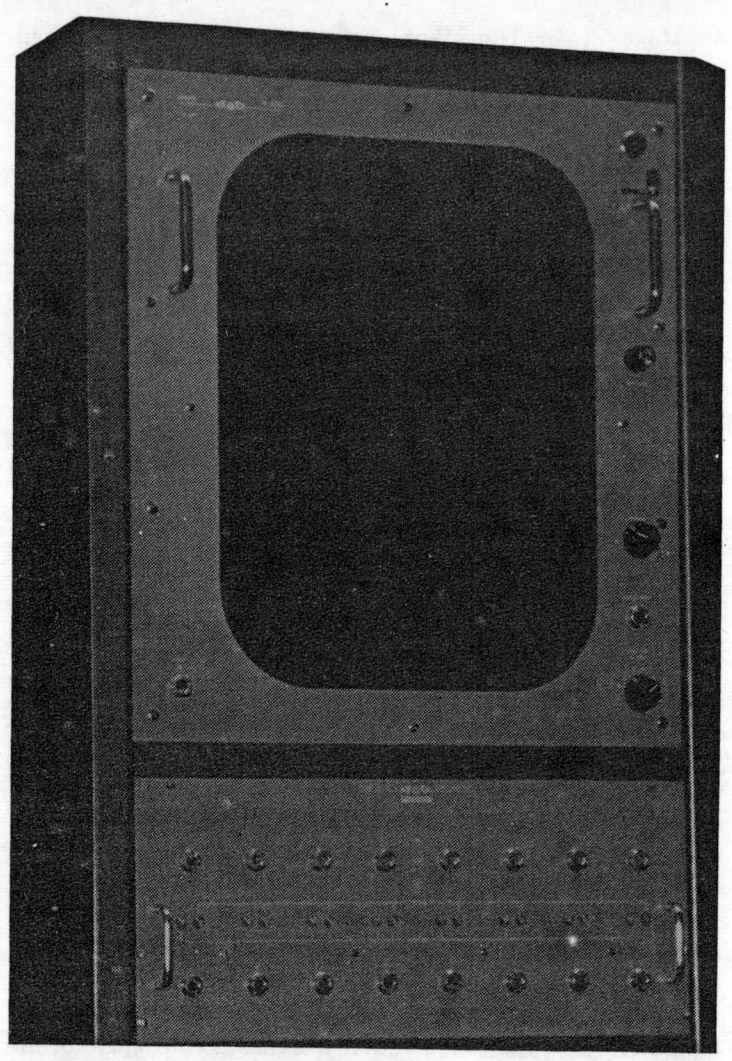

Fig. 4-3. This multichannel Sanborn oscilloscope uses gating amplifiers to display eight vertical input channels.

however, we are going to consider only the eight-channel gating amplifier pictured in the figure.

Each of the eight channels located on the front panel, has three controls: an on/off switch, a sensitivity potentiometer, and a position potentiometer. Both potentiometers, incidentally, are recessed and can only be adjusted using a small narrow-blade screwdriver. In addition, there is a rear-panel connector bringing signals from a remote location for display on the oscilloscope, and power from the main oscilloscope power supply to the gating amplifier circuits. A phone jack is provided for local input to each channel, and this can also be used to bring main channel signals out for routing to an outboard auxilliary instrument such as a strip chart recorder.

Figure 4-4 is the block diagram of a typical gating amplifier medical oscilloscope. Although there may be up to eight independent channels, we shall only consider one in order to simplify the description. There are two separate deflections—horizontal and vertical—applied to the CRT. The horizontal is a linear, low-frequency sawtooth that drags the beam from left to right in about 3 seconds. This rate, incidentally, is low enough that operation of the horizontal system may be checked with a voltmeter to see the sawtooth potential rising.

Simultaneous with the horizontal sweep, there is a high-frequency vertical sweep deflecting the beam up and down at a rate between 15 and 20 kHz. The CRT grids are held very negative by a bias through resistor R2, so the electron beam is normally kept blanked off. You should recognize that this is precisely the opposite of the situation in regular oscilloscopes.

The function of the gating amplifier is to produce high-amplitude positive-going pulses to unblank the electron beam at certain precise and critical times. These pulses are produced in a voltage-controlled pulse generator, consisting of a direct-coupled input amplifier and the R1-C1-D1 network. The pulse repetition rate of the generator is determined by the voltage applied to resistor R1. When there is no input signal present, the applied voltage at the pulse generator will be at a certain quiescent point. Input signals will raise or lower this potential according to the amplitude and polarity of their waveforms. Diode D1 is a tunnel diode, and its negative resistance characteristic is used to generate sharp, fast rise-time pulses of very short duration.

The summing amplifier functions to combine the pulses from all eight gating-amplifier channels into a single pulse channel that is fed to the main oscilloscope chassis. Before being applied to the CRT control grid, the pulses must receive further amplification to boost their amplitude and some waveshaping to increase their rise time. Pulses applied to the grid of the CRT overcome the negative cutoff bias and unblank the electron beam for a very brief instant.

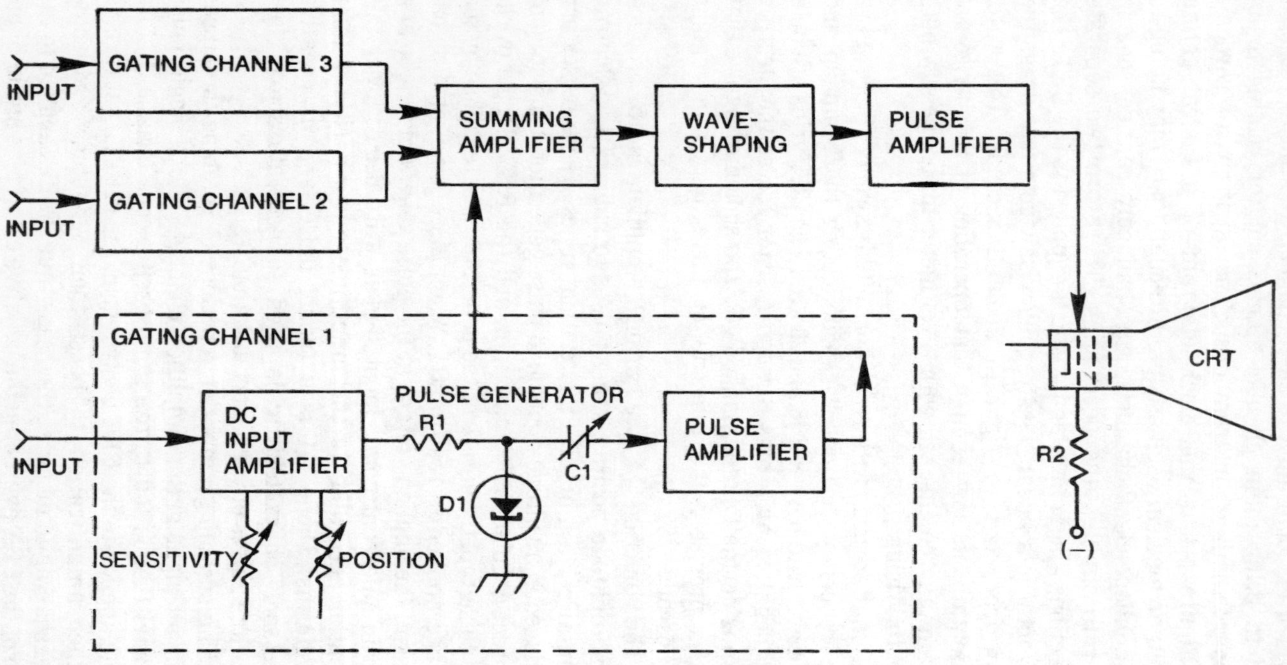

Fig. 4-4. Block diagram of multichannel oscilloscope.

Figure 4-5 shows the timing diagram for this oscilloscope. The waveform at A is the 0.33 Hz sawtooth used for horizontal sweep. At B we have a stylized version of the vertical sweep. In the real oscilloscope, this sweep occurs at a rate as high as 20,000 Hz—which would mean, in the three seconds required

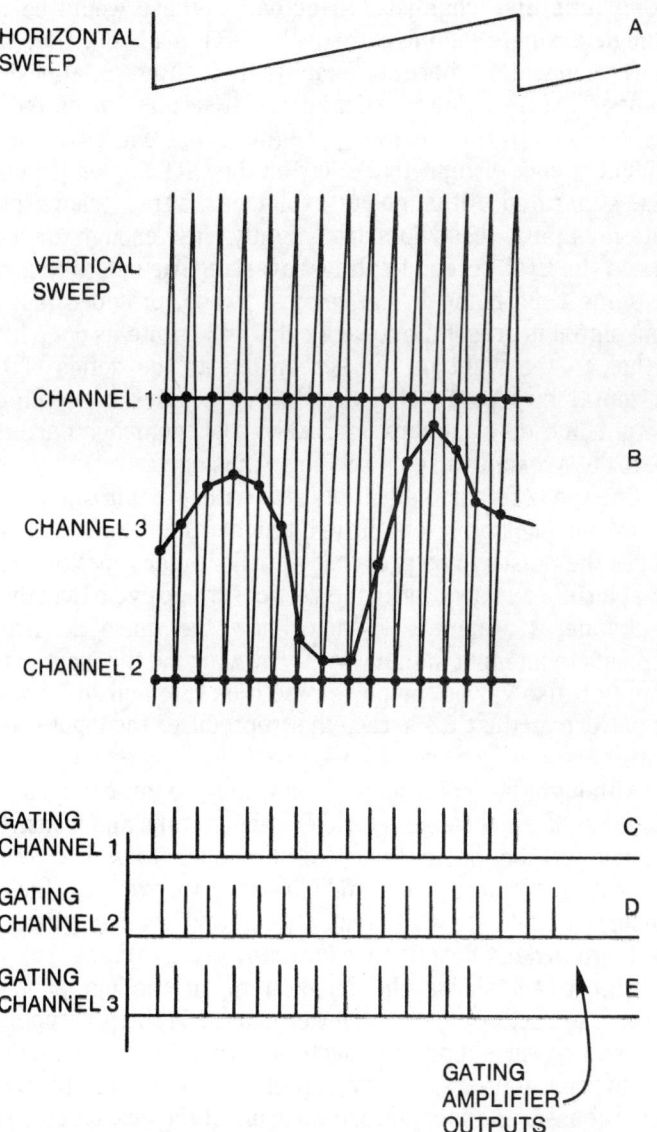

Fig. 4-5. Timing diagram of multichannel oscilloscope.

for completion of waveform A, almost 60,000 vertical sweeps will have been made! Obviously, the limits of printing graphics make it necessary to represent these with only the few sweeps shown at B in Fig. 4-5.

The signals shown at C, D, and E are pulses from the gating amplifier channels. In actuality, these would be fed through a single signal path to the CRT grid, but they are shown separately here to clarify their time relationship. Channel 2 is at a low vertical-position setting, so its pulses occur soon after each sweep begins. This causes them to produce a spot of light that's low on the CRT screen for each pulse generated. Although our expanded diagram shows them quite far apart, these dots are actually close enough for their dots on the CRT screen to almost overlap. The pulses occur at the same time point on the vertical sweep, provided that no input signal is present, but each pulse will create its dot a little further to the right on the screen due to the action of the horizontal sweep. To the viewer this creates a seemingly straight line that appears unbroken; a phenomenon partially due to dot overlap and partially to an illusion.

Channel 2 in our diagram is also without input signal, but its position control is set a little bit higher than channel 1. This causes the pulses to be produced with a similar repetition rate but at a time a little later in the vertical sweep cycle than those of channel 1. Channel 3 shows how the pulse generator responds to an input signal waveform. Varying the input to the amplifier also varies the pulse repetition rate and so causes a dot pattern on the CRT screen that reproduces the input waveform.

Although the oscilloscope from which the foregoing circuit was taken is an obsolete hybrid of vacuum tube and transistor technology, the basic theory still applies to more recent designs. Make no mistake, though—as of this writing, the old Sanborn models are still going strong, and one can expect to find them in daily hospital use for many years to come.

Figure 4-6 shows the inside rear of the old Sanborn workhorse oscilloscope. The lower chassis is the preamplifier rack and power supply. Connectors to mate with those on the plug-in preamplifiers or gating amplifiers are on the other side of this chassis and face toward the front of the instrument. The upper chassis, mounted vertically, houses the sweep circuits and CRT, plus a couple of smaller power supplies. Sweep

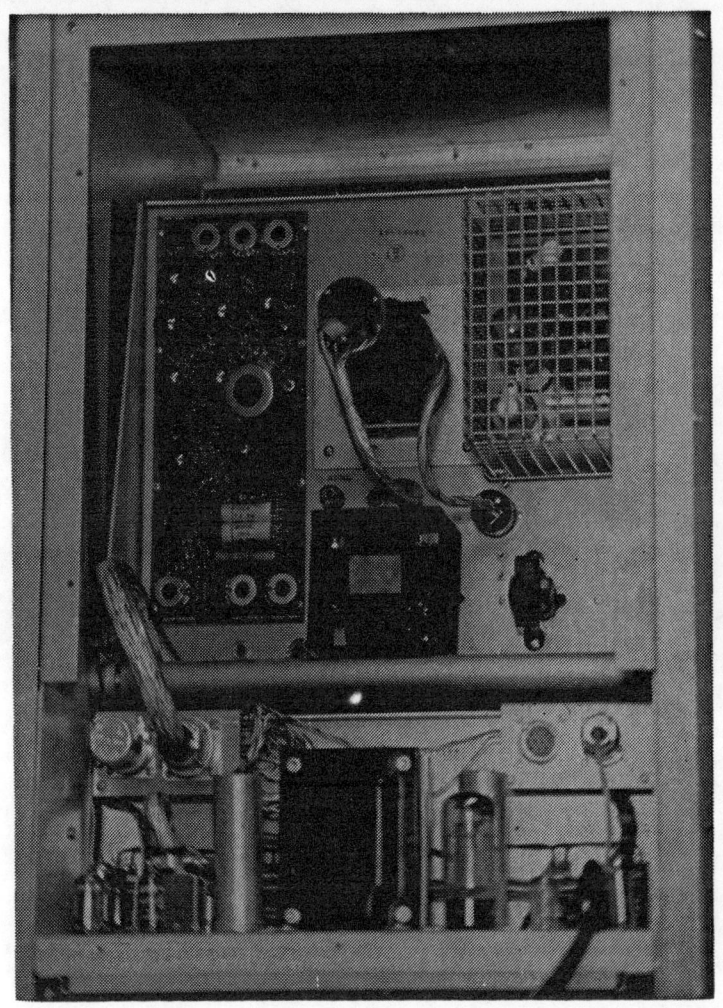

Fig. 4-6. Inside the Sanborn oscilloscope.

oscillators are on the printed circuit board while vertical sweep and the high-voltage power supply are inside the cage.

Some oscilloscopes are equipped with an automatic intensity control circuit, such as shown in Fig. 4-7. If the cathode bias is made more positive with respect to ground, the electron beam will decrease in intensity, since this is equivelent to making the grid more negative. In this circuit, a photocell (PC1) is used to raise and lower CRT brightness in response to changing ambient room light conditions. The

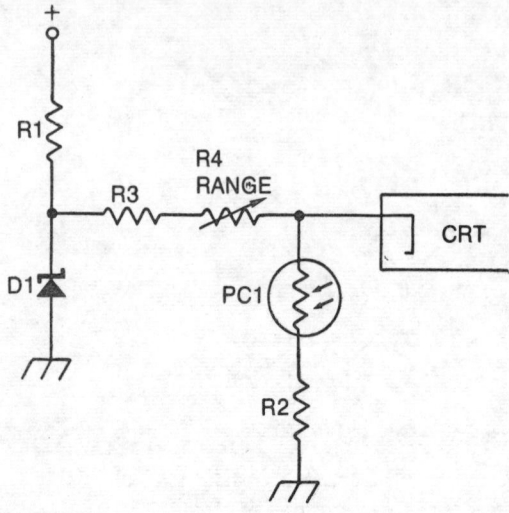

Fig. 4-7. An automatic brightness control uses a photocell to adjust the brightness of the CRT image in response to changes in the level of the room lighting.

photocell in Fig. 4-7 is mounted in such a way that it is exposed to room light, yet it is unobtrusive in physical appearance. The electrical resistance of PC1 will reduce as the room light intensity increases. If the light level decreases, the resistance of PC1 goes up, causing the voltage at the cathode of the CRT to rise. An increase in cathode bias reduces the beam current and thereby reduces the brightness of the CRT display. A potentiometer in the network sets the range of the automatic intensity control, which is usually screwdriver adjustable if only to keep itchy fingers away.

NON-FADE DISPLAYS

Non-fade display oscilloscopes are basically storage types that allow the viewer to see the waveforms in the patient's immediate past history of several seconds duration. Most of these units do not use actual storage CRTs, which is common practice in laboratory and service grade oscilloscopes. Instead, medical monitor storage oscilloscopes are generally equipped with a recirculating shift register, solid-state memory. Circuits of this type can be found in minicomputers and microprocessor instruments. In operation, these circuits are used to store the digitized analog waveform and to refresh the display on the CRT many times each second.

Display Formats

Figure 4-8 shows a Hewlett-Packard model 78304A, four-channel, memory oscilloscope. Others in the 78300 series feature up to eight channels. This oscilloscope is of the stationary display type in which a blanked-out, vertical, erase/write bar travels across the CRT face from left to right. Each ECG signal, or whatever signal is applied, will remain on

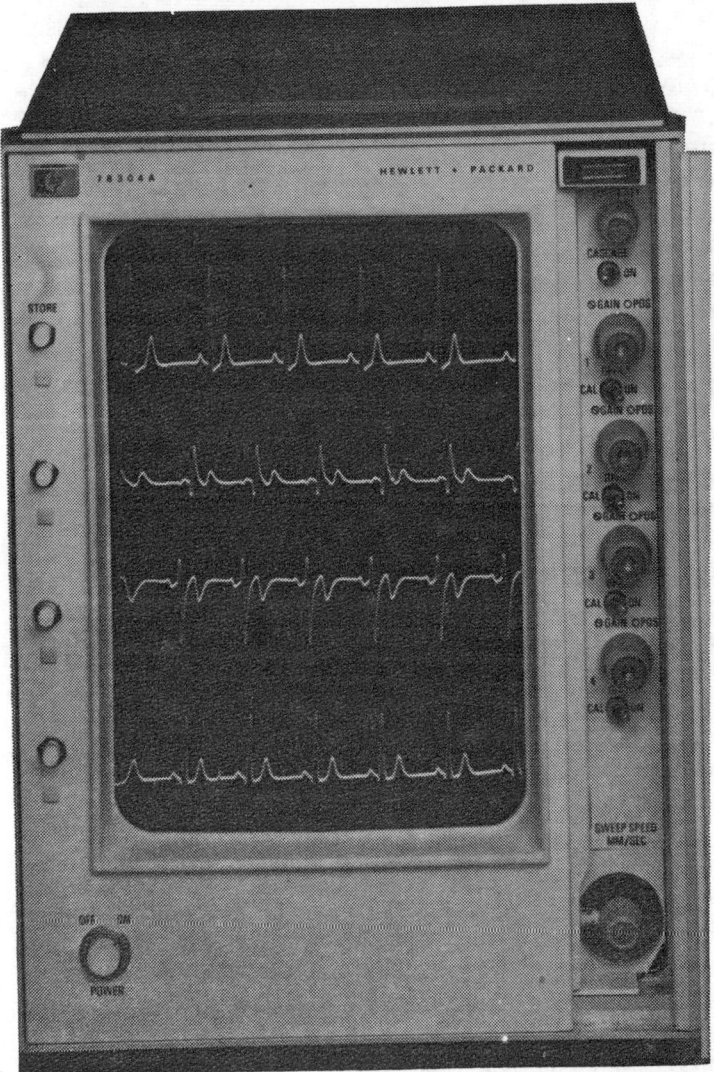

Fig. 4-8. A four-channel medical oscilloscope with memory. (Courtesy Hewlett-Packard)

the CRT screen and will be refreshed from the internal memory many times each second until the erase/write bar once again passes over that spot. Then the trailing edge of the bar will write new information onto the CRT in real time.

These oscilloscopes have several viewing modes, and that makes them very flexible. In one mode, signals from four or eight (as the case may be) patients can be viewed simultaneously, one on each channel. This is the mode preferred in most coronary care units. Alternatively, the user can cascade two or more channels to provide a longer history on any one patient. The trace will begin in the upper left hand corner of the CRT screen in channel 1 and will write onto the screen from left to right. After the erase/write bar retraces to the left, the next signal will be fed to channel 2, which will continue writing the new channel 2 data. The old data in channel 1 does not, however, become erased until the last entry in the last cascaded channel is written. All four channels in this model can be connected in cascade if desired.

Figure 4-9 is another type of non-fade display oscilloscope, but it is somewhat different from the previously discussed model. This model is manufactured by Electronics For Medicine (known as E-for-M). This oscilloscope uses a non-fade display method that is called, in the trade vernacular, a *waveform parade* system. The real-time waveform appears in the upper right as older waveforms move across the screen from right to left. In the H-P system, the location of the real-time waveform changed while the past-history waveforms remained stationary. In this system, the real-time waveform remains in the same location while the past-history waveforms parade across the screen. This E-for-M is not merely a monitor oscilloscope; it is a complete central monitor because it includes alarms and other essential features.

Display Circuits

Figure 4-10 shows the block diagram of a non-fade medical oscilloscope using the waveform-parade sweep method. Previous waveforms can be kept on the CRT screen because they are first digitized and then stored in a solid-state memory. To accomplish this neat trick, it is first necessary to convert the input signal voltage to a digital *word* that can be recognized as representing that particular voltage level. For

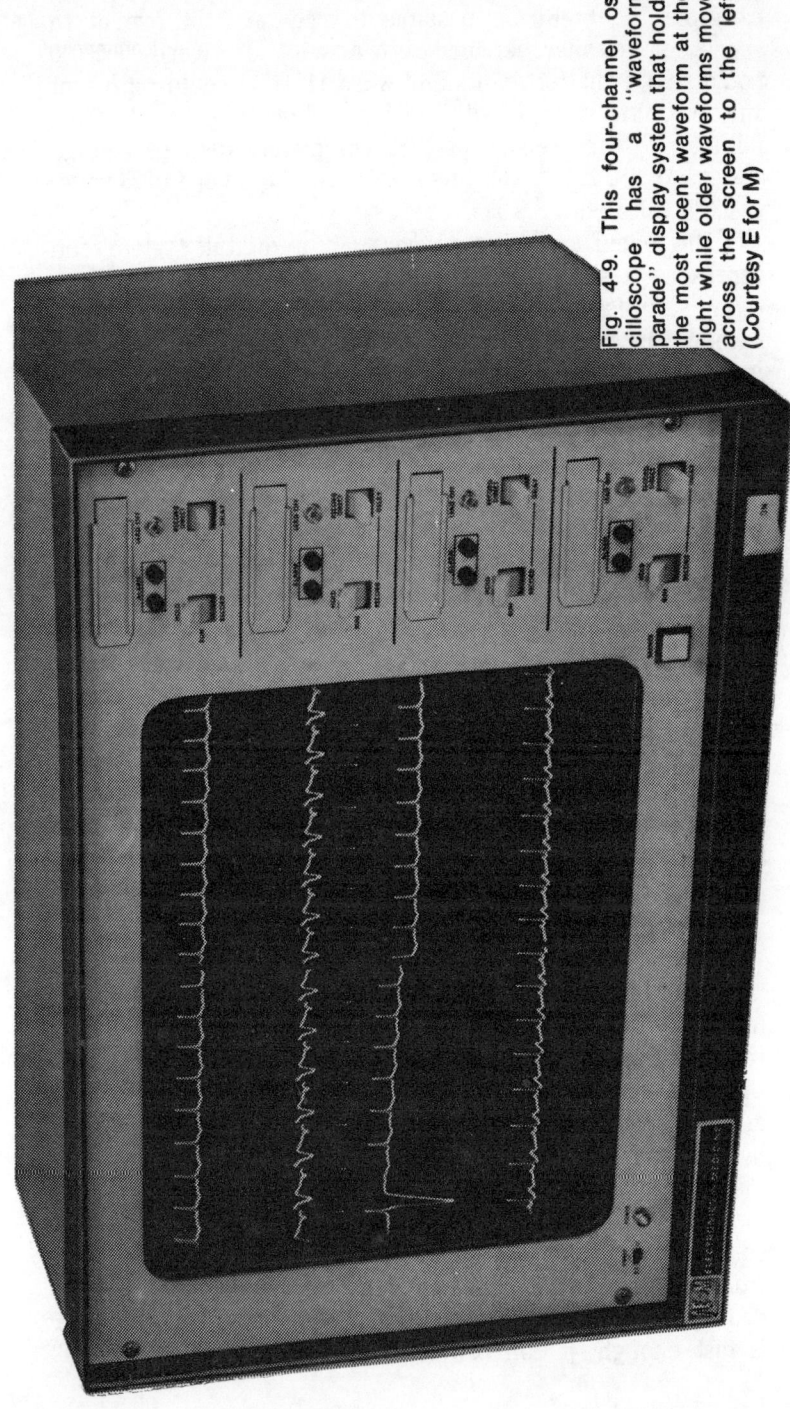

Fig. 4-9. This four-channel oscilloscope has a "waveform parade" display system that holds the most recent waveform at the right while older waveforms move across the screen to the left. (Courtesy E for M)

85

example, it might be possible to use an 8-bit format to represent voltages between zero and 10V dc. Word 00000000 could represent zero volts and word 11111111 could represent 10V, or some voltage within a few millivolts of 10V dc. This number system represents 255 completely distinct voltage states. At 10V full scale, this gives a resolution of 10/225 volts, or 0.039 volts/state.

The accuracy with which such a digital system can represent a time-varying input voltage depends upon how many samples are taken and converted to 8-bit words every second. The minimum number of samples required must be at least twice the highest frequency component of the input waveform.

The analog-to-digital converter (ADC) stage performs the conversion or *digitization* of the analog signal. There are a number of different schemes for implementing the ADC idea, but they are beyond the scope of this book. In medical non-fade oscilloscopes, the ADC might be made of discrete components, or it might be a specialized, plug-in function module or even special integrated circuit. Many different types having various accuracies and resolutions are offered by a large and bewildering number of electronic component manufacturers.

Circuits such as that in Fig. 4-10 operate in a *synchronous* mode—the events in the logic sequence may only occur at the specific times dictated by the arrival of certain clock pulses. In this case, an internal system clock operating at an initial frequency of 131.072 kHz is used. Besides the main clock pulse, there are also memory-bank address, ADC start, and write/recirculate (W/R) pulses.

Two separate memories are used in this instrument. One is a short-term memory, called a *scratch pad*, which holds up to four individual 8-bit words. The other memory is a recirculating shift register holding up to 1024 8-bit words, and this represents the bulk of the data. Such an organization allows updating of the data in the main shift-register memory by replacing the four oldest words with four new words from the scratch pad memory once per recirculation.

Following the main memory bank is a digital-to-analog converter (DAC), and this is used to convert the digital words from memory back into discrete voltage levels that can be displayed on the oscilloscope screen. If the recirculation cycle is fast enough, it can rewrite these voltages onto the CRT

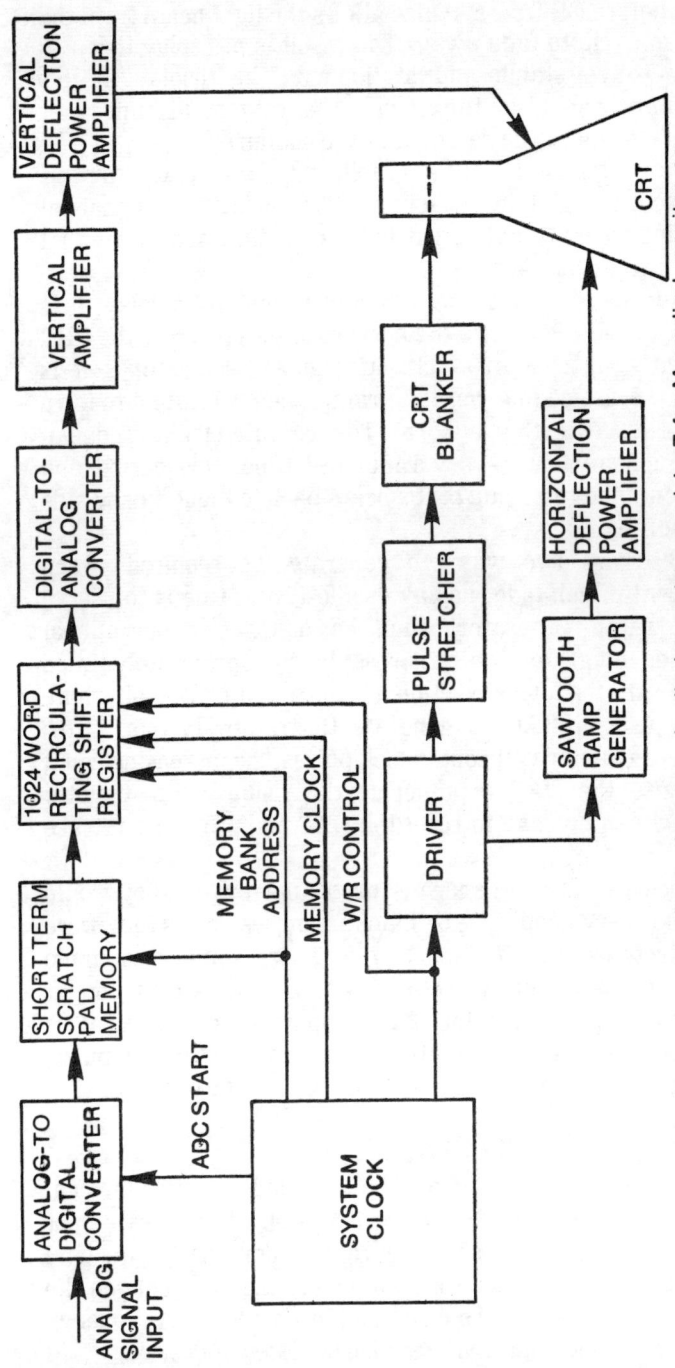

Fig. 4-10. Block diagram of waveform-parade display system used in E-for-M medical monitor oscilloscope. The recirculating shift register is the heart of the display system and is cycled during each sweep of the beam to provide a continually refreshed and updated display. The system clock controls acquisition of new data and enters it into the shift register at the appropriate point.

screen before CRT persistence allows the light beam from the previous cycle to fade away. The result is a display that will appear to be stable and stationary. The display in this particular system is flickering at a rate of 64 times per second—too fast to be detected by the human eye.

The vertical amplifiers following the DAC in this oscilloscope resemble those in regular models. The signals at this point are now undigitized and back in the analog form that is usual to oscilloscopes.

In order to provide an orderly, meaningful display, it is necessary to synchronize the horizontal sweep across the CRT face with the system clock. In regular oscilloscopes it is common practice to generate a ramp, then truncate it to form the classic sawtooth waveform. The truncated trailing edge of the waveform has a very rapid fall time, this period and represents the retracing of the beam back to the left-hand side of the screen.

There are two ways to generate the required sweep waveform in non-fade display oscilloscopes. One is to use an analog ramp generator, such as a UJT or operational amplifier integrator, which is reset by an appropriately timed pulse from the clock section of the circuit. The alternate system uses a DAC to generate the ramp. In this, latter system, a counter will count clock pulses, the increasing count will cause the DAC to generate the rising ramp. Counter overflow can be used to reset the DAC and provide a retrace pulse.

Clock pulses are generally pretty narrow, so they would not make very good retrace blanking pulses unless they were first stretched out. *Pulse stretchers* are sometimes made using one-shot multivibrators, which generate a longer duration output pulse for every input clock pulse that is received. The CRT is actually blanked, not by the clock pulse, but by the stretched-out version produced by the one-shot.

TESTING OSCILLOSCOPES

All oscilloscopes—and that includes the medical variety—should be tested regularly along two lines: input sensitivity and time-base accuracy. Additionally, medical oscilloscopes should be tested for ac leakage currents on the chassis, using techniques discussed in Chapter 16. Frequency response and baseline drift can also be tested, if desired.

The vertical sensitivity can be checked by applying a sine wave of known amplitude and checking the amount of deflection it produces on the CRT screen. Most manufacturers specify these factors with the vertical amplifier gain control set to its maximum position.

The time-base accuracy of the horizontal sweep can be checked using either a time-marker pulse source or a simple square-wave generator. Let us assume a standard 10 cm screen size and a sweep speed of 25 mm/sec. If the unit is a triggered-sweep type, you can get a good idea of time-base accuracy by applying a 0.5 Hz square wave to the input. If the time-base is correct, there will be two complete waveforms visible in the 10 cm space. Alternatively, you could use a pulse time-marker generator to produce a specific number of pulses in a 4-second period. At 5 pulses per second, for example, exactly 20 pulses would be displayed in the 4 seconds required for the correctly adjusted beam to travel from left to right.

Chapter 5

Bedside and Portable Monitors

Bedside monitors are electronic instrument packages used to keep track of certain patient parameters and to sound alarms or take other action should one of these parameters go outside certain predetermined limits. Their purpose is to provide—on a continous basis—medical data that is normally difficult to obtain. They also free the nursing staff for more pressing duties.

Bedside monitors are usually found in intensive care units, coronary care units, operating rooms, emergency rooms, and certain other special or critical care areas of the hospital. Portable monitors are found in all of these places as well as in crash carts, ambulances, and other places where critical care may have to be rendered in an emergency but where there is no convenient source of ac power.

GENERAL FEATURES

An example of one design approach to bedside monitor equipment is shown in Fig. 5-1. These units are manufactured by the medical division of Hewlett-Packard and are good examples of the *modular* approach. The unit on the left is a medical oscilloscope, H-P model *7803B*. Note the relative scarceness of user-operated controls. On this model the user can select a channel (channel 1, channel 2, or both at the same time) and position its beam vertically on the CRT screen.

Users may also select either 25 mm/sec or 50 mm/sec sweep speed. All other controls are located on the rear panel to discourage casual adjustment by the users.

One interesting feature on this model is that each channel is provided with two parallel-connected input jacks so that signals can be simultaneously fed to the oscilloscope and routed to other instruments, such as a strip chart recorder, in a "daisy chain" manner. If the oscilloscope is used for ECG, as is frequently the case, the alternate jack on the oscilloscope's ECG channel might also be sent to a defibrillator's synchronization input for use in cardioversion procedures.

The right-hand units in Fig. 5-1 are an ECG and arterial pressures module housed in a common type *78201* mainframe. Both modules of this instrument can be unlocked and easily removed for servicing or reconfiguring the mainframe with another instrument or pair of instruments. The ECG preamplifier is a three-lead design and has a built-in heart rate meter and alarm capability.

The alarms can be set to certain high and low limits, using the slide scale located immediately below the digital readout of the heart rate meter (also called a *cardiotachometer* by some people). If the patient's heart rate, which is electronically derived from the ECG signal, exceeds the preset limits, then the alarm will trip. On this particular instrument, *high* or *low* panel lights will come on, and a terminal connector on the rear panel will be grounded. In this manner, remote alarms can also be triggered easily.

The criterium for triggering the alarms is the heart rate. This is determined by either counting the patient's R waves over a certain period of time and then multiplying by a factor to obtain beats per minute, or by determining the R-to-R time interval, taking the reciprocal, and multiplying by the appropriate scale factor to obtain the heart rate in beats per minute. In both systems, artifacts can affect the cardiotach and erroneously push the counted rate over the limit to sound a false alarm.

Some electronic pacemakers occasionally used on patient's with certain heart diseases can create a pulse or spike on the ECG waveform. This pulse is often interpreted by the cardiotach as an additional R wave. In such cases, the heart rate meter reading will be almost precisely twice the normal or correct reading taken by the manual methods.

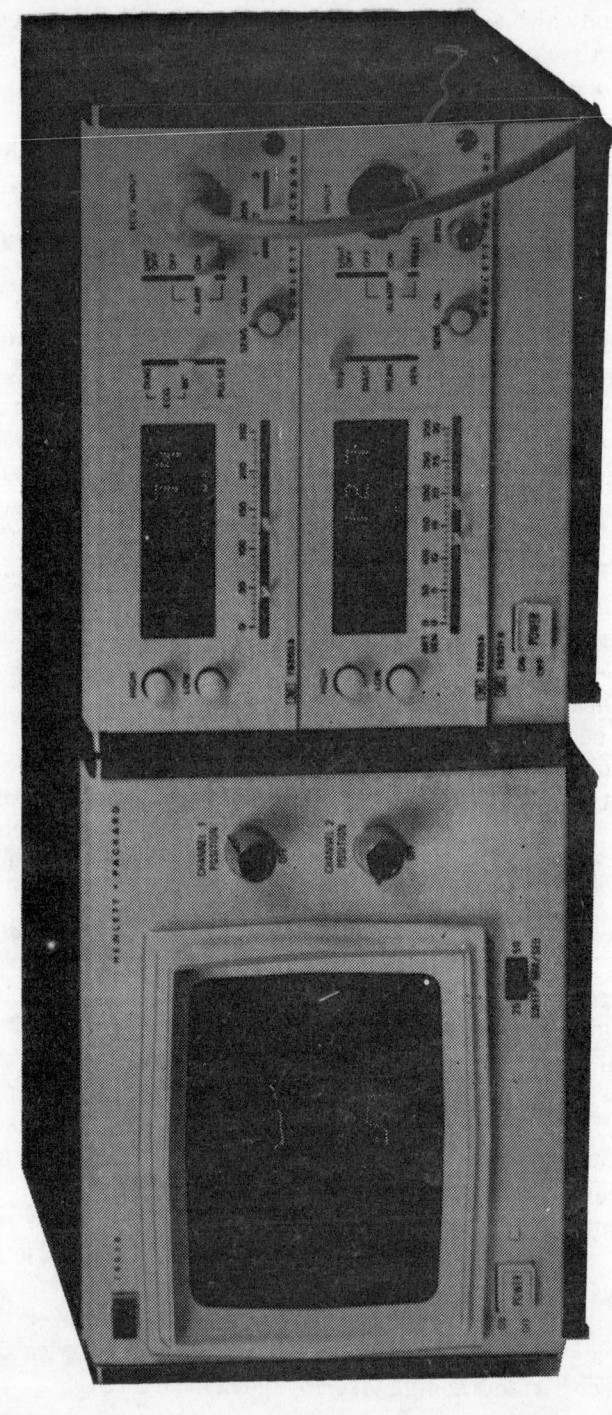

Fig. 5-1. Two-channel bedside patient monitor. (Courtesy Hewlett-Packard)

Hewlett-Packard and some other manufacturers can reduce the artifact problem by building in a short time delay in the alarm enabling circuitry. Fewer false alarms will thus occur if a small delay, say 5 to 10 seconds, is incorporated.

It is sometimes possible to eliminate "falsing" by lowering the gain of the ECG preamplifier. Whenever you examine a false alarm situation, look first to the ECG display and determine if it is of excessive amplitude. If it is high, then back off on the preamplifier gain and note whether or not the "falsing" ceases or lessens in severity.

Some patients have ECG waveforms that are responsible for fooling the cardiotach, and these cannot be helped in any substantial manner. If one of the other wave features is the same height as the R-wave, then some falsing might occur. If the monitor uses a lead selector switch, try going to another lead; if none is used, reposition the electrodes on the patient. There are certain electronic circuit defects that can also cause this problem and these will be covered later in this chapter.

The remaining module in the Hewlett-Packard bedside monitor of Fig. 5-1 is an arterial pressures module. This unit is equipped to calculate the diastolic and systolic arterial pressures, the mean pressure as derived from the arterial pressures, and the venous pressure. A switch on the front panel selects which of these is to be displayed on the single digital readout. The arterial waveform developed in the carrier amplifier is available for display on the oscilloscope. Note that the pressures module is also equipped with limit alarms below the readout display.

The bedside monitor in Fig. 5-2 is manufactured by Electronics For Medicine and represents an example of the "integrated mainframe" approach to monitor system design. The ECG and pressures modules in this instrument are actually subassemblies (as was true in the Hewlett-Packard design) and they can be removed easily for servicing. In this case, however, they are in a common mainframe with the non-fade display medical oscilloscope and share a common ac on/off switch (lower right). The ECG preamplifier in this model is a full 12-lead type and also uses a digital readout for the heart rate meter.

An interior view of an older American Optical bedside monitor system is shown in Fig. 5-3. From an ego point of view, this might be pleasing to electronics people who like to

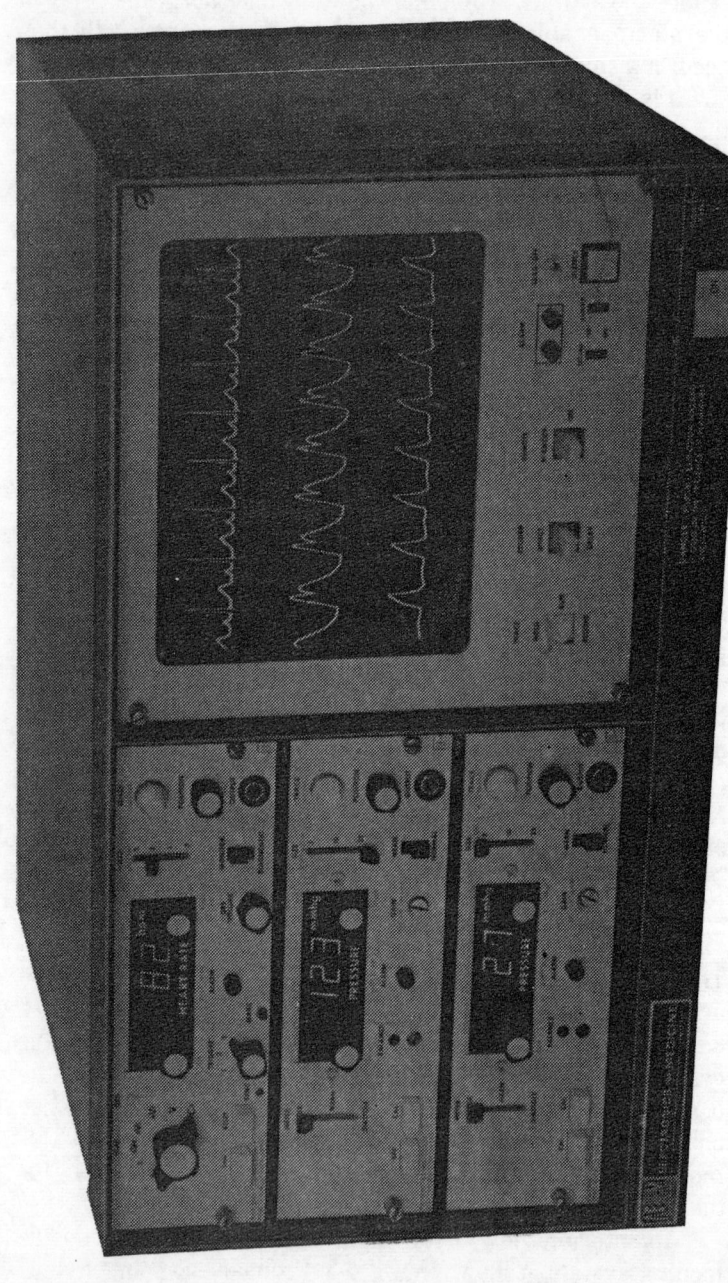

Fig. 5-2. Three-channel bedside patient monitor. (Courtesy E for M)

troubleshoot down to the component level on every job. This matter is the basis of many good-natured (hopefully) putdowns in electronic service circles. Unfortunately, this type of troubleshooting is not always desirable in medical electronic equipment service because it requires too much time to get the unit back into service. Equipment designed along the lines of the A.O. model in Fig. 5-3 place most of the electronic components subject to a high fault rates on plug-in printed circuit boards. The PC boards are arranged by function (e.g. high-voltage power supply, low-voltage power supply, alarms, oscilloscope deflection amplifiers, etc.) so that even relatively inexperienced technicians with limited diagnostic acumen can return the instrument to service with only minimum down time. The approach even lends itself to repair by unskilled persons—on a limited basis, of course—through the use of step-by-step "cookbook" troubleshooting procedures.

TYPICAL BEDSIDE MONITOR SYSTEMS

A block diagram of a simple bedside monitor is shown in Fig. 5-4. Only ECG can be monitored in this example, but other monitors frequently include an arterial blood pressure amplifier or some other form of instrument along with the standard ECG. We have already discussed ECG preamplifiers to some extent and will expand on the theme in due course.

The purpose of the ECG preamplifier is to amplify or build up the 1.0 *millivolt* ECG signal acquired from the patient to a level around 1.0 volt (peak), which is compatible with the oscilloscope input requirements. It is the oscilloscope that is normally used for moment-to-moment monitoring, but if certain waveform features begin to appear or certain changes take place, the staff can easily make permanent records using the strip chart recorder.

The *defibrillator sync* block in the figure may or may not exist in any particular model. Its function is to supply an ECG signal to the defibrillator. In some cases, a monostable multivibrator (one-shot) is triggered by the R wave, and its output is fed to the defibrillator synchronization circuit. In most cases, though, the defibrillator sync signal is just the regular ECG signal buffered by some amplifier stage or resistor network.

The cardiotachometer is used to derive the signal for the heart rate readout. In many instruments this might be a

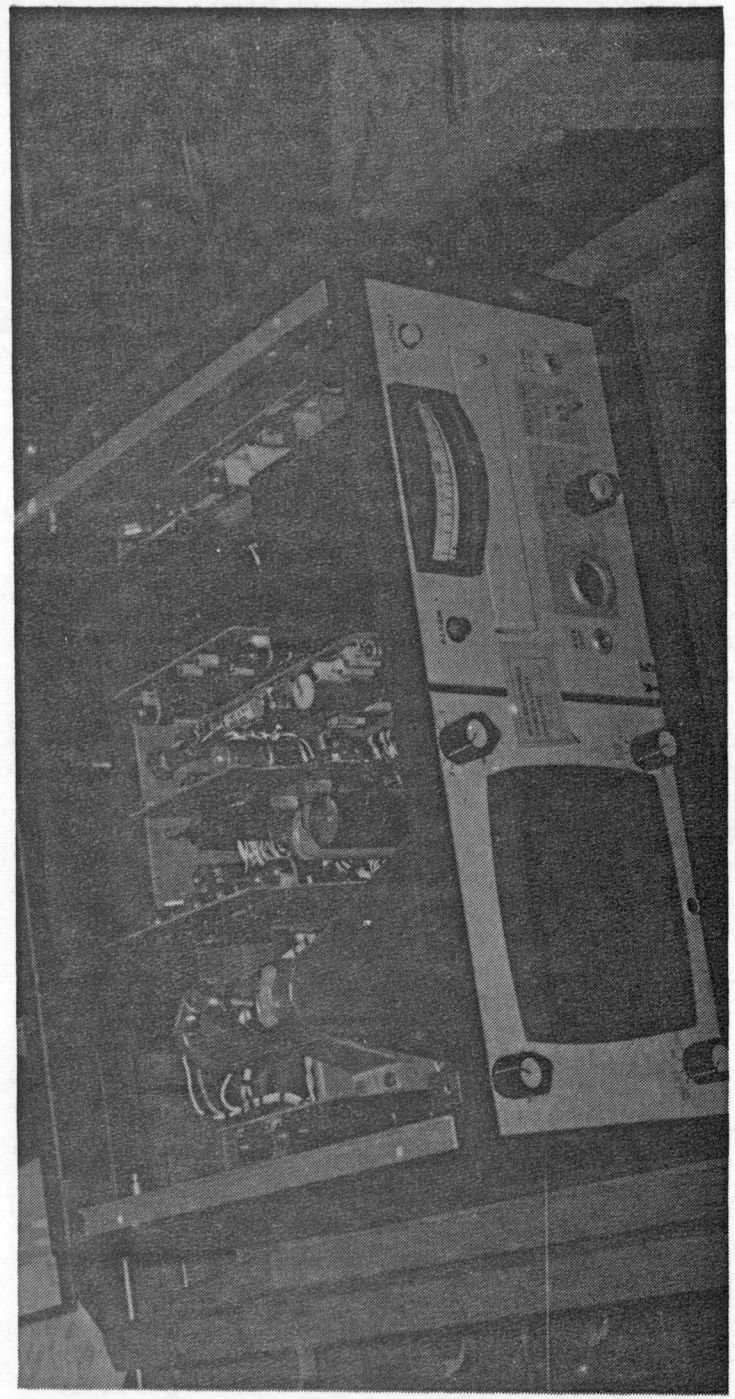

Fig. 5-3. Single-channel bedside monitor.

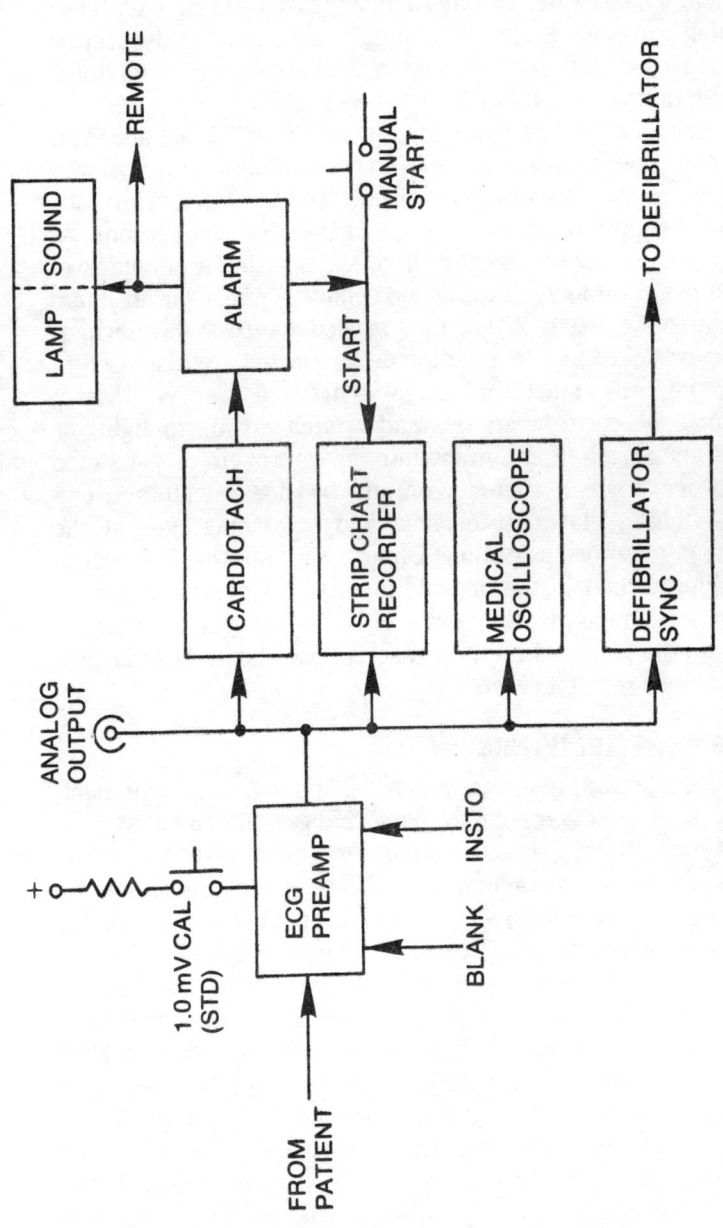

Fig. 5-4. Block diagram of simple bedside monitor.

special circuit such as described earlier. Here, though, the circuit derives a voltage or current that is proportional to the patient's heart rate, and this signal is displayed on a digital or analog readout meter. In some instruments, this section generates a horizontal bar on the oscilloscope screen having a length that is proportional to the heart rate.

An alarm section is used to monitor the ECG rate and to let the operator know if it exceeds an upper limit or drops below a lower limit, both indications of potential trouble. Locally, the alarms generally turn on a lamp or possibly sound a tone. At the remote output connector there will be either a voltage level or, more commonly, a grounded condition whenever an alarm situation is present. This output is used to turn on the alarm at the nurse's station or monitor desk. Alarms are also used to automatically start the strip chart recorder so that a permanent record can be made, latch an alarm light, or possibly put a halt command into the control circuits of a tape recorder cardiac memory. Many bedside monitors use a non-latching alarm at bedside and a latching type at the central monitoring station. Others, such as the H-P, use a latching circuit in the bedside monitor but provide a special reset line on the remote connector so that it is not necessary to go into the patient's room to reset a false alarm. Most alarms will have a manual reset.

ECG PREAMPLIFIERS

ECG preamplifiers used in bedside monitoring equipment, as well as in ECG machines, have changed quite a bit over the past few years. This metamorphosis was given a certain impetus by the advancing technology of electronics and by increased concerns over matters of patient safety. In the earliest instruments, such amplifiers were single ended, so the operators had to tolerate a large amount of 60 Hz interference. Once the differential amplifier became known, its advantages soon became apparent and it was incorporated into ECG equipment design. In both cases, however, the common connection (patient's right leg) was made to the machine's chassis ground, and this was connected to ac powerline ground. Obviously, this could open the patient to danger from 60 Hz leakage currents that always exist on the chassis of ac operated electrical equipment, especially if a ground fault occurred. In later designs, some of which are still seen in older but now obsolete systems, a 5 mA (1/200 ampere) fuse is connected in series with the right leg, common connection.

In newer ECG designs, a common-mode amplifier (called the *right leg amplifier* in ECG terminology) sums the signals from each of the two inputs of the differential pair and uses them to drive a common "ground" line—actually the right-leg signal . This common-mode amplifier produced two extremely useful results. First, it improved the common-mode rejection characteristics of the differential amplifier enough to greatly improve rejection of 60 Hz powerline interference. Secondly, it lifted the patient off chassis ground, thereby reducing the possibility of danger from stray leakage currents or catastrophic component failures within the amplifier itself. Make no mistake—those leakage currents, although small enough to seem harmless, can present a very large danger in certain medical contexts.

An intermediate step, before the use of common-mode amplifiers, used a resistor network to sum the common-mode signals, rather than an amplifier, and such equipment is still in use at some places.

It is often the case that ECG cables are double shielded. The outer shield is terminated only at the machine end (the other end is left floating) where it is connected to chassis ground. The inner shield is concentric to the outer shield and is connected to the output of the common-mode amplifier and to the wire from the patient's right-leg electrode. This inner shield, whether used in ECG work or some other small signal application, is usually called the *guard shield*. Modern low-level and medium-level preamplifiers are usually fitted with input connectors designed to accommodate the guard shield.

The most recent style of ECG preamplifier design, and the one still favored for modern use, is the so-called *isolated preamplifier*. An example of this is shown in Fig. 5-5. This example is from a Hewlett-Packard model, but it can be considered representative of most modern preamplifier designs.

The *isolation* referred to in speaking about ECG preamplifiers is the electrical separation of the patient from the ac powerline system. Some manufacturers are able to boast of connector-to-powerline isolation on the order of 1×10^{12} ohms!

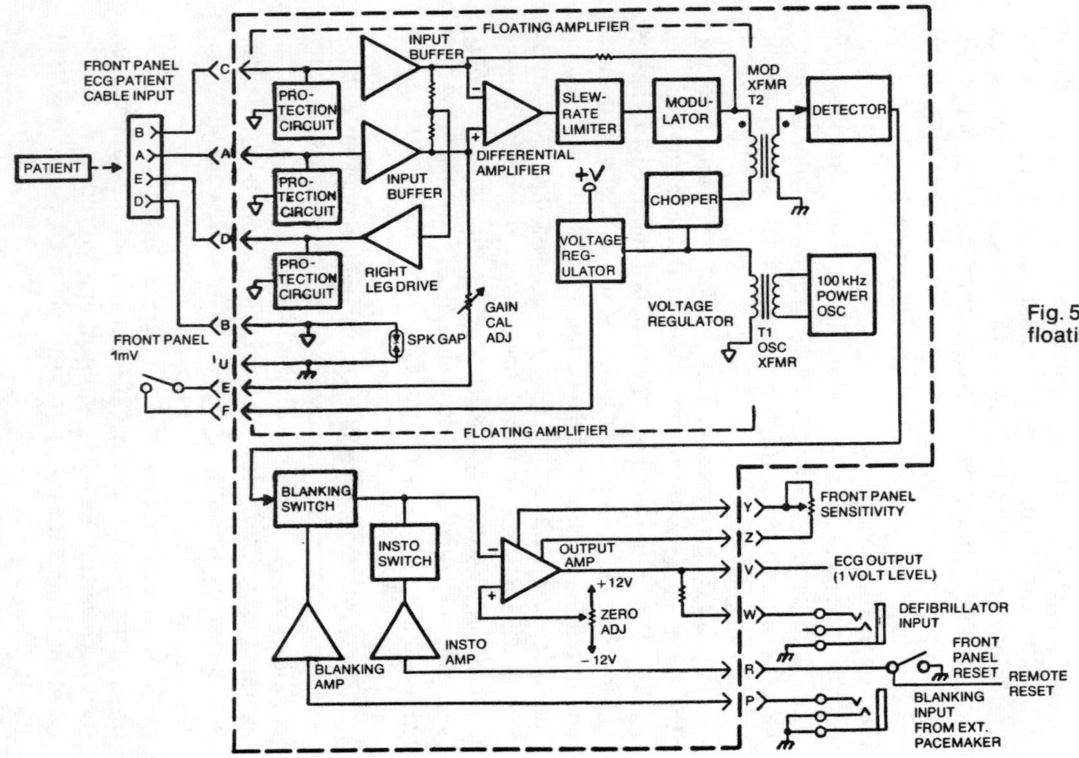

Fig. 5-5. Modern ECG circuit with floating preamplifier.

In order to achieve this level of isolation, it is necessary that the dc power supply for the input stages of the preamplifer be completely *separated* from the normal dc power supplies used to power the remainder of the circuit. In the circuit of Fig. 5-5, this is accomplished by the use of an inverter/rectifier circuit. A two-transistor, 100 kHz, power oscillator obtains its dc power from the instrument's main power supply. The 100 kHz ac signal developed in this oscillator is fed via oscillator transformer T1 to the isolated portion of the preamplifier circuit, where dc power for those few stages in the isolated section is derived by rectifying this 100 kHz signal. The 100 kHz signal is also used to chop the ECG signal so that it can pass through modulation transformer T2 back to the main portion of the preamplifier. Both transformers, incidentally, are specially designed to pass ultrasonic ac signals in the 100 kHz range but to be very inefficient at 60 Hz. This is done to assist in the improvement of isolation to 60 Hz powerline.

The actual front-end preamplifier circuitry is similar, except for the power source, to the circuitry discussed in Chapter 1, so it will not be covered again at this time. The ECG signal is modulated onto the 100 kHz carrier and passes through transformer T2 to the detector, where it is synchronously demodulated. At the output of this stage, the signal is once again in its original form and can now be handled in ordinary dc or low-frequency ac amplifiers. Following the output amplifier, the signal is fed to an oscilloscope or strip chart recorder, as required by the user.

The two remaining features of this circuit are the pacemaker blanking and "insto" (instrument override) sections. The purpose of the blanking is to interrupt the amplifier during the time interval when the pacemaker is firing. The insto circuit creates a short across the amplifier input in order to keep it from latching up during excessive input voltage conditions, such as will exist when a defibrillator is used on the patient. As a result, this keeps the baseline of the display constant so that the ECG waveform will return to view on the screen of the oscilloscope or on the strip chart recorder rapidly after the defibrillator is fired. In some cases, an insto switch is provided that must be manually pushed, but in other preamplifier designs, provision is made for an insto input pulse from the defibrillator. In either event, the insto circuit stabilizes the baseline and prevents amplifier latchup under high input-voltage conditions.

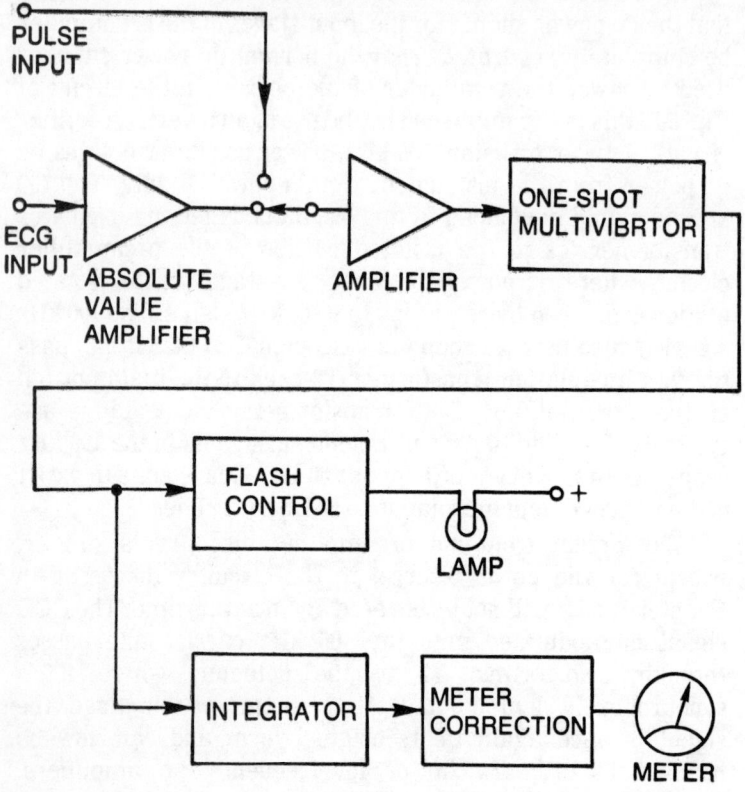

Fig. 5-6. Cardiotachometer block diagram.

CARDIOTACHOMETERS

A block diagram of cardiotach logic is shown in Fig. 5-6. ECG signals from the preamplifier output having a maximum amplitude of about 1 volt are fed to an *absolute-value* amplifier. This is a stage that produces a positive-going output signal, regardless of input signal polarity. If the input signal is already positive going, this transistor stage will pass the signal appearing at its emitter. (In the emitter-follower configuration, a transistor has an output that is in phase with its input.) If, on the other hand, the input signal is negative going, the circuit automatically passes the inverted version appearing normally at the collector of the transistor. Diodes in the collector and emitter circuits are used to prevent signals of incorrect polarity from appearing at the input of the stage following the absolute-value amplifier.

A manual switch, in the line following this stage, allows the user to select, from the front panel of the instrument, whether an ECG signal or an alternate pulse input from a photoplethysmograph is to be used as the trigger signal for the cardiotachometer. The stage following the manual selector switch provides further amplification, and its output is fed to the trigger point in a monostable multivibrator, or one-shot.

The purpose of the one-shot is to generate one pulse of constant amplitude and duration (period) for each and every R wave received from the ECG preamplifier. This, incidentally, is a very common technique that is used in many different types of medical and scientific instruments. You will see this again, especially if you make a career out of such instrumentation, since it permits the next stage, an integrator, to produce a dc level that is proportional to the frequency of the incoming signal. Some service manuals will call this integrator stage a low-pass filter, but that is substantially the same thing.

If the one-shot was not used, if we merely integrated the incoming R waves, we would just get erroneous values. The integrator's output is actually dependent upon the *area* underneath the patient's R wave complex curve, and this can vary considerably from one patient to the next and with the settings of the amplifier gain control. The one-shot is used to normalize the signal for a wide range of input conditions.

The one-shot is also used to trigger a transistor lamp switch so that a flash can be generated for every R wave. This lamp, located on the front panel, is usually referred to as either a *systole lamp* or *pulsometer* by the nurses using the equipment.

If the readout device is a digital readout, such as a digital panel meter (DPM), we can use the integrator's output directly. Only level scaling and perhaps some buffering need be provided, and even that might be redundant. Where analog panel meters are used, however, Hewlett-Packard uses a meter correction circuit that is designed to expand the middle range of 50–120 beats per minute, the normal range for human heart rates.

MONITOR ALARMS

Most bedside monitoring equipment provides alarms to alert medical personnel if certain preset limits are exceeded.

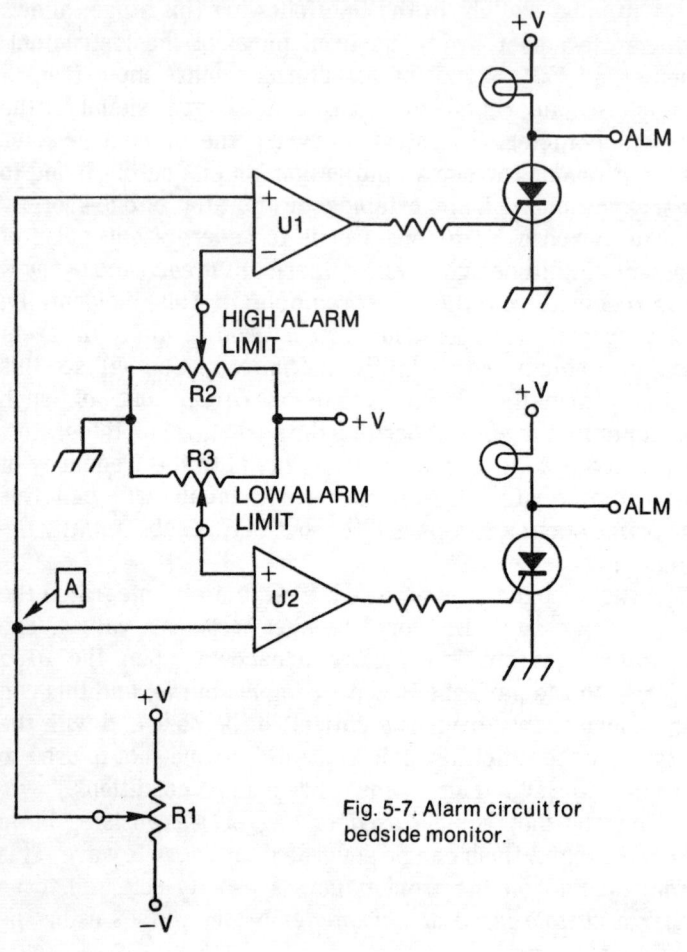

Fig. 5-7. Alarm circuit for bedside monitor.

Figure 5-7 shows a typical alarm circuit. The two integrated circuits used (U1 and U2) are voltage comparators, which issue an output whenever one input voltage exceeds the other. These comparators can be either special integrated circuits such as the LM311 or operational amplifiers connected as comparators (see *Op-Amp Circuit Design & Applications* by Joseph Carr, TAB book No. 787).

In this example, the circuits are merely operational amplifiers connected without the normal feedback resistors. This means the gain of the circuit approximates the open-loop gain of the op-amp, and that is typically 50,000 to 1,000,000. Obviously, then, even a small differential voltage at the op-amp's inputs will saturate the output. In the circuit shown, the comparator output will snap to a positive dc level whenever the plus input exceeds the minus input. This dc level is used to turn on the gate of a silicon controlled rectifier (SCR).

One input to the two comparators, the voltage at point A, is proportional to the patient's heart rate and is generated by potentiometer R1. This variable resistor is located inside of the meter housing and its wiper is gauged to and operated by the meter pointer. The reference voltage to each comparator comes from the appropriate limit potentiometer—R2 for the high alarm limit or R3 for the low alarm limit. These potentiometers may be either separately mounted on the front panel, with scales calibrated in the same units as the meter face, or they may be located inside the meter housing. When inside the meter housing, "set" tabs ganged to the potentiometer wipers would be available to the user outside of the meter housing. The actual meter scale is then used as the alarm scale and the set tabs positioned to coincide with the desired limit points.

An alternate meter-triggering system is shown in Fig. 5-8. This system uses a lamp/photocell assembly inside the meter housing for the high and low limit alarms. A vane attached to a taut-band meter movement blinds the photocell whenever the pointer is beyond the limit point. Normally, light from the lamp will shine on the photocell (a photoresistor) keeping its resistance low. When the meter pointer exceeds the upper limit or drops below the lower set point, the appropriate photocell is blinded. This causes the photocell to assume its "dark" resistance—a value many times higher than its illuminated resistance value.

For our discussion of alarm circuit operation, let's consider only the high-limit alarm section of Fig. 5-8; the low-limit alarm section operates identically, so only one section needs description. The voltage across capacitor C1 is used to trigger the high alarm gate. Diode CR6 will prevent positive voltages from appearing at the gate but will pass negative potentials. This capacitor is charged through resistor R5, a 453K, 1% tolerance type.

When in a no-alarm status, the photocell resistance is very low. The polarity of the charging potential on C1 is governed by the potential polarity at the junction of R5, R7, and the

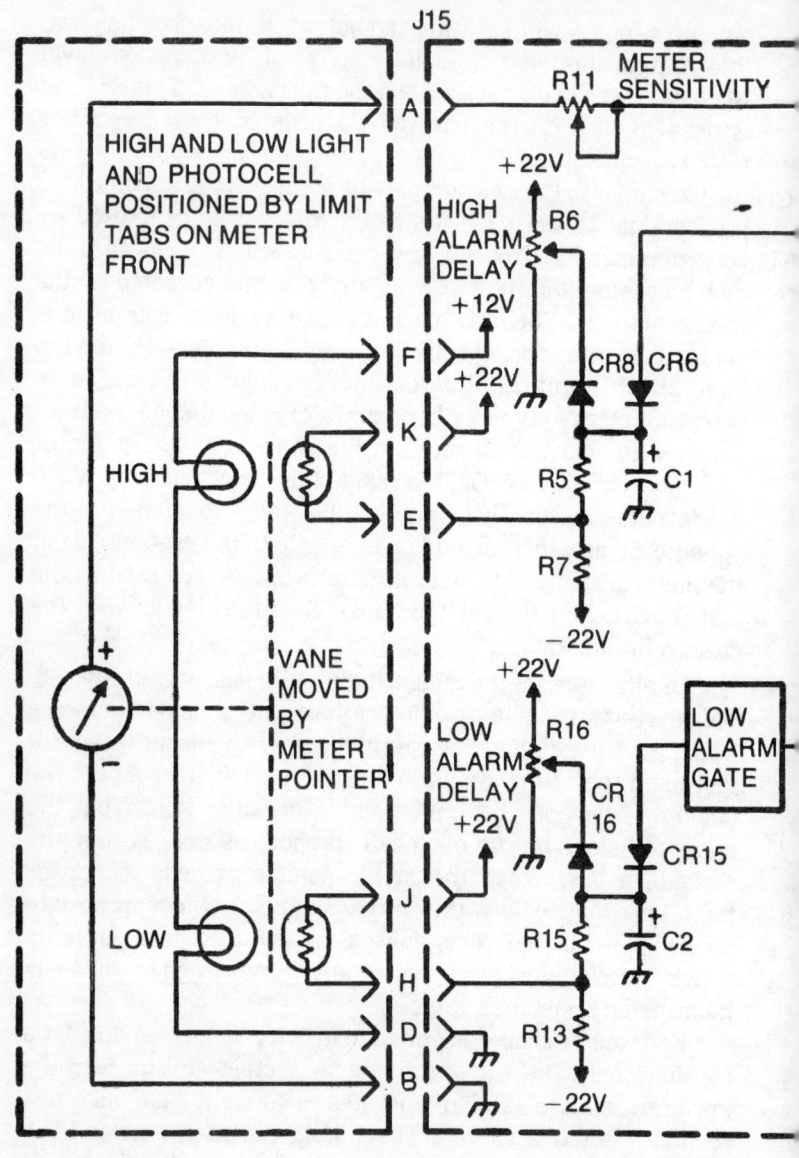

photocell. The other end of the photocell is connected to the +22V power supply while the other end of resistor R7 connects to the −22V supply. When the photocell resistance is less than the resistance of R7, the voltage at the junction is positive. In fact, it will be approximately +18V during the no-alarm

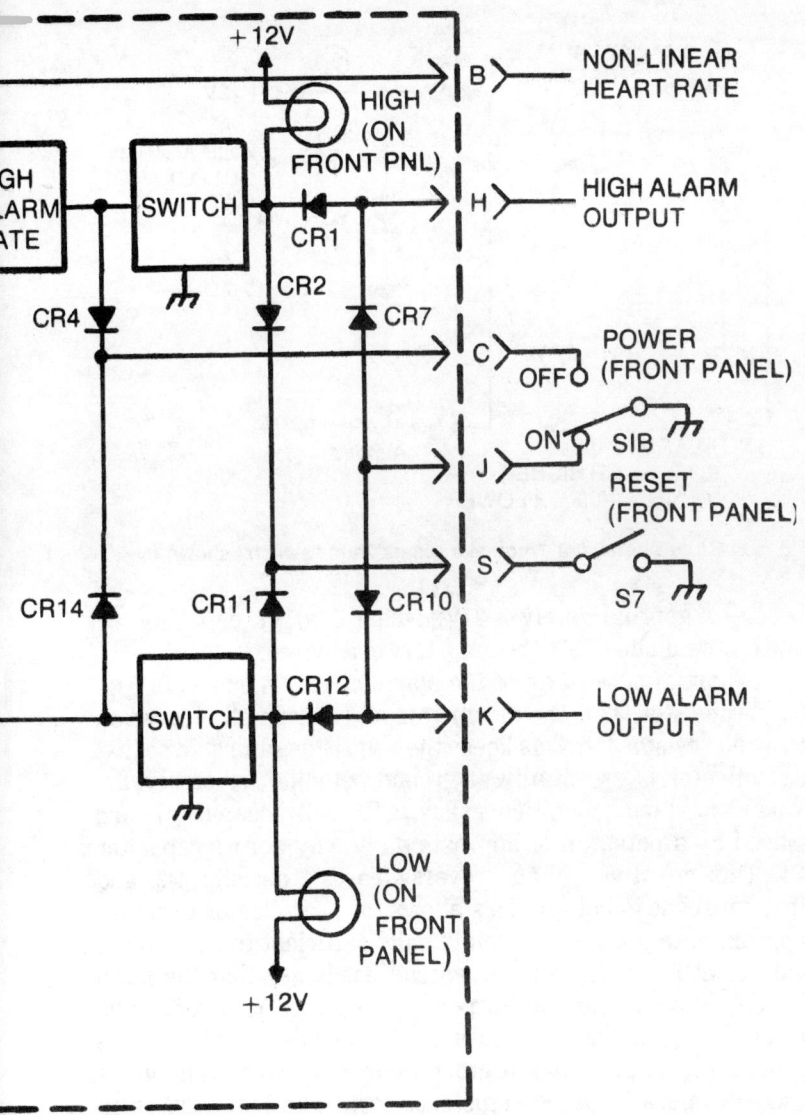

Fig. 5-8. Alarm circuit with lamp/photocell arrangement to set alarm limits.

condition when the photocell is illuminated. If the meter passes this limit and blinds the photocell, a new situation is reached in which the resistance of R7 is less than the photocell resistance. This allows the junction voltage to swing negative. In the alarm condition, then, the potential at this point

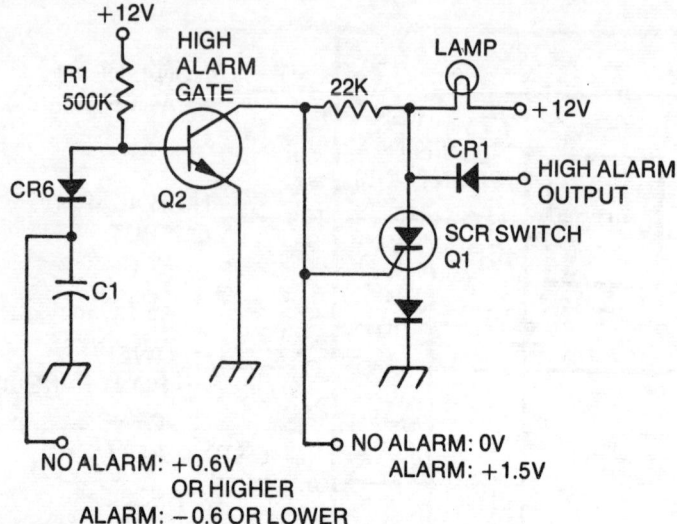

Fig. 5-9. Circuit details of "high alarm gate" and "switch" shown in Fig. 5-8.

becomes approximately −21V, which charges capacitor C1 and allows diode CR6 to become forward biased.

A partial schematic of the alarm circuit is shown in Fig. 5-9. Transistor Q2 is the alarm gate and is normally biased on through resistor R1. This keeps the transistor saturated so that its collector is essentially at ground potential, or zero volts. When an alarm condition exists, CR6 will become forward biased by a potential of approximately −6V across capacitor C1. This negative voltage reverse-biases transistor Q2, and that causes it to cut off. This allows the Q2 collector to rise to approximately +1.5V, which is quite sufficient to turn on the gate of SCR Q1. Of course, we can easily see that the lamp indicating an alarm will turn on at this point. However, a line from the Q1 anode also goes to the outside world (via the remote jack), providing a ground during alarms. This line is used to operate either remote or local aural alarms or to autostart the strip chart recorder.

Photocell alarm systems can exhibit certain problems that can be best described as *peculiar*. Although the circuit just described is from an older vintage Hewlett-Packard *780* series instrument, such circuits were also used by American Optical and other manufacturers, many no longer in the medical electronic instruments business.

The majority of alarm problems originate inside of the meter housing, involving either the photocell or the lamp. If, for example, the lamp burns out, the photocell sees permanent darkness and interprets this as an alarm condition, so the alarm will turn on and be latched.

In older H-P instruments, the lamps were connected in series with each other across the power supply. This means that both will go out if either one burns out. The symptom here will be both alarms turned on. Newer instruments of the same series use zeners across each lamp so only one can go out at a time.

Another problem seen occasionally is a bad photocell. In this case, we usually find the resistance of the cell will be permanently low, thereby creating a situation where the alarm can not come on. This particular problem may often be concealed because the medical staff will not easily notice a *no alarm*. Normally, there is a 5 to 15 second alarm delay to prevent artifacts from triggering the alarm, and this makes the problem even more difficult to detect. Such problems give impetus to the creation of preventive maintenance programs in which alarm circuits are routinely inspected.

One last common fault in the photocell breed of alarm circuit is false alarms caused by lowered lamp intensity. As lamps age, their light output drops. They may well reach a threshold where they sometimes appear turned off to the photocell. Users of the equipment will then report the situation as "frequent false alarms," and they may be quite irritated over the problem. Unfortunately, this can easily become a case where the medical people using the equipment and caring for the patient will learn to ignore the alarm, just as with "the boy who cried wolf." A new alarm lamp in the photocell assembly will cure the problem and restore confidence.

You might be tempted, where a meter assembly is at fault, to replace the entire panel meter, movement and all (Fig 5-10). Although this is the fast way—and may well be the indicated course of action if the instrument cannot be removed from bedside easily—it is extremely expensive. Alarm meters usually cost well over one hundred dollars! It might be best to remove the meter from the equipment and repair it on the spot. If time and logistics permit, take the equipment out of service and remove it to the laboratory for repair. Where situations (that great alterer of cases and facts) demand, or

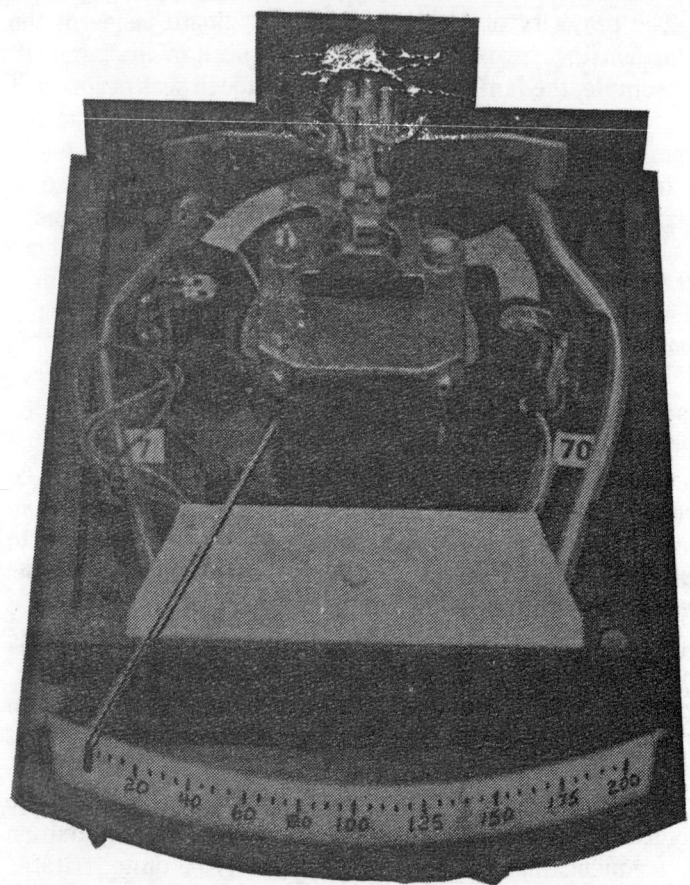

Fig. 5-10. Typical edge-reading panel meter from bedside monitor.

where convenience and common sense suggest, you might be wise to keep a spare meter on hand to allow rapid bedside service. The defective meter assembly can then be taken to the lab for repairs at your leisure.

Hewlett-Packard will sell the lamp/photocell assemblies for most models, and American Optical will sell the individual lamps and photocells. In a pinch, either on obsolete equipment or where the manufacturer is no longer in the medical instruments (or maybe any other) business, you might try to identify the lamps and photocells as to their original equipment manufacturer (OEM). You can then obtain replacements from local industrial electronic distributors or from one of the national parts houses. Even lowly hobbyist-type replacement components might prove acceptable rather than discarding the instrument. Such parts can be obtained from blister-pack displays at most chain store or mail order suppliers such as Radio Shack or Lafayette.

The lamps used in these alarms tend to be the "grain of wheat" type, or even the simple automotive plug-in variety. The photocells tend to be photoresistor assemblies made by well-known manufacturers such as Clairex. In any event, alarm repairs on out-of-date equipment can be made using a small amount of improvisation and only a small amount of redesign in the original equipment.

In older vintage H-P and Sanborn equipment, the front panel alarm lamps can be replaced with little or no ingenuity, despite the fact that the manufacturer no longer stocks replacements. In some models this requires relocation of the reset switch, but even that represents no major problems.

PORTABLE MONITORS

Portable monitors, such as the Tektronix model *414* shown in Fig. 5-11, are compact bedside monitors that can be operated from an internal, rechargeable battery pack or from the 120V ac powerlines. The Tektronix model pictured is a direct descendent of a series which began with the venerable model *410*, a unit numbering among my favorites. Seldom do electronic equipment manufacturers study the needs of their non-engineering customers as well as did the *410* design team.

The model *414* combines a lot of instrumentation in a relatively small package. Primary to any medical monitoring equipment is an ECG capability, and this is provided in a pushbutton choice of leads I, II, or III. The digital readout is also pushbutton selectable to provide arterial pressures, mean pressure, heart rate, or temperature—in either Farenheit or Celsius scales. The arterial pressures setting causes the diastolic and systolic values to flash alternately, so that both are provided even though only one readout meter is used.

Obviously, physical compactness is required of any instrument purported to be portable. Another requirement, though, is a battery pack for operation away from ac powerlines. Models without batteries are, in reality, only semi-portable.

Most medical monitor oscilloscopes use battery packs that have the charger built-in. Manufacturers of such equipment

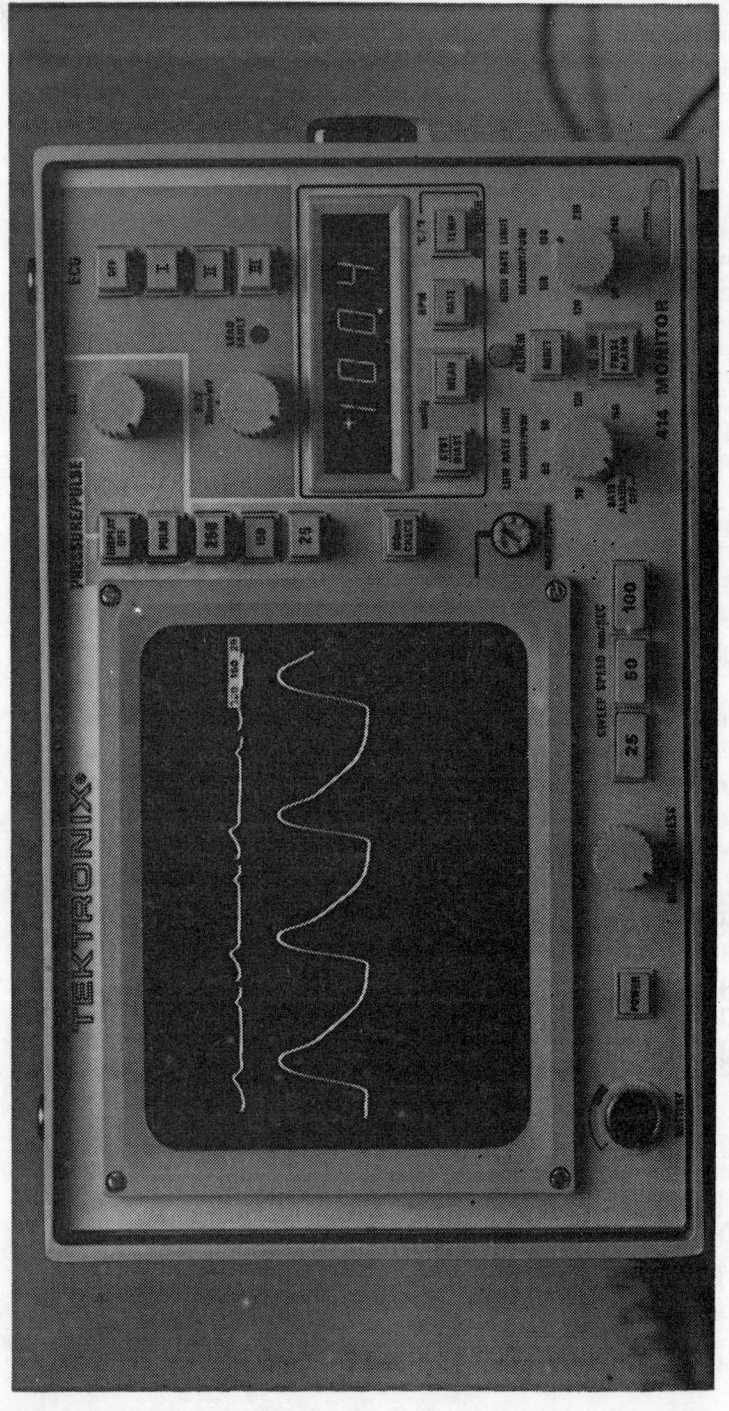

Fig. 5-11. Portable bedside patient monitor containing rechargeable battery pack. (Courtesy Tektonix, Inc.)

often recommend that the battery pack be replaced in its entirety when it no longer takes a charge. However, it is far cheaper to replace the individual cells making up the battery pack. Most often, only one or two of the cells will be the cause of the problem, and these can be detected easily with a voltmeter. Replacement is usually quite easy, but be sure to select a replacement cell with the correct ampere-hour rating.

Most medical equipment uses nickel-cadmium (ni-cad) cells in either plug-in or solder-tab versions. In the event that only plug-in types are available, they can be soldered directly making an impromptu solder tab out of bus wire.

Beware, though, that some of the low-cost ni-cad cells sold through peg-board or blister-pack displays have low ampere-hour ratings to reduce cost and may not be suitable in medical equipment. Typical industrial ni-cads used in medical equipment have a 4 ampere-hour rating in size D and a 2 ampere-hour rating in size C. Many of the blister-pack or "consumer" ni-cads, however, have ratings that are only half those ratings.

Industrial electronic suppliers or battery specialty houses can generally provide battery packs that may no longer be available through the equipment manufacturer. Most such businesses have the nylon or plastic housings and the ni-cad cells needed to custom-fabricate almost any configuration, even a few that are nonstandard.

Diagnosis of a faulty cell is simple and only a simple voltmeter is needed. Normally, for ni-cads (but *not* other types) it is permissible to use no-load readings, but if doubt persists, place a moderate load across each cell. The bad cells will show a voltage reading substantially lower than the rest of the cells in the pack.

It may prove wise to individually charge new cells before installation is made. If no battery charger is available, use a power supply that has both current and voltage regulation. Adjust the current-limiting control for a short-circuit current equal to approximately one-tenth of the cell's ampere-hour rating. For a 2 ampere-hour cell (type C), for example, this would be $2/10 = 0.2A$ or 200 mA of current delivered by the supply into a short circuit. The voltage regulation control is then adjusted, with the output short circuit removed, to produce an open-circuit voltage equal to the voltage appearing across the remaining cells in the battery pack, or if it is intended to fully charge the cell, the rated terminal voltage of the cell, usually 1.36V dc. Once the cell is charged to a level equal to that of the other cells, it can be installed in the battery pack and allowed to become fully charged by the instrument's internal battery charger. This process usually takes 10 to 24 hours, without using the instrument. It is standard practice to charge a ni-cad battery to 140% of its ampere-hour rating.

Ni-cad batteries are often damaged through a process called *deep cycling*—where the battery is allowed to become almost completely discharged. Deep cycling can sometimes destroy the cell and is usually the result of the equipment being left turned on without the charger operating. Some instruments must be plugged in for the charger to operate and medical people often make the error of assuming that it is not necessary to keep it plugged in if no immediate use is planned. If the on/off switch has been left on, however, the batteries may well become damaged after only a few hours. Also, it must be realized that most instruments recharge at a slower rate than the drain rate when turned on. One brand of electronic thermometer, for example, charges at a rate of 80 mA but draws 450 mA when operating; so if the instrument is left on in the charger, there is a 370 mA net loss. Since the batteries are rated at less than 500 mA-h, they are often found damaged. For more information on this subject, see the appropriate article in the Appendix.

Chapter 6
ICU/CCU Multibed Monitoring Systems

Electronic bedside monitoring systems have proven to be a valuable tool in the care of critically ill patients. The usefulness of these techniques is amplified even further by integrating the bedside monitor into a *central* monitoring system that services a group of patients located in a small area. Central monitoring systems are found most often in coronary care units (CCU), intensive care units (ICU), and operating rooms (OR).

TYPICAL SYSTEM CONFIGURATIONS

It seems that there is little agreement among physicians as to which parameters (outside of the electrocardiograph) must be monitored electronically, and which can be monitored on an intermittent basis using manual techniques. Of course, almost every system provides for ECG monitoring and many also routinely provide for arterial pressures monitoring. Also available, though, are monitoring equipment for venous pressures, swan-ganz pressures, temperature, and from at least one manufacturer, on-line blood gases monitoring.

What is to be presented in this section may easily be classed as *typical*, but it is by no stretch of the imagination totally universal to all possible central monitoring systems. Any particular system design will incorporate features that reflect the viewpoint of the medical persons ordering the equipment, the money available to them, and the types of patients being cared for in the unit where the equipment is to be installed.

Regardless of the actual design, however, there are several features forming a common basis for central monitoring. These are:

1—Bedside monitoring equipment provides remote outputs for waveform display on slave monitoring oscilloscopes located at the nurse's station or at a special, central monitoring console.
2—Remote oscilloscopes are set up at the nurse's station or the central monitoring console. One remote unit is used for each patient served by the system, or an all-inclusive multichannel unit might be used.
3—Remote strip chart recorders are used for making permanent records (hard copies) of ECG waveforms. One recorder might serve all patient channels if a suitable switching selector is provided.
4—Alarms respond to both high and low heart rates, and possibly certain arrhythmias. The alarms at the central station should be latching types that must be manually reset.
5—A 30 to 60 second memory capability for the ECG waveform is usually considered nice to have for recent patient history.

SYSTEM CONNECTIONS

Figure 6-1 shows the block diagram of a simple ICU/CCU central monitoring system. The bedside monitor (BSM) would be located in the patient's room, or in many installations, a patient cubicle in a larger room. A bedside monitor is chosen that has a remote output connector, so that the signals developed within the BSM can be connected through wires to a central monitor console, which is usually located at the central nurse's station or desk. The central monitoring console will be equipped with remote or slave oscilloscopes, and meter readouts are provided.

A wire locker, spreading box, or junction box should be located in, on, or near the central monitoring console. In this box, you will connect the wires and cables coming from the individual bedside monitors to a terminal strip or tag block

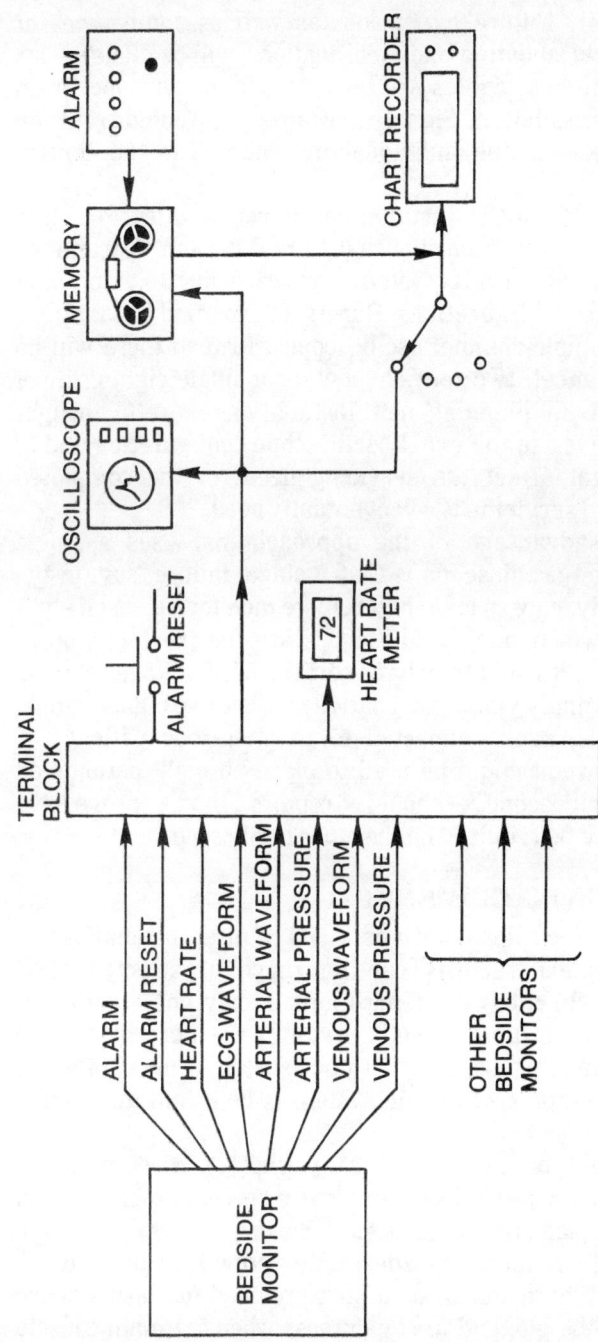

Fig. 6-1. Basic central monitoring system for ICU/CCU applications.

(such as the telephone companies often use in larger installations). Future expansion, as well as some types of system troubleshooting and modifications, will be made easier if *all* BSM remote cables are brought into the wire locker on the initial installation. Signal wires are then routed from the remote locker to the individual instruments in the central console.

Typical ICU/CCU installations have facilities for eight patient beds, so it is not unusual to find remote instruments and central monitoring system hardware in two, four, and eight-channel configurations. Rarely will you find installations with eight single-channel oscilloscopes. Instead there will be four two-channel, two four-channel, or a single eight-channel oscilloscope. In planning new installations, careful thought should be given to the exact oscilloscope configuration and to how it might affect the servicing needs of the completed system...and servicing it will eventually need.

One disadvantage of the approach that uses a single eight-channel oscilloscope is that a single failure, say, in the power supply, causes loss of *all* remote monitoring, on *all* eight patients. Two-channel oscilloscopes are the best solution in this respect, although they have certain disadvantages of their own. A seemingly viable alternative is to use two eight-channel oscilloscopes, each connected to monitor four patients. A switching circuit could be used to place all eight patients on either oscilloscope, should repairs or preventive maintenance be required on the other oscilloscope.

RECORDING INSTRUMENTS

A chart recorder is also provided in most installations so that permanent records can be made of selected ECG waveforms. In many systems there is only one strip chart recorder, so an input selector switch must be provided. In some systems this is a simple rotary switch, while in others a relatively complex switching system is built into the alarms module.

It should be noted that strip chart recorders, being electromechanical devices, have more service problems than most purely electronic devices. This fact makes a certain amount of reduncancy desirable—provided that it is affordable. There should be a jack provided to allow a spare recorder to be plugged in (by nurses) when the main console unit breaks down. The spare could be used on an "as needed" basis in several areas of the hospital.

Certain cardiac arrhythmias may only occur once or twice in a short period of time, but they may still be of critical interest to the physicians attending the patient. Unless some sort of memory is provided, this information is forever lost. Even in installations in which a memory oscilloscope is used, we find that recordings can only be made in real time, so again the past waveforms are forever lost. The use of a memory system will eliminate this problem.

In new and modern systems, solid-state shift-register memories are used that closely resemble the internal memories in most minicomputers and non-fade oscilloscopes. The cost of these memory elements has been reduced markedly, so we can expect to see their use proliferate in the next few years.

In the meantime, you will find many new and most older central monitoring systems relying on magnetic tape-loop memories, which employ a 30 or 60 second, ¼-inch tape cartridge to store ECG information. Of course, ECG signals are of too low a fundemental frequency for direct recording, so FM recording techniques must be used. In this FM system, the ECG signal is used to frequency-modulate an audio carrier having a center frequency typically between 1 and 8 kHz. In most designs, this FM stage is nothing more than a voltage-controlled oscillator (VCO), which derives its control voltage from the output of the ECG preamplifier. The audio frequency output of the VCO is the signal that is actually recorded onto the magnetic tape. Incidentally, a carrier frequency of 1988 Hz is extremely common because it allows compatibility with the Bell Datasets often used to transmit ECG information over telephone lines.

ALARM MODULES

The alarm module may be a simple relay logic box or a sophisticated electronic switching circuit, as is the case in the Hewlett-Packard models *7811* and *7813* patient selectors. Typical alarm modules include a set of pushbuttons or a rotary switch to select which, if any, patient ECG signal is to be applied to the strip chart recorder. The same switch may also be used to select ECG signals from the cardio memory, depending upon the setting of a memory/direct switch (which is the technique used in the American Optical systems).

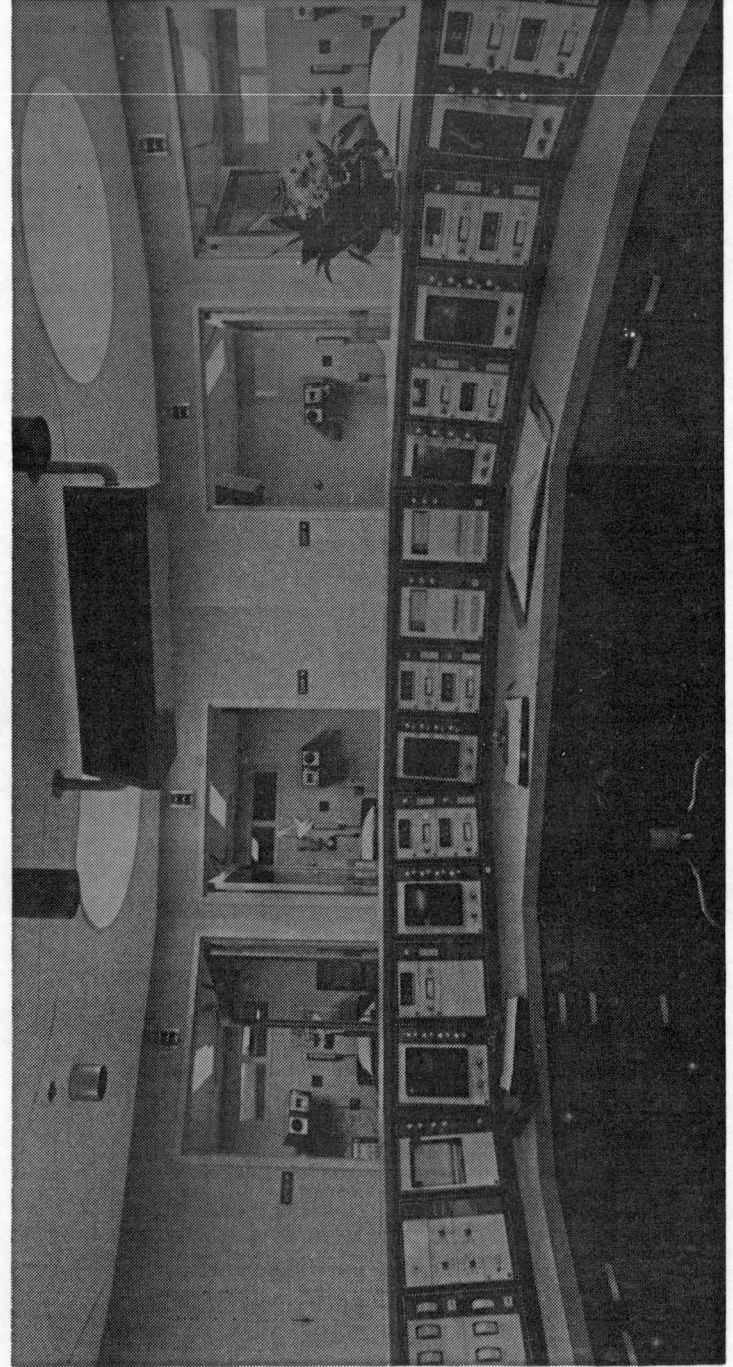

Fig. 6-2. A modern central-monitoring console with essential monitoring, recording, and alarm instrumentation.

An alarm condition from any bedside monitor captures the alarm module and may also autostart the strip chart recorder. The alarm usually locks a relay in the module that keeps the patient's alarm lamp lit until the alarm is manually reset by the operator. This feature is desirable because it alerts the nurses to the fact that an alarm had occured even though it may now have been cancelled at the bedside monitor. A nurse or some other trained person cannot keep their eyes glued to the console all the time, so an alarm memory is very practical.

Most of the alarms do not amount to anymore than a red glowing lamp on the memory console that will prompt someone to examine the memory tape for the past minute's activity. It is common, incidentally, to connect the memory recording logic to the alarm lines so that the recording process can be halted on that channel. This prevents overwriting of new material on the affected channel until an alarm reset has been issued. In relay logic systems, there will be at least one relay per channel (usually more), while in electronic systems the alarm may sequentially scan all eight inputs at a rate of 10 kHz or more.

Figure 6-2 shows an ICU/CCU central monitoring system built along lines just described. This particular console, designed and built by General Electric, is rather extensive and can monitor any patient along several parameters. Such consoles are thought to be effective in reducing nurse/patient ratios by increasing the productivity of the nursing staff.

SELECTING AND DISPLAYING INFORMATION

Another type of central monitoring system is the subject of Figs. 6-3 and 6-4. Such a system might be found in the operating room of a major hospital. In Fig. 6-3 we see the equipment rack, which might be located in either a major operating room or in the central monitoring room close to or between the major rooms. The oscilloscope is an eight-channel model and can accommodate signals from all eight preamplifiers in the rack. Although this particular figure shows only eight preamplifiers (one complete racking subassembly), up to 16 preamplifiers can be provided if a second rack and a suitable switching system is included. The lower unit is a polybeam recorder, which uses a light ray to make permanent records of patient waveforms on a strip of photosensitive paper.

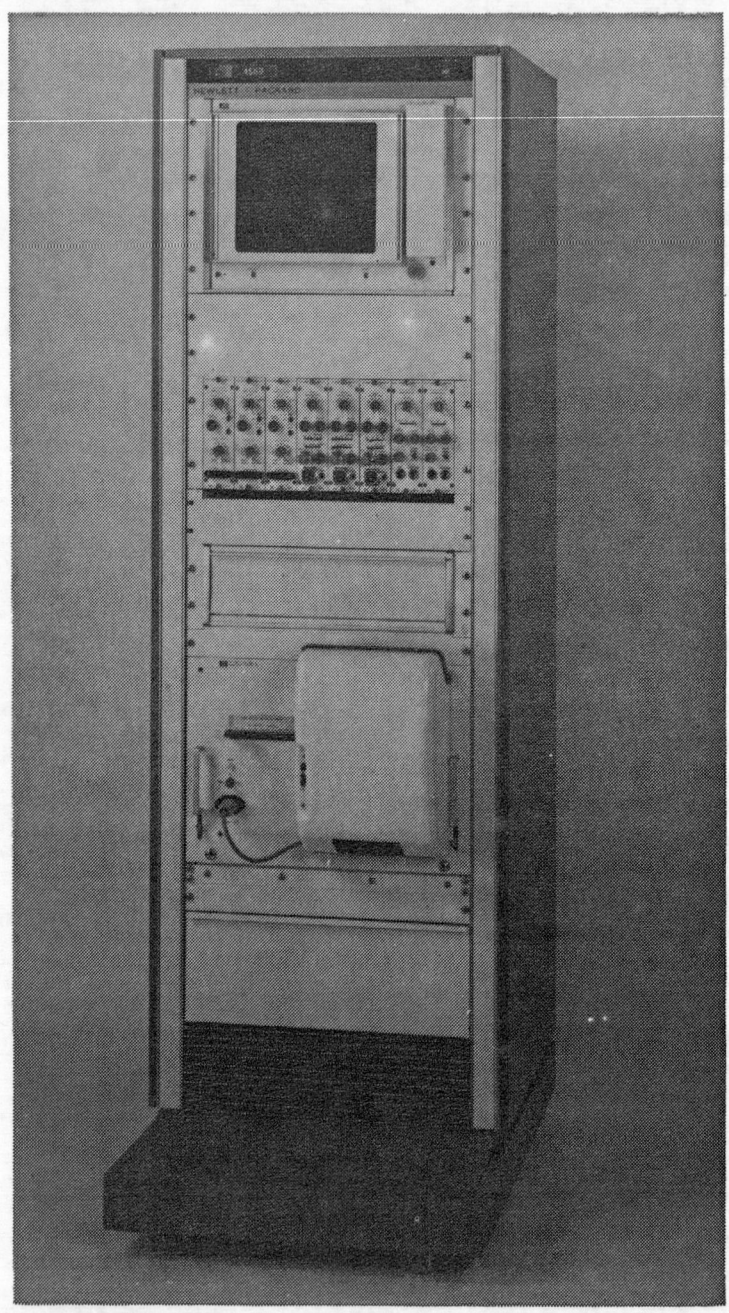

Fig. 6-3. An eight-channel central monitoring system on wheels. (Courtesy Hewlett-Packard)

Figure 6-4 shows a typical circuit layout for an operating room central monitoring system using equipment of the catagory just discussed. Operating rooms located close to the central monitoring room might put the preamplifiers in the control room with the rest of the equipment and feed low-level signals through wires routed through conduit pipe. Other operating rooms located further from the control room will either contain their own preamplifiers or will use regular bedside monitoring equipment. In either event, only high-level (e.g., 1V range) signals are fed to the control room to reduce hum and noise pickup.

A switching system is used to determine which signals will be displayed on the oscilloscope. Crosspoint switching, shown at the bottom of Fig. 6-4 is frequently found and is relatively simple to implement and maintain. Such a system has rows and columns of busbars located on two levels, one above the other. A pegboard cover over the busbar structure allows pins to be inserted that short together any two buses, one row and one column, at the points where they cross over one another. In Fig. 6-4, for example, the oscilloscope inputs are connected to column buses while assorted preamplifier outputs are connected to row buses. Here ECG-1 to channel 1, ECG-2 to channel 2, and so forth. This may well be the normal mode, but should the situation change to demand another configuration, it can easily be selected by merely switching about the crosspoint pins on the pegboard. Also selectable on the pegboard are inputs to remote oscilloscopes, if any are provided.

In one configuration, used at a major university teaching hospital, the eight-channel remote oscilloscope is in the major operating room where doctors can monitor simultaneously EEG, ECG, and two or more pressures. The smaller remote oscilloscope might be located in an observation room or in an anesthesia office where a senior anesthesiologist can keep track of patients under the care of residents or nurse anesthetists. Signals from the recovery room, located near the operating room, can also be routed through the pegboard switching system so they can be remotely displayed, or a hard copy made on a strip chart recorder.

COMPUTERIZED SYSTEMS

Computers are coming into increased usage in ICU/CCU central monitoring systems. But there are more design

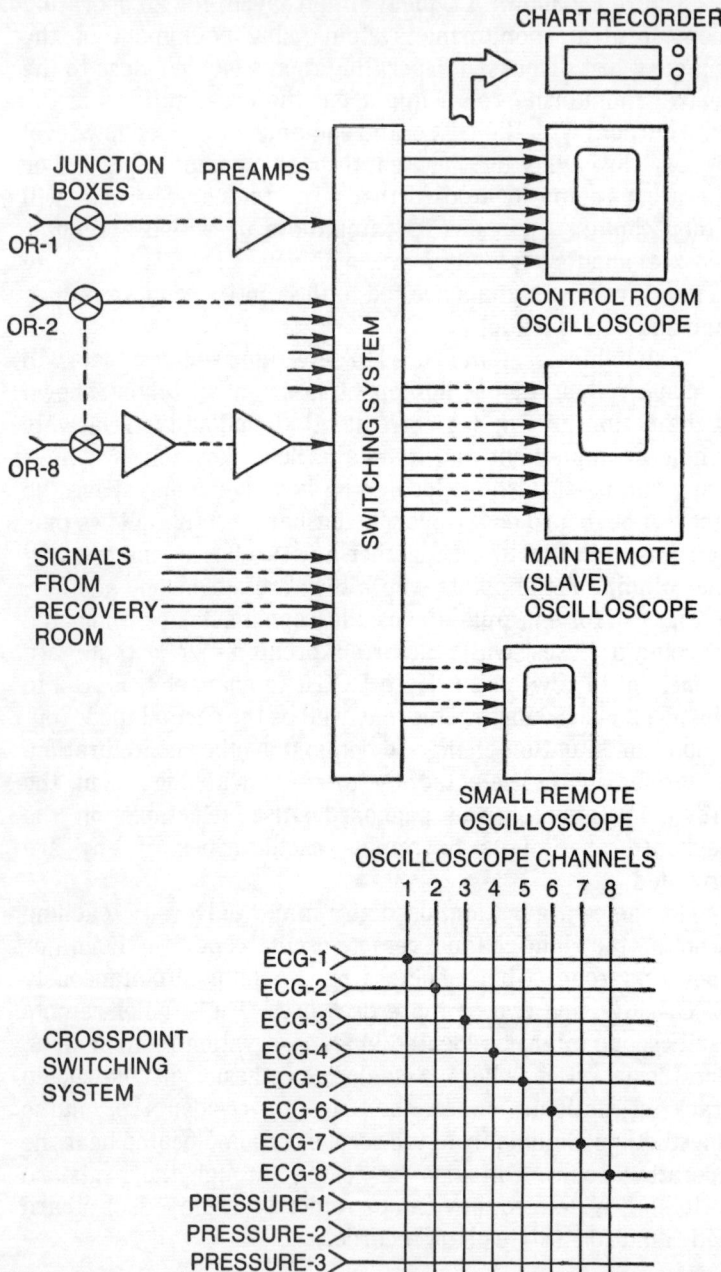

Fig. 6-4. The switching system plays an important role in routing important signals to appropriate—and functional—equipment. Crosspoint switching panels (at bottom) provide a simple way to quickly connect any desired signal to any desired equipment.

philosophies than actually available systems, so expect some degree of confusion to be present when talking about patient monitoring computer systems! Some are mere record-keeping machines, while others use complex programs and advanced techniques to make diagnostic evaluations, or so they claim, for the medical staff.

If the ECG signal is fed through a sampled analog-to-digital converter, its waveform can be processed and stored in a computer. In one pattern-recognition scheme, the computer program examines the digitized ECG signal and compares it with a set of standard patterns stored in memory. If the new pattern differs significantly from the stored pattern, it is then stored in memory for eventual evaluation by a real, live physician. If no significant deviation is noted, the signal is erased and the next waveform is read. Most such systems also provide capability to enter alphanumeric data, and many plot trends over a long period of time.

Two examples of computer terminals used in medical systems are shown in Figs. 6-5 and 6-6. The unit in Fig. 6-5 uses a small video display terminal at bedside and a handheld keyboard for entry of numerical data. Another approach shown in Fig. 6-6 is to use a CRT video terminal at the nurse's station. In either case, it has been found that many of the

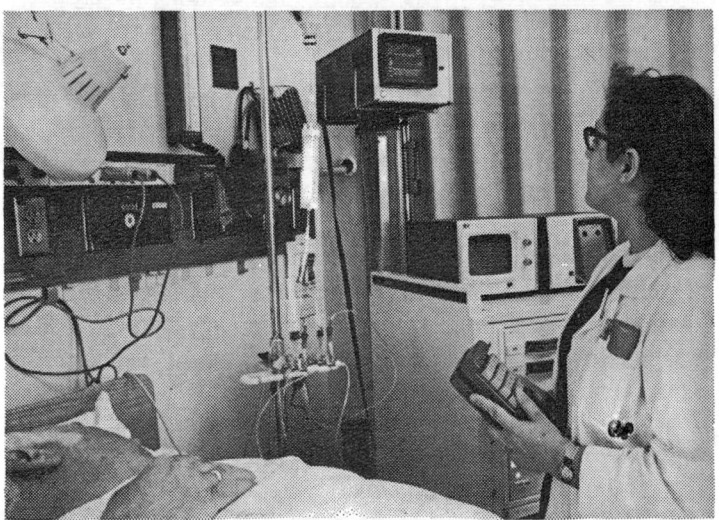

Fig. 6-5. Computerized systems using microprocessors or minicomputers can turn a bedside station into a compete diagnostic center. Here the nurse is keying in pertinent data via a handheld keyboard terminal.

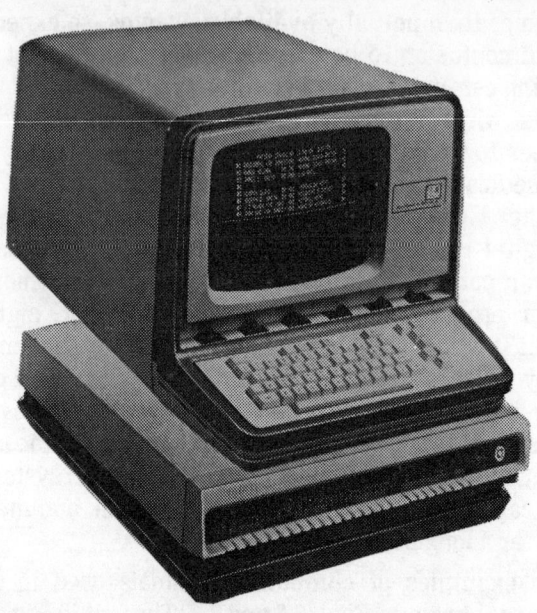

Fig. 6-6. This is a complete computer-aided cardiac arrhythmia monitoring system that can sit on a nurse's desktop. The video terminal can sit on top of the computer terminal, or the two units may be separated. (Courtesy E for M)

problems that beset medical computer systems in the early days of automatic monitoring are alleviated by the use of minicomputers located at the same site as the terminal.

Previously, large and very expensive central computers were used, and these exhibited either excessive down time or exhorbitant rental costs. There were also many problems associated with the communications circuits from the hospital to the computer and from noise picked up in the communications channel.

In the minicomputer market, the cost is now such that it is possible to buy and install a minicomputer with sufficient capacity to do the job for a price that is a lot less than the annual rental on one of the large, number-crunching monsters. Minicomputers are now small enough physically so that the computer, its power supplies, and a disc memory can fit into a single 6-foot by 19-inch standard equipment rack. In case you have not kept up, microprocessors are no longer on the horizon and coming—they are here and can turn the bedside monitor into a complete medical computer system.

SERVICING CONSIDERATIONS IN CENTRAL SYSTEMS

Central monitoring systems always obey one of the most profound (some say profane) laws of physics—Murphy's principle of the uncertainty and perversity of the universe and all physical objects. We should all know this principle, which can be stated as: "If something can possibly go wrong, it will." Applied to the central monitoring system, this reduces to: "The most critical instrument, when connected to the sickest patient, or when it is least convenient for busy nurses, will fail in the worst possible manner or will require an unavailable component."

After a few middle-of-the-night service calls on this type of equipment, you will inevitably discover Thorne's corollary to Murphy's law: "Murphy was a damned optimist!"

Also, if we might be permitted to remain in this digressed mood for a moment longer, let us discourse on the most applicable corollary to Murphy—the law of selective gravitation. This law states that anything that you drop (while working on central monitors in the middle of the night) will land either where it causes or receives the greatest possible damage, depending upon which is worse for the people and situation at hand.

Seriously, though, you might tend to think that old Murphy had us in mind. Almost all central monitor system service is performed on site, maybe in the middle of the night or on weekends. And it will be under conditions of at least some pressure from the users.

Your parts inventory and backup equipment will be critical to any success in the servicing of medical equipment. Keep at least one each of every printed circuit board that can be plugged in. If modular equipment is used, try to arrange for spares. Relays and switches are items that have a high failure rate, a fact that is related to their being electromechanical devices. Keep a generous selection of spare fuses. Memory loops and strip chart recorders are also electromechanical devices, and they employ drive rollers, belts, and other components that wear out predictably fast.

By keeping records of initial demand service on many devices, it is possible to establish the normal failure cycle. You can then take preventive measures to all but eliminate emergency service calls.

Chapter 7

Strip Chart Recorders

It has long been said that Greeks, Jews, and scientists are addicted to writing things down. From the former two we get most of our religious literature, much secular literature, and an extensive view of ancient history. From the latter we get many of the wonders of modern living. So perhaps all of that *writing down* is purposeful after all!

The strip chart recorder is an electromechanical device that facilitates the writing down of information and data from experiments or other activities, in graphical form. This is especially convenient because many of the measurement instruments used in these experiments typically generate a voltage or current analog of the physical parameter being measured, and these can be charted on paper by such recorders.

Three different chart recorders are shown in Figs. 7-1, 7-2, and 7-3. The first of these is a general-purpose single-channel scientific machine made by Mechanics For Electronics (MFE). Although this machine can be purchased as an MFE branded product, many MFE products are actually bare-bones models sold to the original equipment manufacturer (OEM) market. There are a large number of medical and scientific instruments that incorporate a built-in strip chart recorder. Rather than design, de-bug, and then manufacture a strip chart recorder of their own, many OEMs prefer to buy one

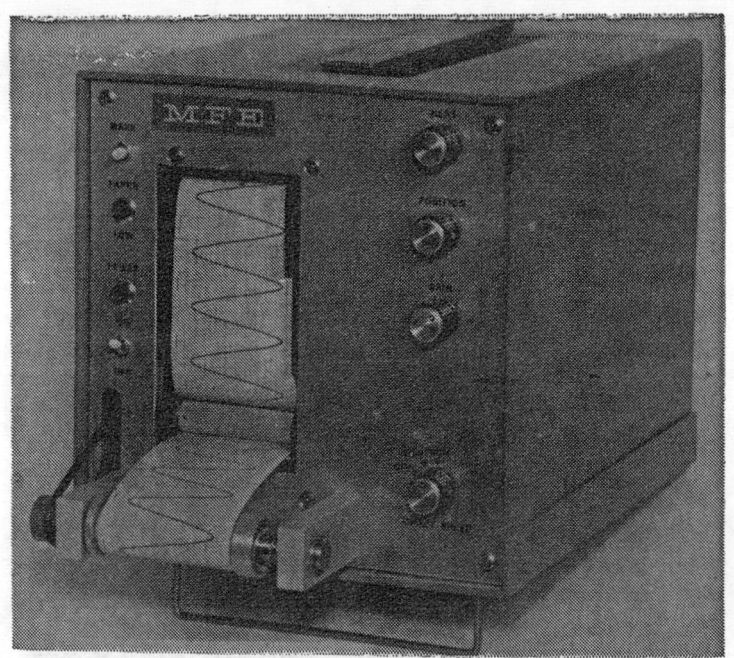

Fig. 7-1. This single-channel, portable recorder comes with a variety of custom speeds and amplifiers. You will rarely see the MFE brand on most units since most wind up being sold to original equipment manufacturers (OEMs) for installation in their products. (Courtesy MFE Corporation)

from a company such as MFE, then drop it into their own product as a subassembly. Consequently, you will see slightly differing versions of the same strip chart recorder popping up in a lot of places. Examples of this approach are the American Optical (AO) cardiotracers in Fig. 7-2. American Optical buys OEM chart drive units from MFE, Parke-Davis, and possibly others, and then integrates them with AO designed electronics to form the cardiotracer product.

The top unit in Fig. 7-2 is a four-channel, single-trace model designed for ICU/CCU central monitoring systems. Electrocardiograph signals from the remote output connectors, on the backs of the respective bedside monitors, are wired to the central monitoring station. The input connector on the back of the tracer accepts these signals and routes them to a selector switch that allows the operator to determine which of the four lines is to be recorded on the strip chart, if any. An alarm at any bedside monitor will capture the circuit, turn on the recorder, and select that patient's input

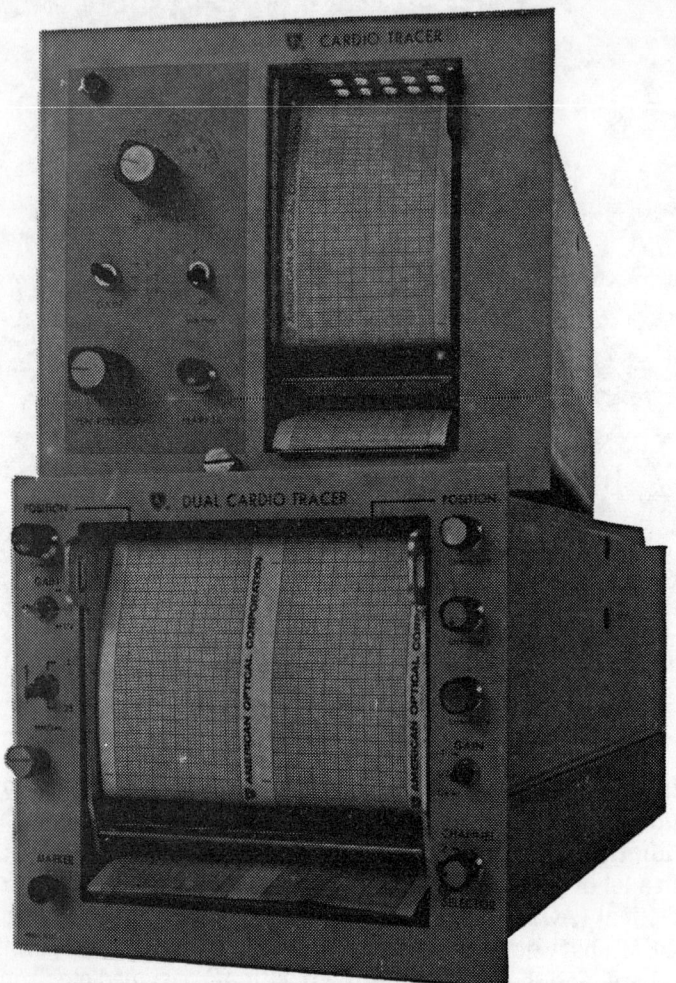

Fig. 7-2. Examples of single-channel and two-channel chart recorders. (Courtesy American Optical)

line. This particular machine is equipped with a chart speed selector that allows either 1 mm/sec or 25 mm/sec time bases. The latter, you should recall, is the normal ECG machine speed while the former is often used for plotting trends of certain slow changing parameters such as blood pressure.

The lower unit in this figure is a two-trace version that allows simultaneous recording of two parameters from the same patient. Rarely would there be any reason to record two different patients simultaneously, but two parameters from the same patient are frequently paired on the same time base. We will, for example, frequently see a patient's ECG and arterial pressures waveform recorded against the same time base from a dual-trace machine. Dual-trace recorders are often used in special instrument packages aimed at surgery, catheterizations, laboratories, and so forth.

The machine in Fig. 7-3 is also a strip chart recorder, but its function is a little different. It is designed to keep a compact record of a single parameter over a long time period so that trends can be spotted. This machine uses a sheet of paper

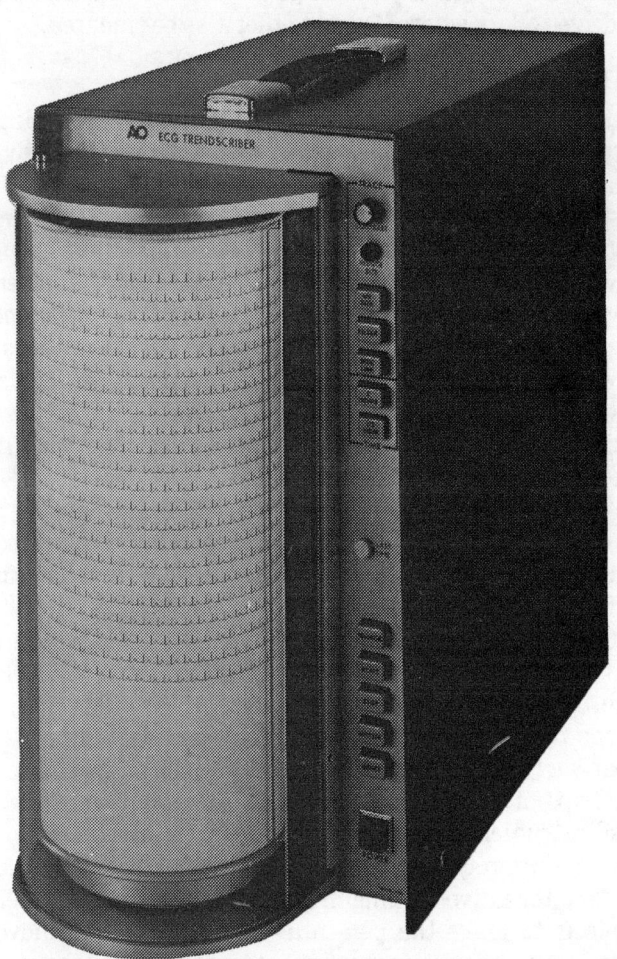

Fig. 7-3. This drum-type recorder is intended for long-term recordings taken over many hours. (Courtesy American Optical)

mounted on a turning drum, and the record is kept on successive lines until the paper is filled.

WRITING TECHNIQUES

There are several methods for actually making the lines on paper. Most obvious, of course, is the hollow pen stylus in which ink is forced under pressure from a storage bottle or reservior to the pen tip. The Brush 220, by Gould Instruments, is a popular two-channel example of such a recorder. When the machine is adjusted properly and when the pen tip is properly lapped, the ink will dry on the paper before the paper reaches the drive rollers where it might otherwise be smeared.

Pen Lapping

Pen lapping is accomplished with a small piece of extremely fine emery paper (usually supplied by the manufacturer when purchasing a replacement stylus). This must be done on initial installation of the stylus and at periodic intervals thereafter. The tip of the pen is raised just enough to allow the emery cloth to slide between it and the paper. Be very cautious in this manuever, since it is easy to permanently warp the pen body, which could be very costly. The pen is then allowed to rest under its point pressure on the emery cloth. Make sure the pen is free to move; this means the power must be off in most machines because a braking current is normally forced through the galvanometer.

There are actually two methods for lapping analog pens, and many technicians can make a case for using either or both. In one technique, recommended by some manufacturers, the free pen is scraped back and forth across the emery cloth about 10 or 15 times. The instructions that come with most pens recommend something like four or five times back and forth, but this is usually not sufficient. The idea here is to abrade the pen tip until it is perfectly parallel with the graph paper surface. This usually requires considerably more than four trips of the tip back and forth through its arc of swing. Most instrument technicians find at least 10 and often as many as 15 laps are required.

An alternative lapping method used by many field service people is to leave the pen in a fixed position and move the emery cloth. The difference in this technique, and the claimed virtue, is that you can move the emery cloth back and forth in the direction of the paper travel. Ideally, this is the direction in which the pen should be lapped. While that is the claim, I find that both techniques seem to produce equally good results. That makes it your choice as to which method is best suited to your work.

Most pressurized ink recorders have a specification as to the drive speed at which ink drying is gauranteed to occur before the paper reaches the drive rollers. A recorder with a properly lapped pen should meet this specification. Incidentally, that speed is often 5 mm/sec. If the ink is still wet when the paper comes out of the machine at the tear-off point, then re-lap the pen tip and keep relapping until the ink dries—regardless of service manual instructions to the contrary.

Frequency Requirements

The most common writing technique used in medical recorders (and one that is also common in purely scientific machines) is the thermal method using a *hot tip* stylus. The tip of the stylus is actually a resistive heating element and is connected to a low-voltage power supply. The graph paper used in these machines is a special paraffin treated type that is sensitive to heat. If a high-temperature stylus is brought in contact with the paper, its heat will turn the paper black at the point of contact, so you will see a line drawn on the paper closely following the stylus tip.

Most medical and scientific applications for strip chart recorders have relatively low frequency requirements, so you can tolerate the usually poor response of the typical permanent magnet moving coil (PMMC) galvanometer/stylus system. A few applications, however, require a higher frequency response than can be provided by the PMMC machines. The inertia of a relatively massive pen assembly produces an apparent sluggishness that attenuates high frequencies. There are, however, at least two writing systems that use low-mass writing mechanisms that offer increased frequency response. Some models can reproduce frequencies to well over 1000 Hz, as opposed to an order of magnitude less for the PMMC mechanisms.

One of these high-frequency systems, popular on some of the European-made instruments, is the high-velocity ink jet. Such machines replace the pen assembly with a lightweight, low-mass, ink nozzle assembly mounted directly to the galvanometer. Ink is placed under high pressure and is sprayed onto the paper in a thin, high-velocity jet. Blinders are provided on either side of the spray path to contain the ink in cases where overrange input signals drive the galvanometer coil past its normal limits. This precaution is necessary to prevent ink from splattering all over the chassis!

An alternate high-frequency recording system (made by Hewlett-Packard, Honeywell, Electronics For Medicine, and others) uses a visible or ultraviolet light beam on a photosensitive strip chart. A lightweight mirror is mounted on the galvanometer, and this is used to deflect the light beam across the paper in step with the input signal. In some versions, the paper must be then passed through a wet developer bath; in others, it is passed under a special developing lamp.

A few models require the paper to be developed in a darkroom as with any ordinary photograph. This produces a longer lasting print of the input waveform at the expense of a somewhat more involved process. This system, incidentally, had cruder forerunners that were popular in the decades of scientific research before electronics entered the picture. Many early experimenters used a small mirror supported by a thin quartz thread. Either magnetic or electrostatic galvanometers were used to create the torque required to deflect the light beam in the mirror.

PMMC Galvanometer

Figure 7-4 shows a top view of the writing assembly used in most recorders, regardless of the writing method. This method is known as the permanent magnet moving coil (PMMC) galvanometer, and it is much like the well-known D'Arsonval meter movement used in many panel meter assemblies. The coil in the PMMC is centertapped (in many cases) so that it can be driven by a push-pull amplifier. In this case, the centertap is connected to either $B+$ or $+V_{cc}$ lines in the power supply. The two coil extremities are connected to the vacuum tubes or transistors of the push-pull amplifier.

If there is no current flowing in the coil, or if the currents flowing in the two coils are equal, then the armature is held at dead center. But if one current is larger than the other, it will generate a slightly larger magnetic field. This interacts with

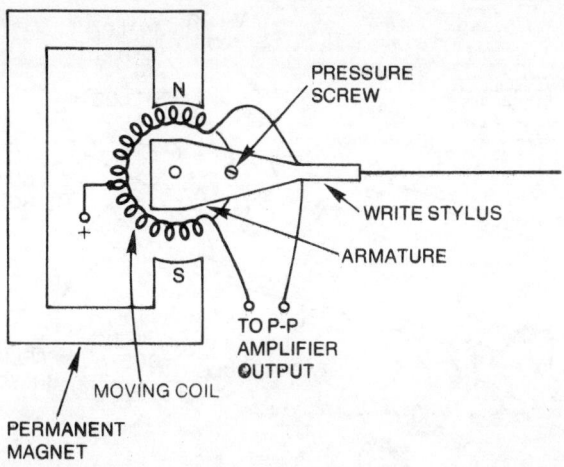

Fig. 7-4. Basic construction of permanent magnet, moving coil (PMMC) galvanometer assembly.

the magnetic field of the permanent magnet, adding to or subtracting from it, depending upon current direction (polarity). A magnetic force is thus applied to the armature in an attempt to neutralize that force. Since the armature is free to move on its jeweled bearings, this will cause the pen to be deflected. Alternatively, if the other half of the coil has the greater current, then the armature will deflect in the opposite direction. Obviously, then, the pen can be swung back and forth through an arc by an electrical signal. Although this mechanism is found in many forms and variations, all units will operate in the manner just described—at least in the essential details.

At low currents, we find that this mechanism creates a small amount of nonlinearity. This is due to the fact that a certain amount of current must be applied before the magnetic field is able to overcome the armature inertia and bearing friction. Consequently, this creates a *dead zone* or *dead band* around the zero input signal. Some recorders have various machine adjustments that reduce the size of this dead zone.

Recorder Mechanics

Although every machine is different, we can still let the diagram in Fig. 7-5 represent the majority of currently used strip chart recorders. The paper is stored on either a roll or in a Z-fold pack that is usually located inside a special

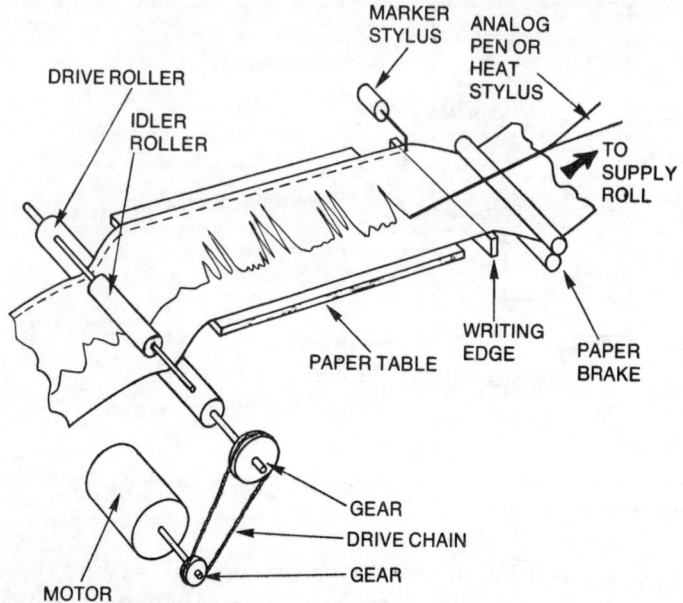

Fig. 7-5. Chart drive system showing principle parts.

compartment on the recorder mechanism. The loose end of the paper is threaded through or across a paper brake: then across a writing edge, paper table, and finally between the idler and drive rollers. Generally speaking, the brake, writing edge, and table form one assembly, which pulls out when paper is loaded into the machine (see Fig. 7-6).

The paper brake is used to supply a back tension to the chart paper. The brake and the two rollers operate together to stretch the paper firmly across the writing edge so that the paper will stay steady under the tip of the stylus or pen.

Marker Stylus

There are actually two pens on most recorders, and that includes most single-channel machines. The first is the analog pen connected to the PMMC galvanometer that makes a recording of the input waveform. The second pen does not actually contact the paper under most circumstances, but it will drop down to mark the edge of the paper on command from a timer circuit or user-operated external marker switch. This marker stylus is used to mark certain events in the experiment or to give an indication of a patient code number, time of day, ECG lead selected, or whatever the user requires.

The marker stylus can be operated either manually or by some internal logic circuitry. In ICU/CCU central monitoring systems, the marker is often found connected to a patient code generator, which is turned on by the alarm circuitry. If an alarm on a bedside monitor comes on, and no one is at the central monitor console to see which patient it is, they can tell by counting the number of dots in each group printed onto the paper by the marker stylus.

The Paper Drive System

Paper drive power originates in the electric motor and is coupled through a gear train or chain to the drive roller. Where chains are used, they sometimes resemble miniature bicycle or motorcycle chains. The drive roller is cylindrical and may be made from either hard rubber or serrated aluminum. MFE, for example, often uses aluminum drivers, while Parke-Davis and Hewlett-Packard seem to prefer large rubber rollers. You will, however, almost universally find that the idler roller is smaller than the drive roller and will be made from rubber.

There are no further mechanics actually required after the roller pair, but some machines are equipped with a paper take-up spool to eliminate the annoyance of coping with a long

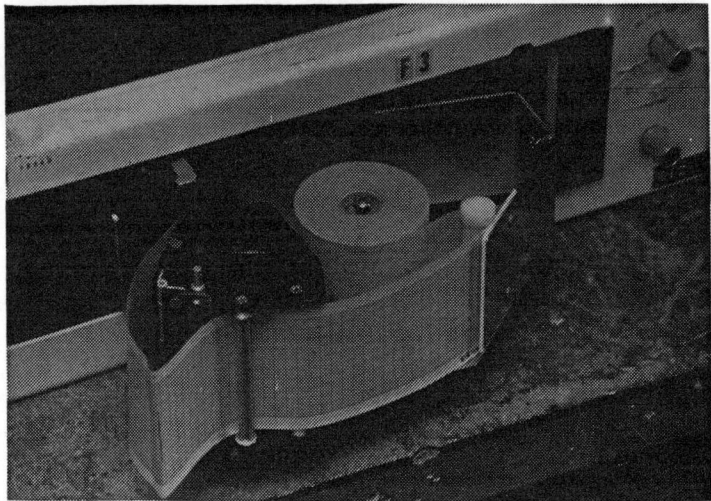

Fig. 7-6. The chart paper compartment usually swings open for easy reloading. Note the correct threading of the chart paper and compare with Fig. 7-9.

run of paper spilling out onto the floor. Simple ECG machines do not usually have this feature, but most central monitor medical machines and the scientific machines do. During a medical emergency, for example, there might be a central monitor recorder that is autostarted by the bedside monitor alarm. Under these circumstances you can expect that the medical and nursing staff will be very busy and will not have the time required for a lot of housekeeping as the recorder continues to spill paper out onto the floor.

The time base of the recordings made on these recording machines is determined by the speed of the chart paper as it is dragged through the mechanism and across the writing edge. In some machines the speed is regulated electrically by changing the voltage applied to the drive motor. In other cases, this is done mechanically by changing gear train ratios. Most chart recorder paper is divided into some sort of standard graticule, such as millimeters.

You can check speed on slow machines by using a stopwatch to time a paper run. It is common, for example, to time a run for 10 seconds. You can then count the number of divisions on the paper required to pass a certain point. You can usually find a convenient point on the writing table, then make a mark on the paper at the beginning and again at the end of the run. It is then a simple matter to divide the number of millimeters passing that point by the time required for the run. For example, suppose on a 10-second timed run, a total of 250 mm of paper passed under the chosen point. This means the speed was 250/10 or 25 mm/sec, which is the correct speed for a typical ECG machine.

Another tactic is to use a precise 0.5 Hz square wave applied to the input. At that frequency, the stylus deflects to opposite sides of zero once per second. It is then a simple matter to count the divisions between deflections. Personally, I prefer the first method when accuracy is important because you can easily use a longer time period to obtain more accuracy.

Most of the drive problems occuring on strip chart recorders can be traced to the two rollers. Frequently, the complaint is slipping paper—the strip chart paper will either fail to pull through the rollers or will intermittently slip. This last condition is particularly bad on medical machines because it can sometimes lead readers of ECG strips astray. This situation can usually be traced to either the drive or idler rollers, or both, being worn out.

In rarer cases, the slipping can be caused by a defective or worn-out gear train or chain. In some gear-train models there is a centrifugal clutch assembly, and this sometimes will wear out and cause slipping. Rarer still are motor failures.

Pen Problems

One other class of mechanical faults involves the stylus or pen. When pen recorders stop writing, look first for adequate pen pressure against the paper. This can be checked by *lightly*—they are delicate—touching the pen while the machine is running. If insufficient pen pressure is the problem, the pen will make a line on the paper when this is done. Keep in mind, though, that it is easy to damage delicate pens, so this test must always be performed with gentleness. A spring-loaded pressure gauge is also useful, and this is the preferred method if such a gauge is available.

The next point to check is a clogged pen or vacant ink reservoir. If a pen is found to be clogged by dried ink, as might easily happen if the machine has not been run in some time, it is often possible to unclog it by squirting some solvent (or even plain water) down the tube inside the pen under pressure from a hypodermic syringe and needle. Choose a needle size that will just fit inside the pen tube and hold it firmly against the back end of the stylus, at the point where the ink capillary attaches.

Thermal pens also suffer from a loss of pressure, but it is not recommended that you try the "touch test" using bare fingers! This type of stylus has a *hot* tip that will burn you. Use a tool to gently press the stylus tip against the paper. If the stylus still refuses to write, look for the low voltage that is supposed to appear across the stylus wires. If it is found, assume a defective stylus and replace it.

Thermal pens also suffer from a buildup of wax (from the paper) that may cause a poor trace. In that case, try cleaning the tip with an alcohol swab before attempting replacement—it saves a lot of money.

RECORDER ELECTRONICS

Figure 7-7 shows the block diagram of a typical chart recorder electronics section. Transistors Q1 and Q2 drive the

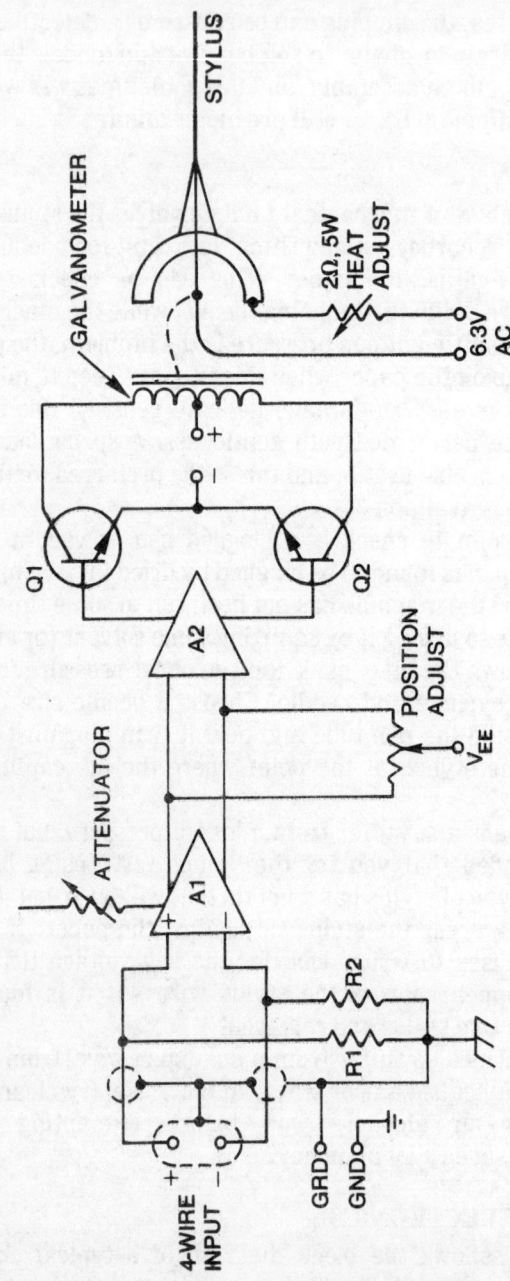

Fig. 7-7. Typical block diagram of PMMC type recorder with push-pull output.

galvanometer in the manner discussed earlier. These transistors are driven in push-pull by driver amplifier A2. This amplifier is, in turn, driven by preamplifier A1. A variation of the output circuit is shown in Fig. 7-8, which is a design used with single-ended galvanometers. If there is no input voltage, the net current through the galvanometer coil will be zero. A positive-going voltage turns Q1 on, while a negative-going voltage will turn Q2 on.

The *position* control in Fig. 7-7 is a potentiometer that upsets the balance of amplifier A2, thereby biasing either Q1 or Q2 harder than the other. Preamplifier A1 will have a differential input and possibly some type of guard-shield protection to reduce deterioration of the common-mode rejection figure. An attenuator sets the input voltage sensitivity of the circuit, but not the gain of the individual amplifiers. Typically, the amplifiers will respond well down to 10 mV or less, and the attenuator is used to reduce any input voltages to this level.

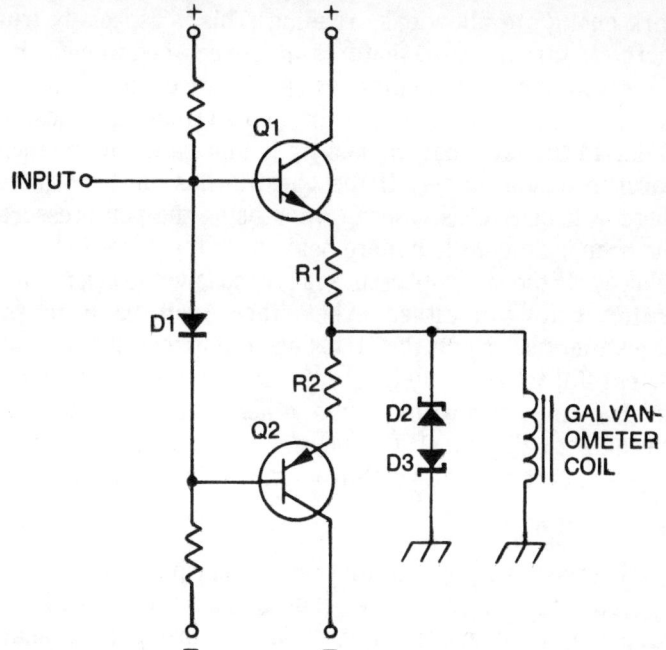

Fig. 7-8. Single-ended outputs are often used instead of push-pull today because of the availability of better high-voltage transistors. This type of complementary output stage is now in most hi-fi equipment. The zeners across the galvanometer coil prevent the stylus from being pegged and damaged by the application of too much voltage.

Some machines are designed for use in a limited number of applications, or for use by people not sophisticated in scientific instrumentation. These types of instrument will not use a calibrated range-selectable input attenuator. Instead, they will have a variable input sensitivity control that is often adjustable only with a screwdriver. These machines are typically designed to accept a 1V signal for full-scale deflection. They may be found as "barebones" OEM models, or as a mainframe in a cabinet that accepts plug-in preamplifiers or special-purpose modules.

ADJUSTMENTS AND TYPICAL FAULTS

There are several minor faults occurring in chart recorders. These are relatively easy to remedy in most cases. One fault that is seen frequently is incorrect stylus pressure. If the pressure is too great, there will be excess drag on the paper, causing the stylus to distort the input signal. If the pressure is too light, on the other hand, the tracing will not be dark enough to allow easy reading. This is especially true if there are fast rise-time features on the recorded waveform.

Also—and this comes as a surprise to many—light pressure can cause excessive drag on thermal machines! This is due to the fact that the pen tip is lubricated by the melted paraffin on the paper. If the paraffin has not been melted, there will be excessive drag. Increasing the pen pressure to the *proper* amount lets more heat reach the paper in the time allowed. If the stylus pressure is far too low, the pen might not write at all. In either event, there will be a pressure adjustment screw on the stylus or on its mounting assembly. Be careful to correctly locate the pressure adjustment screw or you may throw off some other aspect of the stylus' mechanical alignment. It is usually quite sufficient to turn the pressure screw only an eighth or quarter turn at a time.

Paper Loading

There is one problem that proves exasperating because of its frequency of occurrance—that is incorrectly loaded paper. Although there are endless variations that are peculiar to specific models, most of the time its the same error. People bypass the paper braking system located prior to the writing edge when loading the paper. This is the case in Fig. 7-9. The result is to produce a poor quality tracing that is smeared

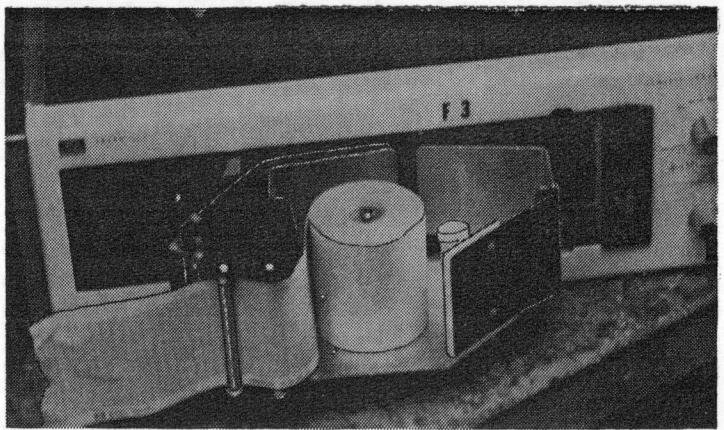

Fig. 7-9. An all-to-common problem. The paper feed on this chart recorder will not function properly because the chart paper was not fed around the paper brake on the right side (compare with Fig. 7-6). Despite the fact that most recorders provide easy-to-understand instructions for loading the paper, including arrows and other printed guides in the paper compartment, rest assured that medical personnel will find a new and unique way of installing the paper.

because of lack of back tension. The paper slips and skews sideways under the psn tip as it is recording. In fact, the action of the pen makes this phenomenon even more pronounced. Although the user almost invariably complains of a bad stylus, this is not a correct diagnosis.

Stylus Damping

One other common problem area involves the damping response of the stylus on fast rise-time waveforms. When hit by a square wave or step function, the stylus may tend to overshoot the mark, and that action leaves a spike-like artifact at the top of the leading edge, or at the bottom of the trailing edge if it is also a fast fall-time transition. This situation is caused by an underdamped stylus. An overdamped stylus, on the other hand, causes the pen to undershoot and approach its final value slowly—as if the high-frequency response was limited.

Both damping symptoms can usually be corrected with the damping control. This is adjusted for best overall appearance of an input square wave. It is usually better to allow a tiny amount of overshoot if the perfect square wave cannot be obtained. In any event, overshoot is usually specified to be not greater than 0.1 division. Under-damping and overdamping are often a tradeoff, but many quality recorders can come extremely close to producing a perfect reproduction of the input square wave.

Stylus Protection

The stylus or pen assembly is the weakest part of the chart recorder. A thermal stylus will burn out and get too dirty to transfer heat to the paraffin paper, while an ink pen will dry up and clog. Both types will bend or break if allowed to slam against the high- or low-end stops. It will prove wise to stock a modest supply of the more commonly used styluses and pens... just to be prepared for the inevitable.

Some manufacturers protect their delicate stylus or pen with special design features that prevent the sort of violent mechanical overshoot that breaks so many. One simple trick used by several companies is to connect a pair of zener reference diodes across the galvanometer coil as in Fig. 7-8. Since a current flows in that coil, a voltage drop will appear

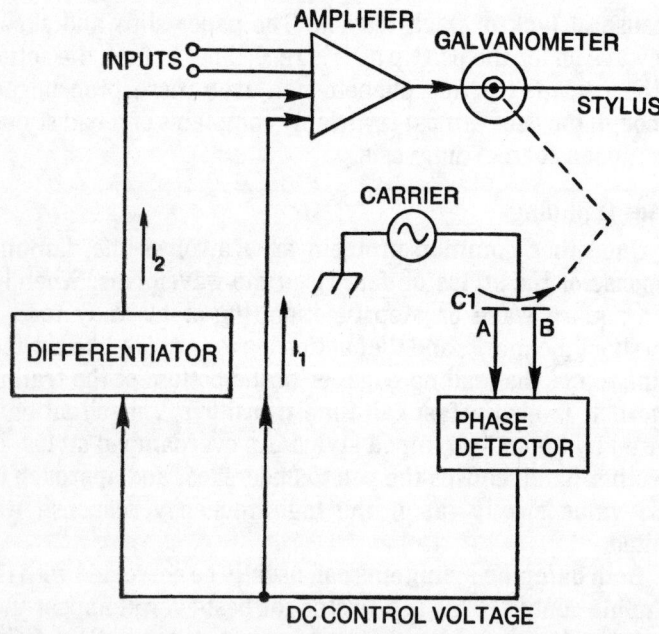

Fig. 7-10. This stylus protection system uses both position and velocity feedback to the galvanometer amplifier. The position feedback information is used to accurately position the stylus on the chart paper, while the velocity feedback is used to control the damping response and to protect the stylus from extreme motions.

across the coil, and this voltage is limited by the zeners in cases of overshoot. If the current pulse is high enough to drive the pen too far off scale to be consistent will stylus safety, then the coil voltage will exceed the breakdown voltage of the zener. When this occurs, the zener limits any further increases in applied voltage level. Thus, a limit is placed on the system to keep violent destruction by overshoot to a minimum. For normal safe operation, the zeners have no effect on stylus response. This technique, incidentally, is often added to older recorders as a field modification. In the absence of any specific manufacturer's instructions, try to ascertain the correct zener voltage by making measurements of the coil voltage for extreme deflections.

A somewhat more sophisticated stylus protection system is shown as a block diagram in Fig. 7-10. This circuit uses a position feedback signal developed in a transducer ganged to the galvanometer armature. In this case, the transducer is a differential capacitor, C1. When the stylus is exactly in the center position, the two halves, C1A and C1B, will have the same capacitances. As a result, the ac carrier signal fed to each section will have equal phase and amplitude relationships. Under these conditions, the dc control voltage output and current I_1 will both be zero.

The control voltage will vary and assume a value and polarity proportional to the amount and direction of any deflection. If either the upper or lower voltage limits is exceeded, a "sift" turnoff occurs due to current I_1, and this prevents the amplifier from allowing any further increases of output level.

We know from calculus and physics that velocity is the first derivative of position. If the stylus position changes too fast, then, we also know it will have too high a velocity. When this happens, it must be slowed down fast or damage will result. So an electronic differentiator is included to receive the transducer signal and generate a second current, I_2, that carries velocity information. When I_2 becomes too large, the amplifier slams on the brakes and halts the stylus excursion before damage can occur.

SERVORECORDERS

One popular class of chart recorder uses a servomechanism to drive the pen assembly. An example of

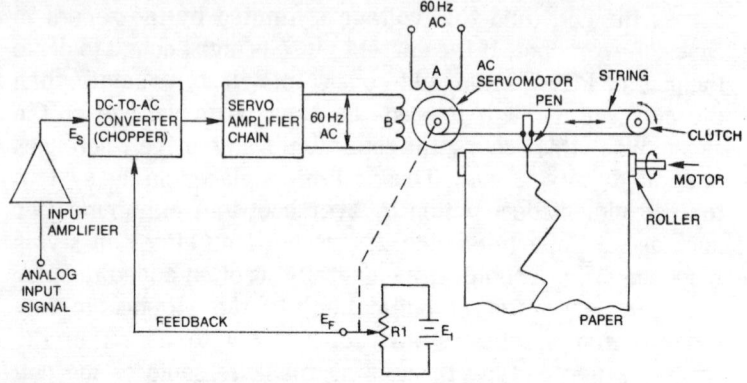

Fig. 7-11. Basic operation of servorecorder. An X-Y recorder would have two such circuits to control both vertical and horizontal movement of the pen across a stationary sheet of graph paper.

such a system is shown in Fig. 7-11. The heart of this instrument is the two-phase low-power ac induction motor. The pen, in this case, is attached to a string or cord looped around a motor pulley and clutch assembly. As the motor turns the pen travels back and forth across the surface of the paper. Also ganged to the motor shaft is a potentiometer, R1. This resistor generates a feedback voltage (E_F) that is proportional to the position of the pen. This potential becomes the feedback signal used in a servo loop.

If the two windings of the two-phase induction motor are fed simultaneously with in-phase voltages, they will produce a stationary magnetic field that cannot cause any shaft rotation. Out-of-phase voltages, on the other hand, produce a rotating magnetic field, and this does generate shaft motion in the motor. The servoamplifier will turn on and drive the pen whenever the quantity $E = (E_S - E_F)$ is not equal to zero volts. If the quantity is zero, the pen will be stationary. If E_S input signal voltage is greater than E_F, the pen will move in one direction, and if less, the pen will move in the opposite direction. The pen will therefore follow the analog input signals with only a small amount of dead band.

Several varieties of servorecorder are commonly seen. The type shown in the figure uses a motor to drive chart paper, so it is little more than a strip chart recorder. You might be tempted to ask why anybody would go to the trouble of making a servomechanism chart recorder when galvanometers are easily available and generally have a higher frequency response. The answer lies in the fact that the galvanometer and pen size become unwidely when chart widths become large. For wider charts (10 inches is very common) the servomechanism is easier to implement and is more convenient.

Another popular servomechanism is the *X-Y plotter*. This class of instruments uses one servomechanism to drive the pen in the X direction (horizontal) and another to drive it in the Y direction (vertical). This allows the recorder to produce graphs, vector figures, drawings, and even lettering on a piece of standard graph paper, which is held stationary. This is especially convenient in some scientific work where you don't want to be held to some standard graph chart selected by the recorder manufacturer. With the X-Y recorder, you can use any standard graph paper or even make your own custom design!

With the X-Y plotter, you can plot two different parameters against each other on any type paper—linear, log-log, semi-log, or even a Smith chart. In the event that one parameter is to be time, you can make a time base by applying a linear ramp voltage to the X input. In fact, many models have an internal ramp generator and a switch that selects either X-Y or T-Y modes. If a nonlinear time base is desired, an exponential time base for example, it is only necessary to generate a ramp that has the desired shape and apply *it* to the X input.

Chapter 8
Defibrillators and Cardioverters

Defibrillators are instruments used in resuscitation of certain heart attack victims by delivering a large electrical shock to their heart. These instruments are well known to viewers of television medical shows—they can be used by script writers to very good dramatic effect. Such machines are designed to deliver a large but controlled current, which is stored in a capacitor and discharged through a set of paddle electrodes applied to the patient's body.

Ventricular fibrillation is a condition in which the cells of the ventricle depolarize in a random manner, not with their normal synchronous rhythm. Cells beating in this chaotic manner do not "pull together" and this impairs the heart's ability to pump blood effectively, so much so that the victim will die within a few minutes if the condition is not corrected. The purpose of the defibrillator is to electrically stimulate the heart cells simultaneously so they all enter their refractory periods together. Hopefully, the heart will begin beating in step with its own internal pacemaker after this is done.

BASIC CONFIGURATIONS

Several different configurations are popular, and these are shown in Figs. 8-1, 8-2, and 8-3. The instrument in the first illustration is a semiportable model manufactured by American Optical. This class of machine might be permanently stationed in an emergency room, coronary care unit, intensive care unit, operating room, or strategically located points on the floors. In this last instance, the instrument is used to service a larger area of the hospital, and it is carried to the scene of an emergency, anyplace in the hospital. This approach is common in smaller hospitals that have lesser resources. The patient paddles for this machine are attached to the front panel through a high-voltage connector made of a plastic material that has a high dielectric strength.

The meter in Fig. 8-1 is actually a kilovoltmeter, but it is calibrated in *watt-seconds* units of electrical energy, abbreviated W-sec. Older machines are calibrated according to *stored* energy, but all machines of more recent vintage must be calibrated in terms of *delivered* energy, a figure that tends to be somewhat less optimistic, much in the manner of hi-fi power ratings! A number of instruments are calibrated in terms of both stored and delivered energy, in order to reduce any confusion arising from medical persons being more familiar with the older systems.

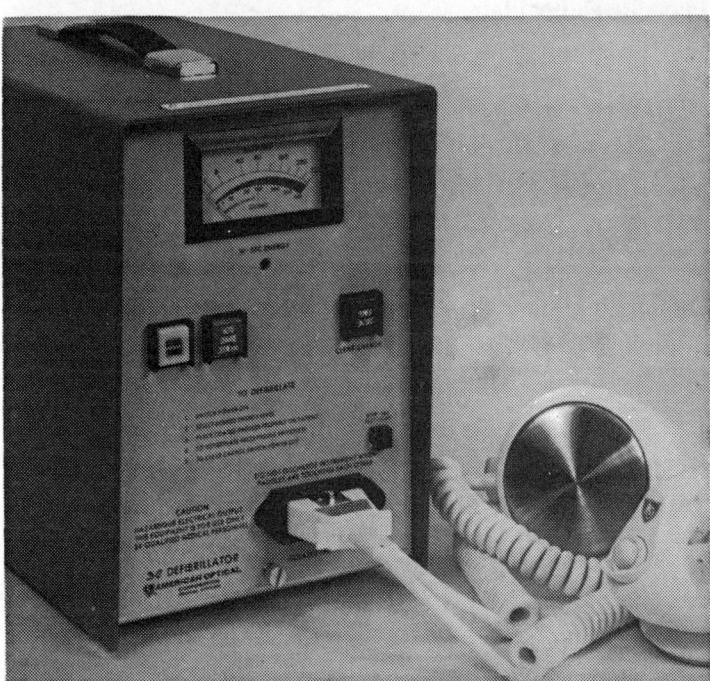

Fig. 8-1. Semiportable defibrillator for use near standard ac power receptacles. (Courtesy American Optical)

The usually accepted—but unofficial—standard is that a defibrillator must be capable of delivering at least 70% of its stored energy to the patient. The remaining "lost" energy is burned up in the coil resistance of an internal inductor and in the wiring and relay contacts.

Operation of defibrillators such as this requires first that power be turned on, then a selection be made for either manual or automatic charging modes. In the manual mode, the capacitor will charge as long as the button is depressed or until a stored energy of 400 W-sec is reached. If the button is released prior to the full charge level, the capacitor will only be charged to whatever energy level that had been reached at that point in the cycle. The automatic mode allows the unit to charge to the full 400 W-sec level with just one press of the button. This is a setting used for dire emergencies where rescuers will have a lot on their minds besides fiddling with a defibrillator setting. Thumbswitches on the patient paddles energize a high-voltage vacuum relay that transfers the capacitor charge to the patient via the paddles.

Portable Defibrillators

The American Optical machine in Fig. 8-2 is a truely portable defibrillator that is intended for use in ambulances or whatever ac power may not be readily available. The package includes a defibrillator, medical oscilloscope, strip chart recorder, and ECG preamplifier. All of these instruments are powered from either ac power, if available, or an internal rechargable battery pack. Besides their obvious use with rescue squads and ambulance teams, battery portables also find application inside hospitals during patient transportation from emergency rooms, operating rooms, and other units to critical care areas. Similarly, heart attack patients entering the hospital's emergency department may be transported to a coronary care unit facility. This could be a very dangerous period should additional problems arise. A portable defibrillator can be mounted on the stretcher for use in such a case.

An interesting feature of some defibrillators in this class is that the patient's ECG signal can be acquired either with a regular patient cable or through the defibrillator electrodes. Placing the paddles against the patient's chest automatically picks up the ECG and displays it on the oscilloscope screen or strip chart recorder paper.

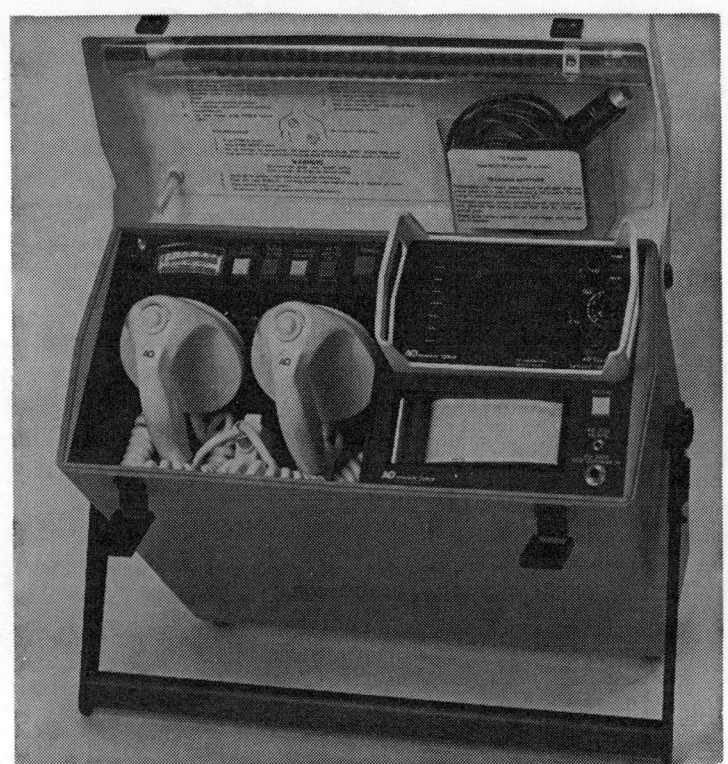

Fig. 8-2. Fully portable defibrillator for all-around use, anywhere. The unit is equipped with rechargeable battery pack and portable carrying case, and it also contains a medical oscilloscope, strip chart recorder, and ECG preamplifier. (Courtesy American Optical)

Stationary Defibrillators

Figure 8-3 shows a defibrillator that is decidedly not portable but is, instead, a heavy duty machine intended for a fixed location. It is the Hewlett-Packard model 7802. These instruments are intended for use in either a fixed location or in a semiportable manner on a roll-around cart, mainly in ICU, CCU, ER, and OR service. The controls on this machine are essentially similar to those of the others so will not be covered here. We will, however, examine the circuitry of this machine in some detail, if only by block diagram analysis. But that is for a little later in the chapter.

Defibrillator Circuits

Figure 8-4 shows the simplified circuitry of a basic defibrillator. Energy is stored in capacitor C1—in most cases a

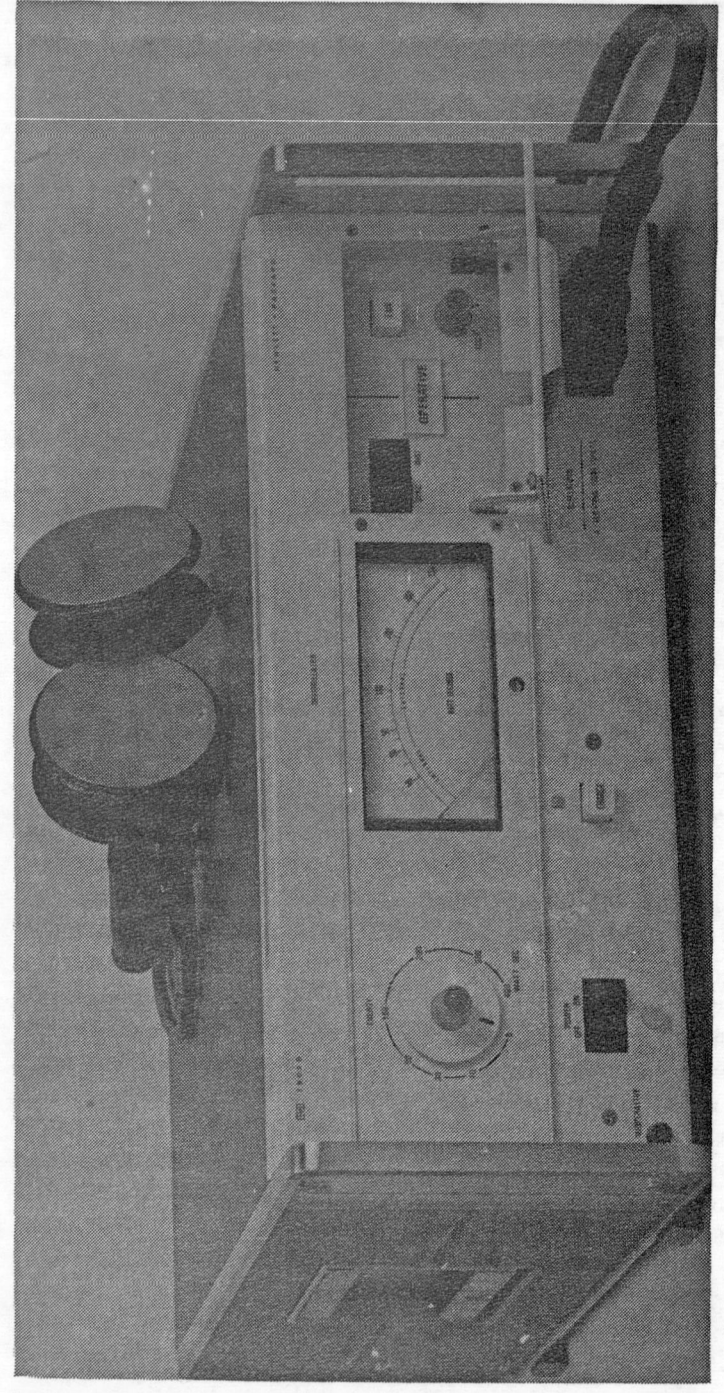

Fig. 8-3. Heavy duty defibrillator for stationary use. (Courtesy Hewlett-Packard)

16 μF, high voltage, oil-filled type. In the charge mode, 120V ac power is applied to the primary of variable transformer T1, which energizes the primary of high-voltage transformer T2. Diode D1 is used to rectify the ac from the high-voltage side of transformer T2 so that capacitor C1 can be charged. K1 is a high-voltage vacuum relay. In the charge condition, K1 is de-energized with one side connected to ground and the other side connected to the high-voltage supply at diode D1. This condition causes C1 to charge, and its charge level is indicated by the kilovoltmeter (calibrated in watt-seconds) connected in shunt with C1. Energy stored in the capacitor can be found from the formula

$$U = \tfrac{1}{2}CV^2$$

where U = stored energy in watt-seconds (or joules)
C = capacitance in *farads* (e.g., 16 μF = 1.6×10^{-5} F)
V = voltage across the capacitor in volts

Note that joules and watt-seconds are equivalent units that can be used interchangeably. The defibrillator, however, will have its energy meter calibrated in watt-seconds rather than joules.

Most defibrillators are designed to charge to a stored level of 400 W-sec. These normally use a 16 μF capacitor but some

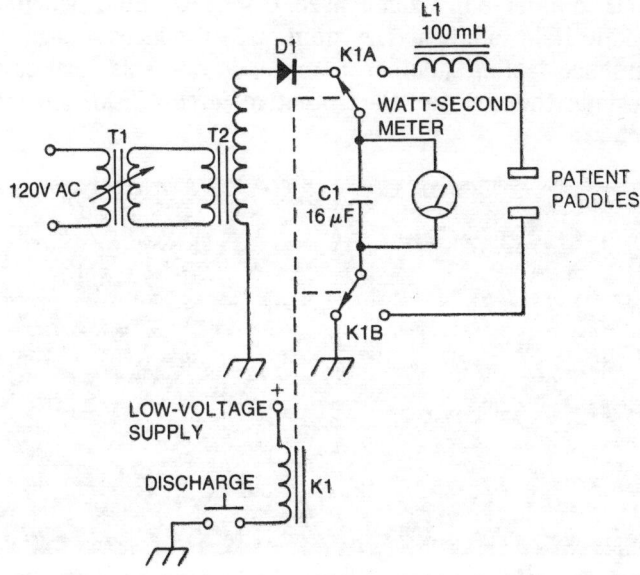

Fig. 8-4. Basic difibrillator circuit.

units use a different value. The voltage across that capacitor is then

$$V = \sqrt{2U/C}$$
$$= \sqrt{(2)(400)/(1.6 \times 10^{-5})}$$
$$= 7071 \text{ volts}$$

Clearly then, a defibrillator is no toy and can be very dangerous if played with or handled in a manner seemingly oblivious to the high level of energy it can deliver!

The output waveform (Fig. 8-5) produced by this circuit is called the *Lown waveform* after Dr. Bernard Lown, a cardiologist at Harvard. The waveform has a rise time of less than 500 μsec and a peak amplitude of a bit less than 3000V. This waveform is due to the nature of the capacitor discharge path in the defibrillator circuit of Fig. 8-4.

When the operator presses the discharge switch, relay contacts K1A and K1B close and place the capacitor across the output circuit, and the patient. This is a series RL circuit path consisting of a 100 millihenry (mH) inductance and a resistance that is the sum of the coil resistance of the inductor, relay contact resistance, and the patient's body resistance. This RL circuit is designed to make the capacitor discharge follow the highly damped Lown waveform. The main positive pulse is completed in about 5 msec. Discharge of the inductor's magnetic field following the main pulse produces a negative undershoot lasting another 5 msec or so. This last pulse represents the counter electromotive force (CEMF) of the inductor.

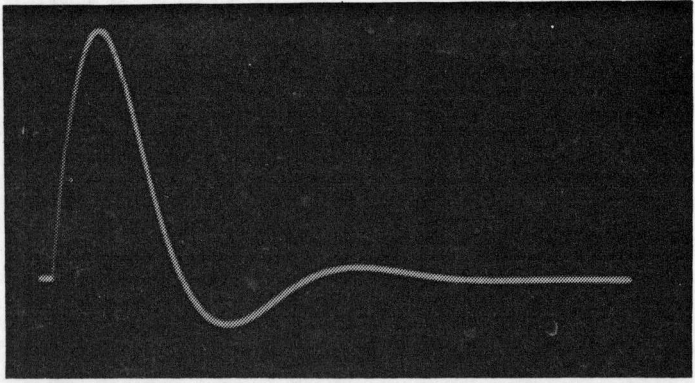

Fig. 8-5. Oscilloscope trace of defibrillator discharge waveform, the so-called Lown waveform.

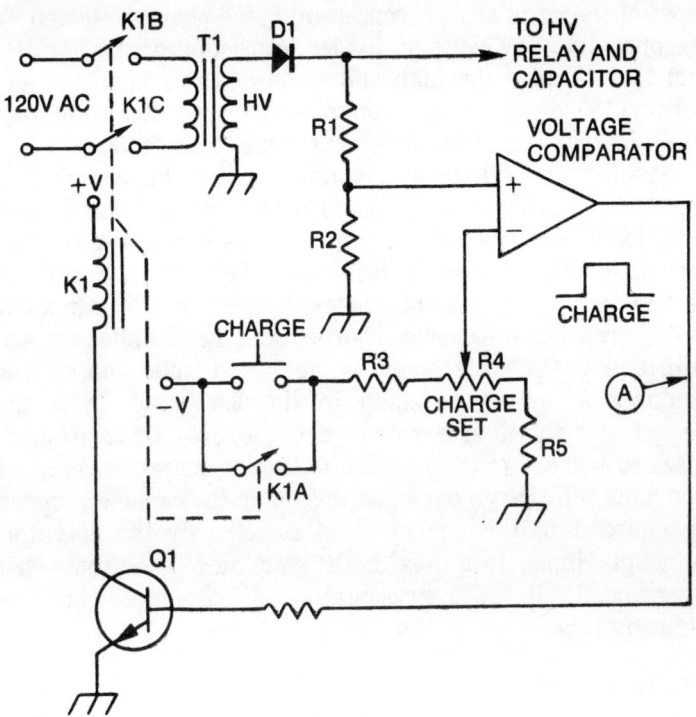

Fig. 8-6. Charge control circuit for automatically charging storage capacitor to desired energy level.

Control Circuits

Figure 8-6 shows one type of control circuit used in some defibrillators. Transformer T1 and diode D1 were seen also in the circuit of Fig. 8-4. The *charge* switch places a negative voltage at the inverting input of a comparator circuit, which causes the comparator output to switch from a zero (ground level) output to a logic high. If TTL logic is used, this will be approximately +5V dc. This potential forward-biases NPN transistor Q1, causing the coil of relay K1 to become energized. Contacts K1B and K1C close and apply power to the primary of high-voltage transformer T1. A third set of contacts, K1A, shorts out the charge switch so the charge cycle is latched on for the duration of the change cycle latched.

Resistor R4 is part of a voltage divider and is mounted on the front panel. This potentiometer is calibrated in watt-seconds and will be set by the operator to the level of charge desired. This puts a reference voltage on the inverting

155

input of the comparator, representing the charge selected by the operator. The voltage divider, consisting of resistors R1 and R2, samples the high voltage across the capacitor and delivers a scaled down, proportional representation of that potential to the non-inverting input of the comparator.

As long as differential voltage across the comparator inputs is greater than zero, its output remains high. This situation occurs when the voltage from the sampling circuit on the high-voltage side is less than the voltage from the reference source, potentiometer R4. When the capacitor voltage reaches the desired charge level, the sampling voltage will equal the reference voltage, and this causes the comparator output to snap to the low state. With the comparator output at ground level (logic zero), Q2 is no longer forward biased, so it will cut off. This de-energizes relay K1 and halts the charge cycle. At this point, the capacitor should be charged to the energy level selected by the operator. Although this circuit is both simplified and somewhat generalized, it is representative of a large class of defibrillators.

CARDIOVERTERS

Defibrillators fire instantly when the operator presses the *discharge* button. This mode is used when the patient is in ventricular fibrillation. Electrical shock is also used, however, in other procedures in which the patient has a QRS complex. Timing is very important, since if the capacitor is discharged at a time coincident with the ECG t wave, the patient may actually go into ventricular fibrillation.

A cardioverter is nothing more than a defibrillator with a built-in synchronization circuit that inhibits firing until the next R wave to occur following the command from the discharge button. Hewlett-Packard's model 7802 shown in Fig. 8-3 is a combination cardioverter/defibrillator, as are the other machines.

A stylized and very much simplified block diagram of the 7802 circuitry is shown in Fig. 8-7. The defibrillator portion of the instrument is pretty much the same as the simple machine discussed earlier in this chapter. K1 is the high-voltage charge-transfer relay. Switch S2, located behind the front panel trap door, determines whether the 7802 operates as a defibrillator ("inst" for *instantaneous*) or a cardioverter

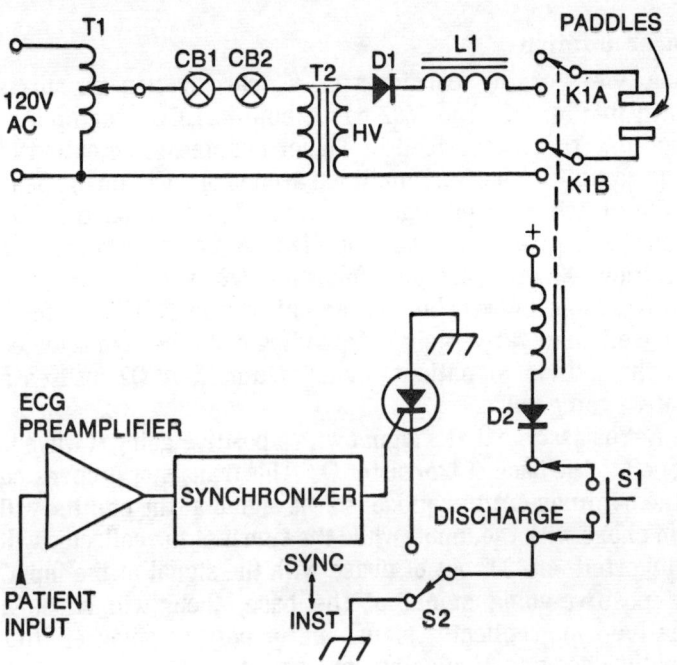

Fig. 8-7. Basic timing circuitry of Hewlett-Packard model 7802 cardioverter.

("sync" for *synchronous*). In the instantaneous position of S2, the relay coil will energize and fire the defibrillator as soon as discharge switch S1 is pressed.

When S2 is in the synchronous position, firing of the transfer relay is inhibited until SCR1 is gated on. In this condition, the firing is AND-gated by switch S1 and the SCR. So both S1 and SCR1 must be conducting current before the machine will discharge. SCR1 is gated on when a pulse is received from the synchronizer circuit. This section will issue one short-duration pulse every time an R wave is received from the ECG preamplifier. When the thumbswitch is depressed by the operator, the machine will pause, that is to say remain dormant, until the occurrance of the next R wave in the patient's ECG signal. The R wave creates a pulse in a one-shot multivibrator and that pulse fires the SCR. When both thumbswitch operation and the R wave sync pulse are coincident, the machine will deliver the capacitor charge to the patient cable.

Synchronization

A view of the cardioverter synchronization circuit is shown in Fig. 8-8. The 7802 has a built-in ECG preamplifier much like those described in earlier chapters. The output of the preamplifier has an amplitude around one volt on the peak of the R wave. This signal is amplified to around 5V in transistor Q1 and is then applied to polarity correction amplifier Q2. The circuits following Q2 want to see only positive-going pulses, but the actual human ECG waveform may well be negative-going, depending upon the lead selected and the individual patient. Polarity amplifier Q2 insures a positive-going pulse.

Let us assume that a signal with a positive-going R wave is applied to the base of transistor Q2. This transistor is operated in the common-emitter mode, so the signal at the emitter will be in phase with the input, while the signal at the collector will be inverted, or 180° out of phase with the signal at the input. The positive-going signal at the base, then, will cause a negative-going collector signal and a positive-going emitter signal. The negative-going pulses at the collector will reverse-bias diode D1, so it is blocked. The emitter signal, on the other hand, is positive-going and will forward-bias diode D2, passing onto the following circuitry.

Alternatively, suppose an ECG is presented with a negative-going R wave. In this case, the emitter signal will be negative-going and the collector signal will be positive-going. The emitter diode is then blocked and cannot pass a signal, while the collector is forward biased, passing the signal onto the following circuitry in a manner similar to the previous case. In the latter case, the stage operates as an inverter while in the former it is simply an emitter follower.

R-Wave Detection

The discharge criteria in the cardioverter must include the ability to decide whether any particular input feature is or is not a genuine R wave. Examination of the typical R wave reveals two properties that can be used to decide: higher amplitude and faster rise time. Unfortunately, simple circuitry using only a threshold detector to find the highest amplitude feature is not sufficient. Other features sometimes equal or exceed the R wave in amplitude. It is also true that the operator might turn up the preamplifier gain so far that

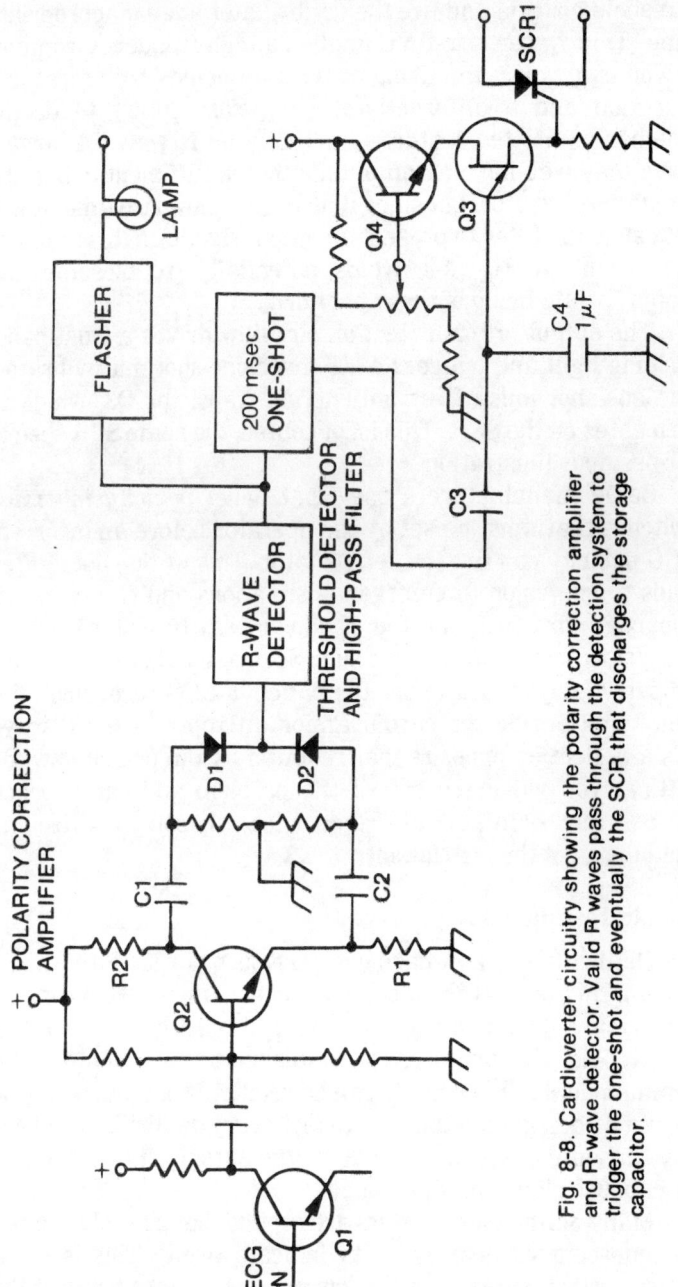

Fig. 8-8. Cardioverter circuitry showing the polarity correction amplifier and R-wave detector. Valid R waves pass through the detection system to trigger the one-shot and eventually the SCR that discharges the storage capacitor.

several features in the ECG waveform might exceed the threshold criteria and fire the defibrillator at an inappropriate time. That faster rise-time implies a high frequency content, so you can expect the firing criteria to include both threshold detection and a differentiator (high-pass filter) to decide whether or not the feature is actually an R wave. A large t wave may well have an amplitude that is sufficient to trip the amplitude detector, but since it also has a slow rise time, it will not cause the filter to present an output signal. In this manner, the circuit in Fig. 8-8 avoids potentially troublesome and inappropriate firing of the capacitor.

The output of this detection circuitry drives a front-panel flashing light and triggers a 200 msec one-shot multivibrator. The one-shot pulse fires unijunction transistor Q3, which in turn gates on the SCR. This is, of course, the same SCR seen in the previous illustration.

Some manufacturers use front panel *polarity inversion* switches that must be set by the operator before an incorrect ECG polarity can fire the defibrillator. This works, but it often leads to confusion in emergency situations and can cause an apparent "misfire" of the cardioverter. If you receive a request to service a machine such as this, but it seems to work properly for you, ask to see the patient's ECG recording (if it was taken during the cardioversion attempt). If the R wave has a deflection opposite that required by the polarity switch setting, you will have solved the problem and can proceed to—as the commerical electronics shops say—fix the customer, not the instrument.

Simple Testing

Defibrillators and cardioverters seem to have the nasty habit of misfiring at the most inopportune times, like during an emergency. This is always serious and must be avoided if at all possible. Fortunately, the avoidance or detection of most common defibrillator faults can be relatively simple. Someone should be designated the "it" to test every defibrillator, every day. In some cases this is done by the nursing staff; in others by in-house electronics personnel.

Many defibrillator testers are around that use only a small incandescent or neon lamp to indicate firing. This is not a satisfactory test because the low current requirements of the tester can indicate the instrument is in fine working order, yet the patient cable is wide open. The high voltage can ionize the air in the gap across the break to pass enough current to fire the bulb, but not enough to actually defibrillate the patient. In cases of open cables—and they occur frequently in certain brands of defibrallators—a lot of the stored energy is burned up ionizing the air in the gap at the break, and this deteriorates the level actually delivered to the patient.

Fortunately, qualitative daily checks can be made using a special gas cell as the load. A good policy is to first set the machine to store 400 W-sec of energy and see if it can handle this level. After discharging the machine into the load cell, reset the charge level to a point between 1 and 5 W-sec and retest by again firing the instrument into the load cell. If the cables or relay are in poor shape, the load cell will not flash when the machine is discharged.

QUANTITATIVE TESTING

The testing procedures just described are merely qualitative, but they can be the first line of defense against malfunctions that are well on the way toward being a serious incident. If defects are found routinely, not during an emergency, they can be corrected before the machine is critically needed. A secondary level of testing can be even more sensitive, but it need be performed only on a weekly or monthly basis. This testing is usually performed by trained electronic personnel.

A defibrillator is one of those instruments that might be needed badly at any moment, so an acceptable test procedure should not take the instrument away from its assigned station and should be done quickly without disassembly of the machine. This means that all of your instruments and procedures must be totally portable and totally external to the defibrillator/cardioverter package.

A high-impedance kilovoltmeter can be used to calibrate the watt-second meter. We know how much voltage should be present across the capacitor at any given watt-second setting by solving the equation presented earlier in the chapter. A spare high-voltage connector can be used to attach the kilovoltmeter to the machine in a safe manner, with a switch installed on the kilovoltmeter to fire the high-voltage charge transfer relay. Keep in mind that most common kilovoltmeters are not too accurate, so you must decide what tolerances are actual machine problems and what is merely a measurement error.

In the test equipment chapter, we will discuss the type of defibrillator testers often used by medical service personnel and will give an example of one popular model. These are actually little more than integrating voltmeters calibrated in watt-seconds. Keep a record of the readings obtained on a weekly or monthly inspection basis. Look for trends where the output level seems to be dropping. This can spot dying rectifiers, a wornout charge transfer relay, and other defects.

An oscilloscope equipped with a Polaroid camera is often used to examine the output waveform produced by the machine. This is probably the most sensitive test that can be performed on the instrument. Many hidden problems will show up on the photograph that cannot be seen on the testers, and problems may show up on the photograph long before they are capable of producing other symptoms, such as reduced energy output.

In the oscilloscope method, the defibrillator is discharged into a 50Ω power resistor, shunted by a 60 dB voltage attenuator consisting of a series combination of a 1M and 1K resistor. The oscilloscope input is connected across the 1K resistor and should display a waveform such as Fig. 8-5. This procedure should be followed whenever a machine is inspected or whenever repairs are made. It is also a good idea to include an oscilloscope photograph as a part of the analysis when troubleshooting a malfunction report.

Figure 8-9 shows a waveform photograph from a machine with a badly pitted relay contact. This machine will probably function for a while, but it is headed for trouble in the *near* future. It had also just passed the tests using the load cell and integrating voltmeter! Ergo...use an oscilloscope camera if at all possible.

SPARES AND REPAIRS

Repairs to defibrillators must be made rapidly and your parts stock should reflect an effort to keep turnaround time to a minimum. Few hospitals have sufficient equipment for the servicer to be able to take his time and order parts on an "as needed" basis. Spare parts to stock for the defibrillator include spare paddles—and these should be kept with the machine. The nursing staff should be trained to look for those

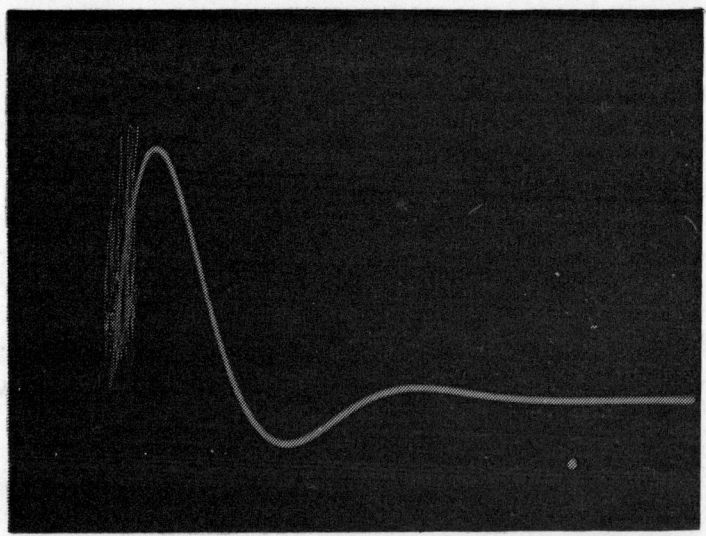

Fig. 8-9. An oscillograph can reveal a badly pitted relay contact like this long before a noticeable drop in output power occurs. A camera can catch and record this type of detail, which might otherwise go unnoticed. Alternatively, if you have access to an oscilloscope with storage capability, you can also capture and hold the waveform for closer examination.

paddles and change them in the event of a malfunction. Also stock, where available, parts for the patient paddles so that they can be repaired locally. New paddles cost an arm and a leg, so repair can be attractive if it is done effectively.

Other mandatory spares include small relays, switches, and rectifiers, including the high-voltage rectifier. Transistors and other semiconductors should also be kept in stock. If your budget permits, or if you are a commercial servicer handling a number of hospitals, also stock any plug-in printed circuit boards and a vacuum relay.

Some out-of-date equipment cannot be serviced with components purchased from the defibrillator manufacturer. In those cases, you can use parts from one of the others. Many defibrillator designers used, for example, the Torr Laboratories TMR-10 vacuum relay for the charge transfer relay. If the coil voltage of this type is compatable, or if the power supply can be easily modified to make it compatible, then use one of these to replace obsolete numbers. Of course, it must be kept in mind that a defibrillator that old might be better replaced.

Bedside troubleshooting should not be to the component level on plug-in boards. Replace the board and then troubleshoot it back on the workbench. Even if you lack a test jig (one can be made easily in most cases), it is usually feasible to "shotgun" the board or test each component separately.

The turnaround time and the quality of the repair job are quite critical, much more so than in other areas of electronic servicing. Who really cares, for example, if a just-repaired television set conks out in the midst of the Super Bowl? Only the irate customer. But you cannot joke about a defibrillator being used to save someone's life. It is never excusable to knowingly produce poor quality work because in medical instrument servicing, sloppiness can easily cost someone their life! If a technician or engineer cannot produce high-grade service on these machines, they should stay out of medical electronic service!

Chapter 9
Electrosurgical Generators

Surgeons often use high level, but controlled, radio-frequency currents as an electronic scalpel of sorts. Besides being able to cut tissue and make incisions with this current, the physician can also cauterize any bleeding blood vessels that may have been cut. Normally, this would have to be done by tying them off with short pieces of suture. Interestingly enough, electrosurgery machines in daily use today span the technology spectrum from the ancients to the astronauts! You can still purchase brand new machines built around the same circuitry used by Guglielmo Marconi and Heinrich Hertz in their early pioneering "wireless" experiments.

Medical people frequently refer to *all* electrosurgical machines by using the word *Bovie* as a generic term. Properly, though, Bovie is a brand name, a credit to one of the inventors of electrosurgery, and is used to designate those machines manufactured by Liebel-Flarsheim and sold through The Ritter Company, of Rochester, N.Y.

Figures 9-1 through 9-3 show some typical electrosurgical machines. Figure 9-1 is a full-size general surgery machine, while Fig. 9-2 is a small, wall-mounted (or tabletop) Bantam Bovie by Liebel-Flarsheim. These latter machines are often found in surgeon's offices for minor work and in certain light procedures areas of hospitals. The machine in Fig. 9-3 is a modern, all solid-state model with several options not available on the other models.

165

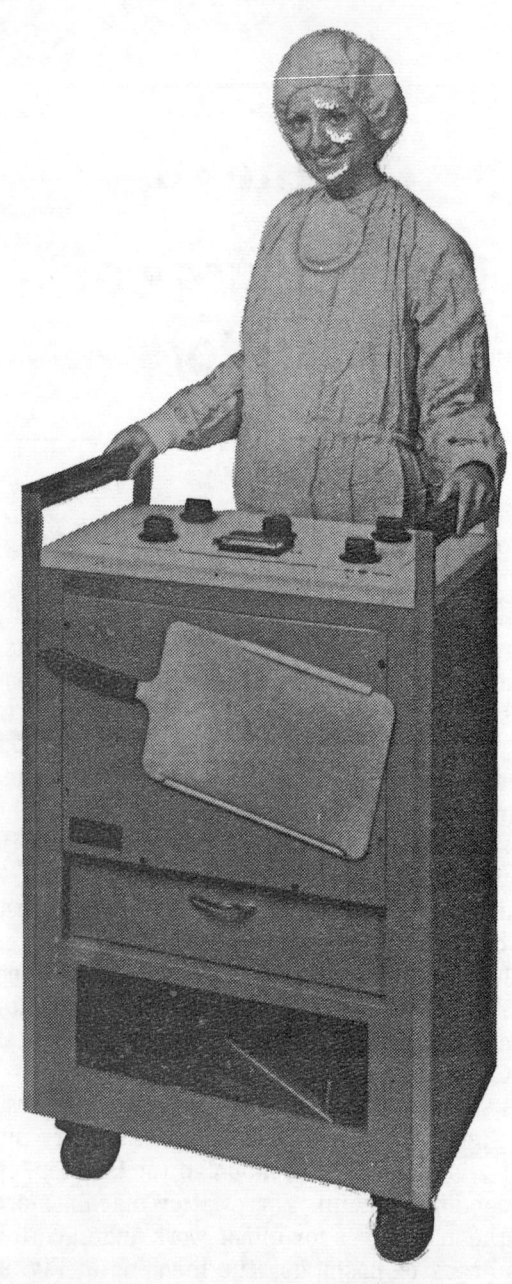

Fig. 9-1. A Bovie CSU II electrosurgical machine. (Courtesy Liebel-Flarsheim)

HOW THEY WORK

Anyone who has worked with radio transmitters or transmitting antennas is probably well aware of the fact that radio frequency currents can burn tissue! In surgical uses of radio frequency current, the patient is electrically placed between the two output poles of the current generator, the electrosurgical machine.

In *unipolar* systems—the most common in general use—the patient lies on a large-area metallic grounding plate such as that hanging on the machine pictured in Fig. 9-1. The

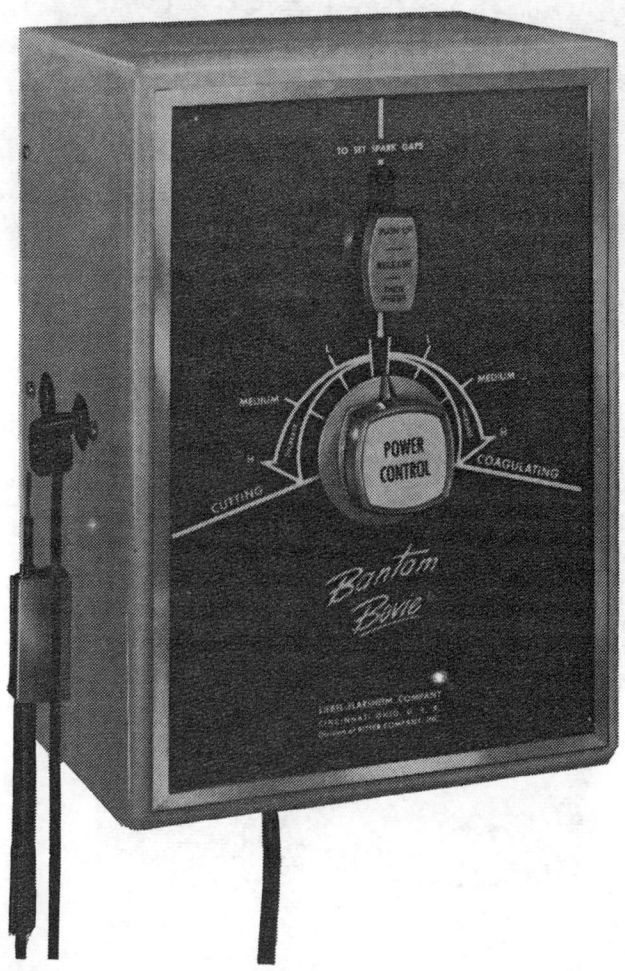

Fig. 9-2. A Bantam Bovie for less demanding electrosurgical uses. (Courtesy Liebel-Flarsheim)

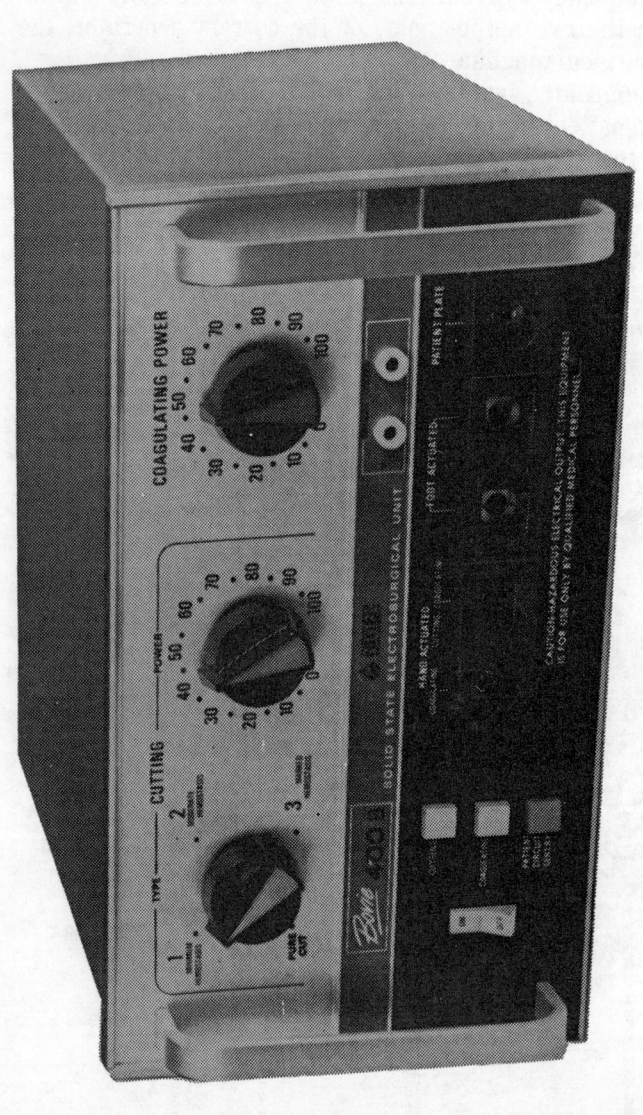

Fig. 9-3. An all solid-state Bovie 400 with special features like patient protection circuitry. (Courtesy Liebel-Flarsheim)

"scalpel" is a handheld electrode with a small-area tip. The tip might be either pointed or rounded off and blunt. The ground plate is connected to the designated "cold" or actual ground side (as the case may be) of the rf output, while the "active" electrode is connected to the "hot" side of the generator.

When the surgeon places the active electrode against the patient's skin and steps on the footswitch controller, an rf current is generated, which then oscillates back and forth between the two electrodes through a path completed by the patient's body. The current flowing in the patient grounding plate is diffused over a relatively large area, so it is not of sufficient intensity at any given point to cut tissue. It can, though, cause burns if the plate is improperly prepared or if it is positioned under a bony point on the patient's body.

The same current flowing in the ground plate also flows in the active electrode. Since the active electrode surface is of small area, the current density is very high, so cutting and burning can occur. This action is analogous, if you torture reality a little, to the difference between a flat pane of glass and a magnifying glass. If sunlight is allowed to pass through the pane of glass to a point on your skin, there should be no pain or burning since the light energy is diffuse. But replace that glass with a lens, and place the lens so that the light falls on your skin in a focused dot, and it will become painfully burned in a very short time.

Figure 9-4 shows some of the common current waveforms used in electrosurgical generators of classic design. Most efficient cutting occurs when the applied waveform is a sine wave, as in part A, with a frequency between about 500 and 2500 kHz. Cauterization or *hemostasis* is best with a current that is highly damped such as the two waveforms shown in part B (moderate) and C (heavy). The generator circuits required to produce these waveforms in classical, nonsolid-state machines differ considerably and will be treated separately.

The *cut* current is a sine wave with a power level of 50 or 60 watts at low settings and going up to several hundred watts on high settings. In the higher power condition, these machines are very similar to medium-wave shipboard radiotelegraphy transmitters and the rf decks in some low-powered AM broadcast transmitters. If you are already familiar with these types of equipment, then there will be little trouble in learning to service electrosurgical machines.

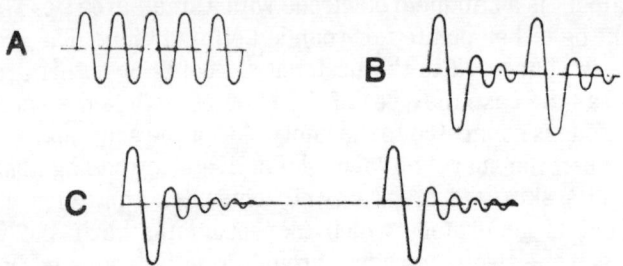

Fig. 9-4. Typical electrosurgical waveforms. (A) continuous sine wave cutting current, (B) moderately damped sine-wave pulses closely spaced. (C) heavily damped sine-wave pulses widely spaced.

CUT OSCILLATOR

Figure 9-5 shows a circuit, simplified only a little bit, from a Birtcher model 770 electrosurgical generator. The *cut* oscillator is a push-pull design using a pair of UXCV-11 power triode vacuum tubes. These tubes, incidentally, are used in several different machines and by many different manufacturers. The tuned tank circuit is resonant at a frequency that is determined by the capacitance of C1 and the inductance of the primary winding of transformer T1. Power output from this tank is fed directly to the patient with no need for further amplification. The current in the secondary of transformer T1 flows through capacitor C3 to the active electrode. Radio-frequency current is returned to ground through the coil in the *coagulate* generator output circuit. The power level for the cut function is set by selection of various output taps on the inductor via switch S1, which is mounted to the front panel.

The DC power supply for this section (not shown) uses a full-wave rectification system using mercury vapor, high-voltage rectifiers, type 966A/866AX. If these are not readily available, you can usually substitute the high-vacuum type 3B28 for this set of rectifiers, although you will miss the beautiful blue glow of the mercury types, which light up nicely when energized.

The 120V ac primary of the plate transformer feeding the push-pull tubes is connected to the powerline through a footswitch that is controlled by the surgeon. Note that no filtering is used in these machines. Capacitor C2, which might be mistaken for a filter in the schematic because of its position, is a low value type and is used only to decouple the rf—it has no effect on the 120 Hz ripple component riding on the dc voltage.

SPARK GAP COAGULATOR

If your father or grandfather was in radio during its early days, especially as a "ham" (amateur) or merchant marine radio-telegrapher, he would probably be more at home and familiar with the *coagulate* generator than even the best engineer or technician educated in these technologically more sophisticated times. The *coagulate* current is generated by a spark gap! These spark gaps create an electrical arc that is very rich in energy. This fact was put to use in early radio's pioneering days as the only practical means of generating large amounts of rf power. Almost all shipboard radiotelegraph transmitters of that era were spark gaps, although a few used Alexanderson alternators. Both were made illegal for communications under the regulations established by the F.C.C. In fact, the bright arcing and ozone smell of early marine radio rooms (radio shacks) is the origin of the nickname *sparks*, given almost universally to the ship's radio officer ever since those days.

The same rf property that made the spark gap no longer desirable for radio communications is exactly what makes it useful for electrosurgery. Figure 9-6 shows a typical spark gap

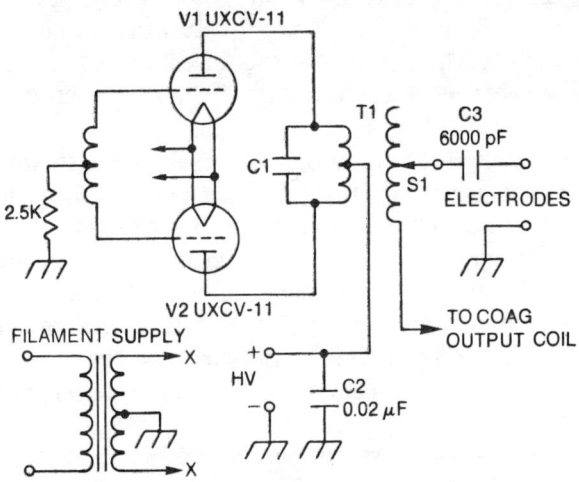

Fig. 9-5. Simple push-pull oscillator circuit provides sine-wave cutting current for electrosurgery.

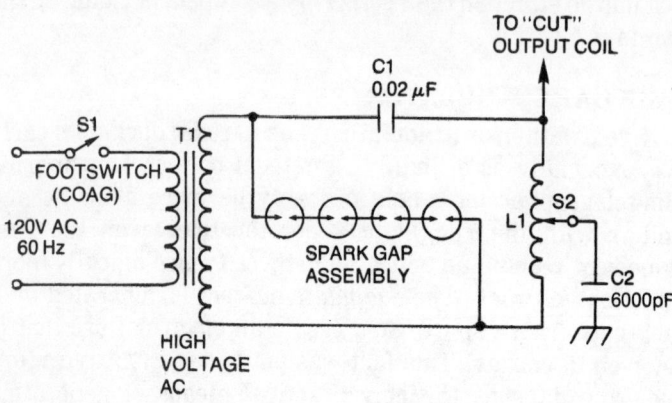

Fig. 9-6. The four spark gaps provide bursts of rf energy for coagulation in electrosurgery. Since no regenerative power is added, the spark gaps naturally deliver the desired damped sine waves.

rf generator, also from the Birtcher 770. The spark gap assembly is not a single pair of points, but rather four pairs in series.

The primary of transformer T1 is energized by the *coag* footswitch operated by the surgeon. This places a high-voltage 60 Hz ac potential across the gap and that ionizes the air in the gap. This ionization creates the arcing that is used to produce rf power. The rf oscillatory path consists of the spark gaps, capacitor C1, and inductor L1. The power level is set by switch S2 on the front panel. This switch is returned to ground through capacitor C2. The hot side of this circuit is fed to the active electrode through the secondary of the *cut* generator output transformer (see Fig. 9-5).

The inner works of the Birtcher model 770 is shown in Fig. 9-7. On the right are the UXCV-11 power triodes used to generate the cut current sine wave. Behind these tubes is the cut-current generator's output transformer, and above, the capacitor tuning the primary of that transformer. The mercury vapor rectifiers are on the left; these are normally types 8-66AX, 966A, or if substitutions have been made, 3B28. In some of the more recent models, a solid-state rectifier stack is used.

The spark gap assembly is just behind the vacuum tube rectifiers (also see Fig. 9-8). The oscillator tank consists of the two series-connected open-frame mica capacitors and the coil above the spark gap assembly. The ac power connector and footswitch connector are located on the rear apron of the rf deck chassis.

You will soon learn that most electrosurgery equipment repairs involves either the footswitch or its connectors. Typical faults actually encountered will include bad or misadjusted microswitches, open cables (use 4SS-16-Black wire for replacement), or bad (physically broken) connectors. Most older machines are fitted with rugged size 18 or size 24

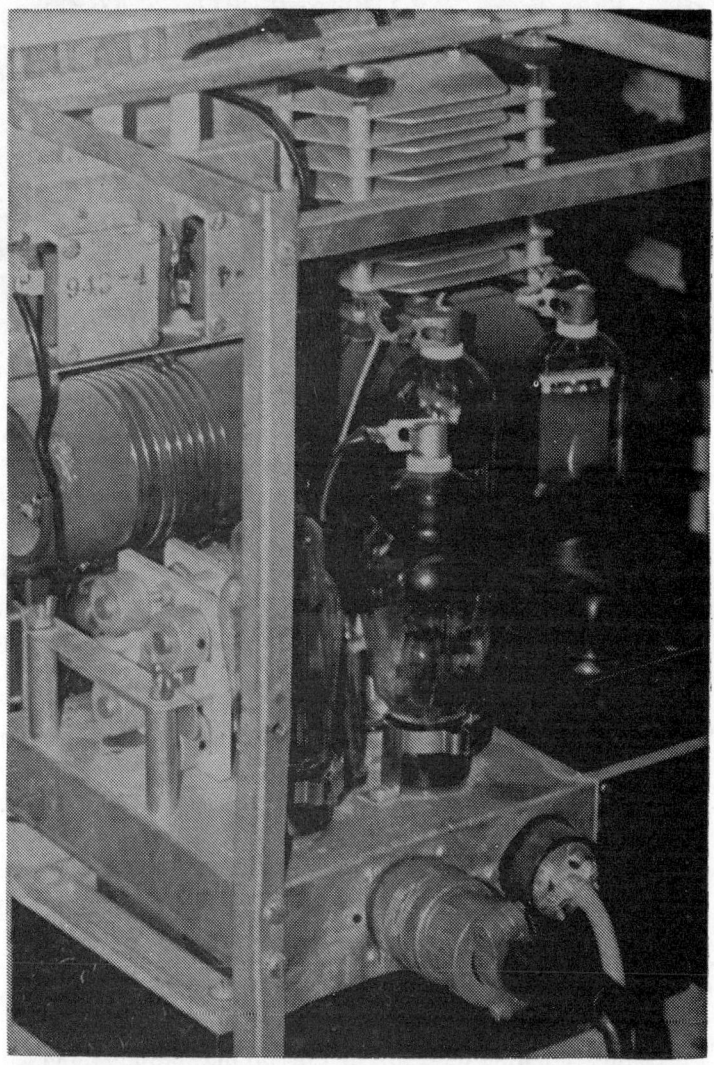

Fig. 9-7. Rear view of Birtcher model 770 electrosurgical generator.

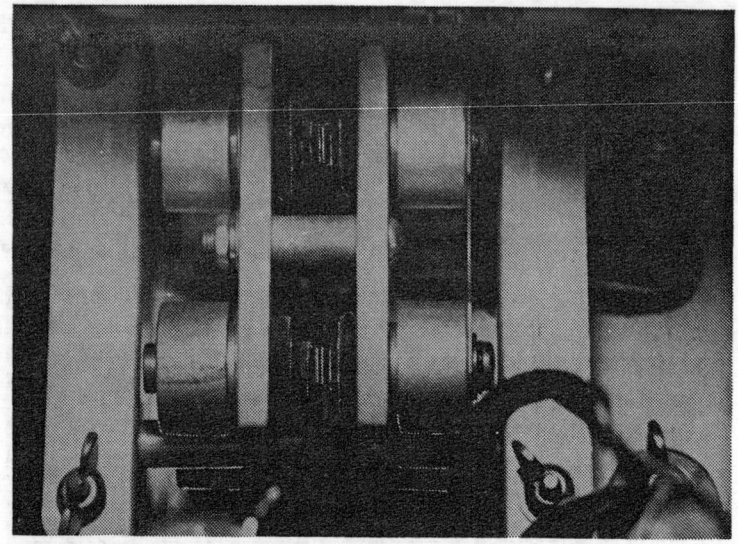

Fig. 9-8. Close-up of spark gap assembly in Birtcher unit.

AN-series military connectors intended for application in combat zones. Incredulous as it might seem, these tough connectors are occassionally broken into several small pieces by operating room usage. Stock a few AN connectors of appropriate size and type for footswitch repairs!

MODERN DESIGNS

Figures 9-9 and 9-10 show some electrosurgery machines of a more recent design. That of Fig. 9-9 is the rear view of the ACMI model C-650. Although of more recent vintage than the types discussed earlier, it is essentially similar in most details that are important. The coagulate current is not, however, generated in a spark gap but in a special gas-filled vacuum tube called a *thyratron*. This type of tube must be allowed to heat up, which takes a few minutes from turn-on, before it can begin to generate current. This fact leads to a relatively large number of erroneous complaints from operating room personnel who are not familiar with this peculiarity. The ACMI C-650 may also be equipped with a high-intensity light source for use with fiber-optic endoscopy equipment. The photograph in Fig. 9-10 is the inner workings of the solid-state Bovie shown in Fig. 9-1 earlier in the chapter.

Solid-state machines are fast becoming dominant and will soon overtake and pass the older types in actual total hours of

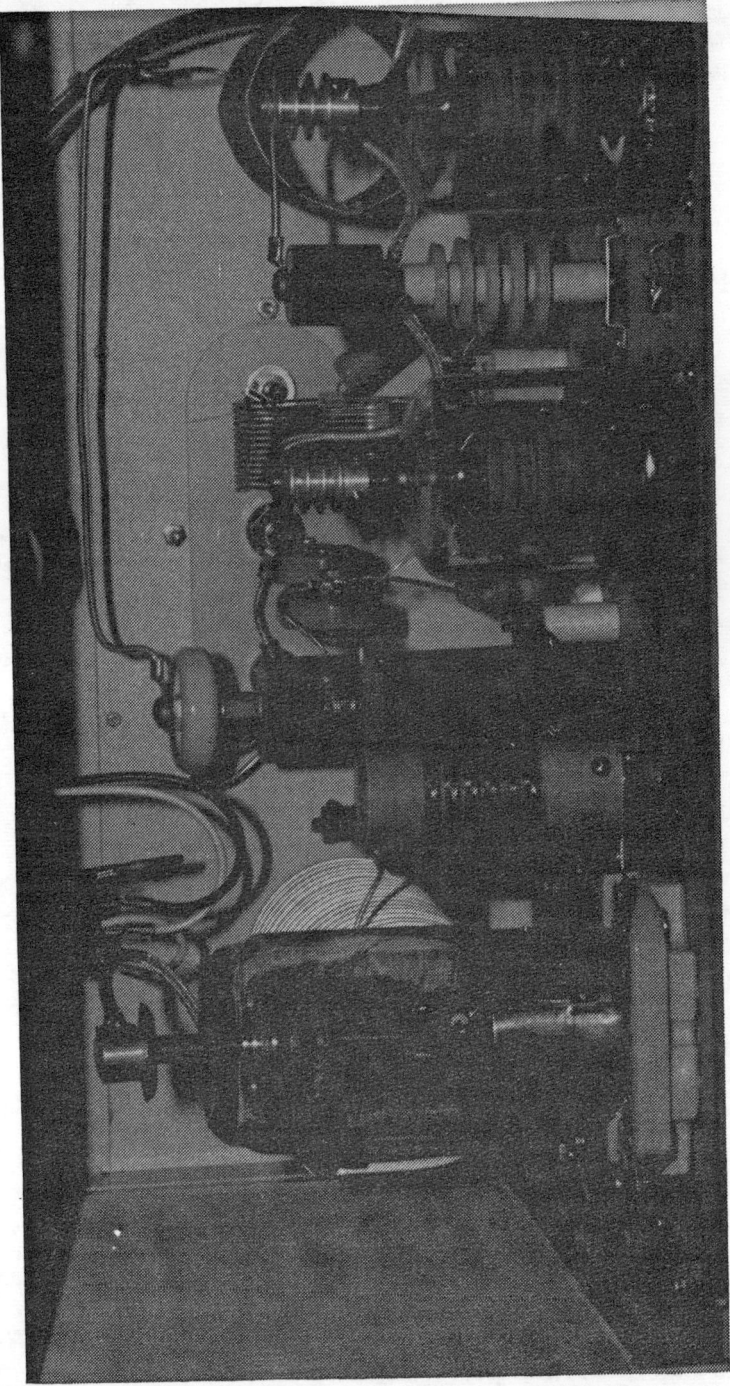

Fig. 9-9. Inside the ACMI model C-650 electrosurgery machine.

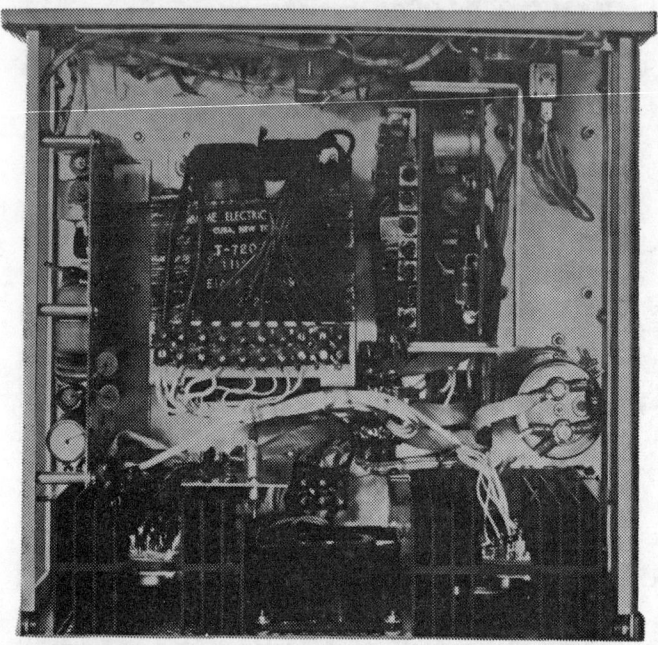

Fig. 9-10. Inside view of Bovie CSU II shown in Fig. 9-1.

weekly usage. But do not expect to see a large housecleaning of the old warhorses—they were well built and have an extremely long life expectancy. Most solid-state machines use a somewhat different technique to generate the sine-wave current. The sine-wave oscillator in tube machines operates at a high level, meaning that it delivers power directly to the load. In most solid-state machines, the sine-wave signal is generated at a low level, and this signal is then amplified to the required power level.

The 500 to 2500 kHz sine wave is generated in a simple transistor oscillator circuit and is then fed to the multi-transistor power amplifier. In the cut mode, this signal is fed, unmodified, to the patient electrodes. In the coagulate mode, though, the sine wave must be chopped (Fig. 9-11) at a rate between 20 Hz and 15 kHz, depending upon the manufacturer. Although other techniques exist, this is the one most commonly found.

MAINTENANCE

One of the primary points to preventive maintenance of solid-state electrosurgical machines is to keep the dust cleaned out. Most of these machines use a small whisper fan to cool the rf power amplifier transistors. If dust builds up on the blades of this fan or covers the TO-3 transistor cases, poor heat transfer may cause the transistors to overheat and burn out.

Measuring RF Power

Although most electrosurgery machine suppliers will sell you an rf power meter for the testing of these machines, you can easily fabricate your own. All that is required is a dummy load resistor and an rf ammeter. You will need a resistor with a value of either 250 or 500 ohms, and it must be capable of dissipating upwards of several hundred watts of rf power for a short time. Furthermore, the resistor or combination of resistors used for the dummy load must be *non-inductive* if they are to perform correctly. Since some manufacturers specify 500Ω while others use 250Ω as the dummy load, it might be wise to use two resistors that can be switched in as needed for the different brands of electrosurgical machine.

The best indicator of output is a thermocouple rf ammeter connected in series with the dummy load resistor. Most modern instruments of that type are frequency independent to well over 50 MHz, so no compensation is needed at low electrosurgery frequencies. Actually, two ammeters are required, and these can be selected by a high/low switch on the front panel of the tester. For low-powered machines, use a 0.5A (500 mA) rf meter; but for high-power instruments, use either a 1.5A or 2A rf meter. These ranges actually complement each other rather nicely because thermocouple meters tend to be nonlinear and will crowd and scale on the lower ends of their respective ranges. The high-current meter

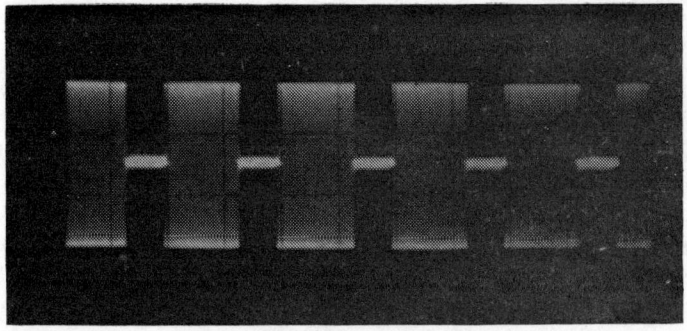

Fig. 9-11. Chopped rf waveform.

will become all but unreadable in the same region where the low-range meter is at its best.

The tester should be housed in a metal-shielded container. Switches and jacks used for this application should be capable of handling rf at a high power level, or trouble will surely result. The output power can be computed from the formula

$$P = I^2 R$$

where P = output power in watts
R = dummy load resistance, either 250 or 500 ohms
I = current read from rf ammeter.

Example—An electrosurgical generator operating at 2500 kHz delivers 1.22A to a 250Ω dummy load resistor. What is the output power of this machine?

$P = I^2 R$
  $= (1.22)^2 (250)$
  $= (1.49) (250)$
  $= 373W$

An alternate technique involves measuring the rf voltage across the dummy load, which in high-power units can be up to several hundred volts. Using Ohm's law, the power is then equal to E^2/R. To be accurate, however, you should use an rf voltmeter. Although it is possible to use an attenuator, a peak rectifier circuit, and an ordinary dc voltmeter, this approach is highly prone to error because the stray circuit capacitances become quite significant at the radio frequencies employed in this equipment.

Checking Specifications

If the manufacturer's specifications are known, you can check electrosurgical machine performance relatively easily by comparing readings with published specs. In those cases where no information is available—which is rare because electrosurgical machine manufacturers tend to publish decent service manuals—it is still possible to do a preventive maintenance service by checking outputs when the machine is believed to be working properly. Subsequent preventive maintenance checks would be made to compare recent readings with the "known good" readings made in the past. A subjective technique in an objective world, perhaps, but effective none the less.

Electrical Shocks

From time to time, medical people report electrical shocks to either the surgeon or patient from electrosurgical machines. All such reports should result in an inspection of the machine involved. Even though most shocks to surgeons result from getting holes in their sterile gloves, it is still necessary to check the machine. And it is a whole lot easier to check a machine right the first time than it is to explain to an authority later why you didn't.

In any electrical shock case, check the power wiring for open grounds or paths from the powerlines to ground. Shocks to patients are usually reported as twitching or convulsions of the body when the active electrode touches the body. Several defects can cause this phenomenon. One is a misadjusted spark gap width. Another cause of patient shocks is shorted or leaky capacitors in the rf output circuitry. These can be checked using an ohmmeter. Set the ohmmeter to its highest scale and connect the probes across the capacitor. If there is no other path for current, you will see a sudden drop in resistance, followed by a slow return toward infinite resistance as the capacitor charges. Replace any capacitors that have some resistance after charging up.

Chapter 10
Cardiographic and Catheterization Lab Equipment

Cardiac catherization laboratories and cardiographics organizations use some rather specialized medical instruments to perform sophisticated diagnostic studies on patients.

CATH LAB INSTRUMENTATION

Figure 10-1 shows a portable roll-around instrument package by Hewlett-Packard. This instrument is made up to customer specifications from a set of basic H-P modular instruments. The lower unit is an eight-channel, multi-speed, thermal strip chart recorder. This particular instrument is a rack-mounted model with its inputs permanently wired to a preamplifier rack that is mounted in the upper portion of the cart. The preamplifier rack is a standard piece of hardware and includes dc power supplies and at least one carrier oscillator to drive the preamplifiers, where needed. The ac power distribution to the preamplifier rack and the strip chart recorder is provided by the cart, so a single toggle or pushbutton switch can be used to turn on the entire system.

The modules in the rack can be selected by the customer to suit the application at hand. Items that might be included in a typical H-P rack up for a catheterization laboratory might include one or more of each fo the following:

- low-gain preamplifier (5 mV), model *8801*
- medium-gain preamplifier (1 mV), model *8802*

- high-gain preamplifier (1 μV), model *8803*
- carrier amplifier (pressures), model *8805*
- ECG preamplifier
- low-frequency ac amplifier (to about 2500 Hz).

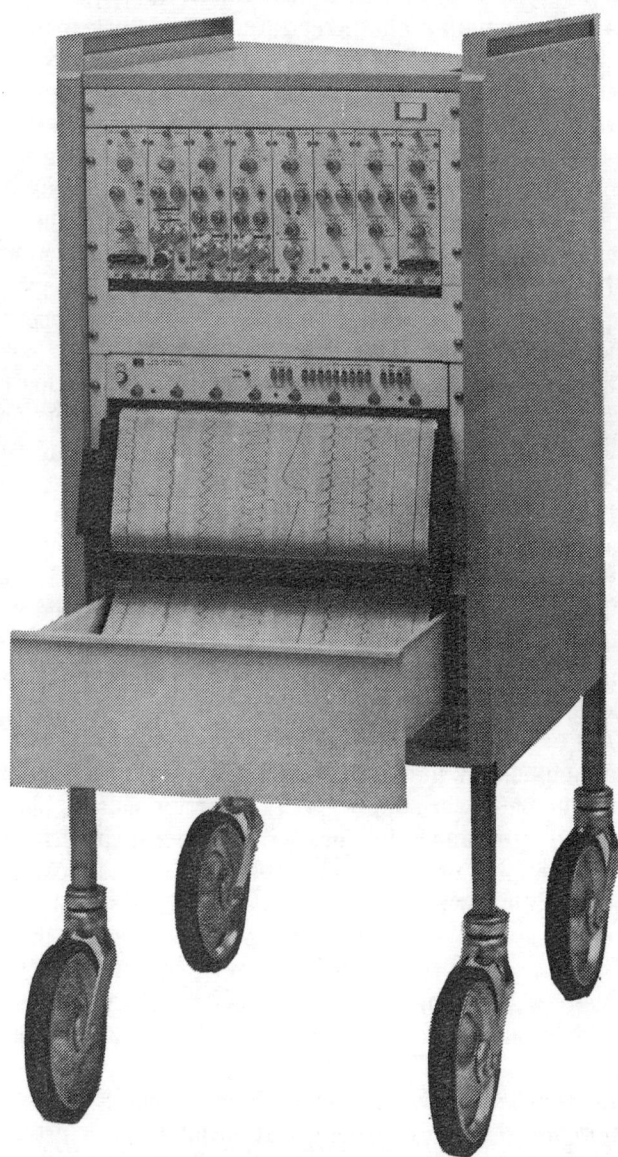

Fig. 10-1. Cath lab instrumentation package in a roll-around cart for portable operation. (Courtesy Hewlett-Packard)

Additionally, there might be a four-channel (*7806*) or eight-channel (*1309*) oscilloscope mounted on top of the cart. In some systems, using a side-by-side tandem cart, they will rack-mount either the oscilloscope or a *7802* defibrillator. The remaining instruments will be mounted on top of the cart.

Another popular chatheterization laboratory instrument package is the Electronics for Medicine (E-for-M) model *VR-6* Simultrace recorder shown in Fig. 10-2. The lower unit in the *VR-6* is called the "camera" by most users; it is a high-frequency light-beam chart recorder that uses a special photosensitive chart paper. The upper section houses the oscilloscope, its input and time-base controls, and the signal acquisition and processing modules (the items in the left half).

The *VR-6* is a six-channel recorder and is specially designed for both research and catheterization laboratory application. The oscilloscope has an unusual 12-by-15 centimeter format and includes circuitry that allows the operator to superimpose timing and baseline markers on the tracing. Every trace on the oscilloscope is also fed to the light-beam oscillograph in the lower housing. Both the housing and the oscilloscope can be made to perform in A-scan or loop (Lissajous figure) presentation modes.

The chart paper is a daylight-load variety, but it can be developed in either a darkroom or in the built-in Rapid Writer developer. The darkroom-developed charts have a greater premanency than those machine developed, but even the latter are long lasting enough for many purposes.

The preamplifier section houses all of the signal-acquisition and processing modules. The mainframe houses the dc power supply ($\pm 15V$), carrier sources (5 and 20 kHz), and interconnection for oscilloscope and camera inputs. A direct-coupled preamplifier (model *DCV*, the lowest unit in the preamplifier rack) is used with a variety of signal sources, including several different types of transducer. It has two differential inputs to accept high (1V) and low (1 mV) level signals. This preamplifier has a switch-selectable filter to provide frequency response from dc to either 25, 250, or 2500 Hz.

A modified dc ECG preamplifier, model *ECV-20*, is an absolute must in any catheterization laboratory instrument package. This item is the second from bottom module in the preamplifier side of the *VR-6* shown in the figure. It is very

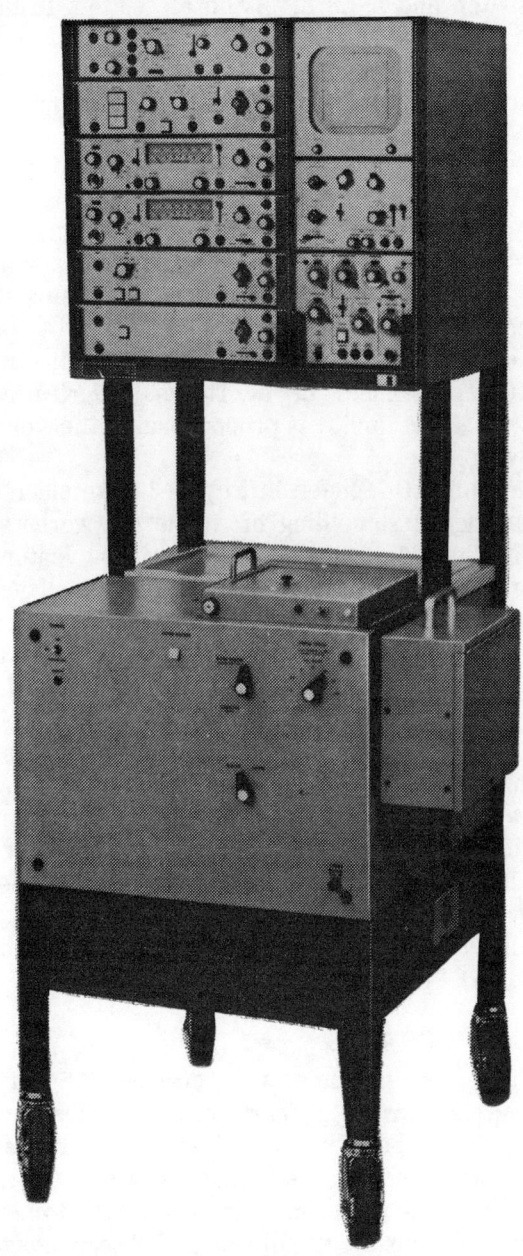

Fig. 10-2. Multichannel physiological monitoring system popular in cath labs and physiological research. (Courtesy E for M)

similar to the dc preamplifier except that it has an ECG-lead selector switch and a 1.0 mV calibrate button. In the ECG mode, the frequency response is limited to 0.5 Hz on the low end.

Another popular plug-in for those versions intended for catheterization laboratory application is the dc excitation pressure amplifier (model *PDV*, third and fourth in the rack shown). Most instrument packages for this market include at least two pressures, and many include up to three or four. These instruments operate like other pressure amplifiers discussed in Chapter 3 and, in fact, use the same types of transducers as any dc-excited system. The *PDV* pressure amplifier does, however, have one unique output that makes it desirable for researchers: dP/dt. This is the *derivative* of the pressure waveform, and it is proportional to the slope of the pressure wave.

The instrument depicted in Fig. 10-3 is an older version and is considered something of a fine old warhorse even though it is of the 1950s vintage. One interesting feature of the old E-forM is that pressure-transducer balancing is accomplished by nulling the resistance and capacitance of the transducer (as is usual on any pressures system) using a Lissajous pattern displayed on the lower oscilloscope.

In my experience, the main problem area found when servicing this instrument is the power supply, at least in the older vacuum tube versions. A clever designer, though, has provided the servicer with a row of neon lamps and tip jacks for measuring each critical voltage point in the power-supply section. These are located along the rear apron of the power supply chassis in the lower half of the rack. Expect to occasionally replace a 6AS7/6080 tube and one or both associated 47Ω, 2W resistors.

PHONOCARDIOGRAPHS

This class of instruments is designed to graphically display heart sounds on a chart recorder. Physicians have used the stethoscope (from the Greek words for *examine chest*) to listen to chest sounds that are within the range of human hearing. The phonocardiograph is an electronic device that not only extends the useful range of observation to those frequencies below the range of human hearing but also provides a written record of the heart sounds.

Several versions of this instrument exist, but they all depend upon a sensitive microphone that has a frequency response from 5 Hz to either 1000 or 2000 Hz, depending upon manufacturer. This microphone is placed at critical points on the patient's chest. The principle differences between various versions of the phonocardiograph is in the galvanometer type used in the chart recorder.

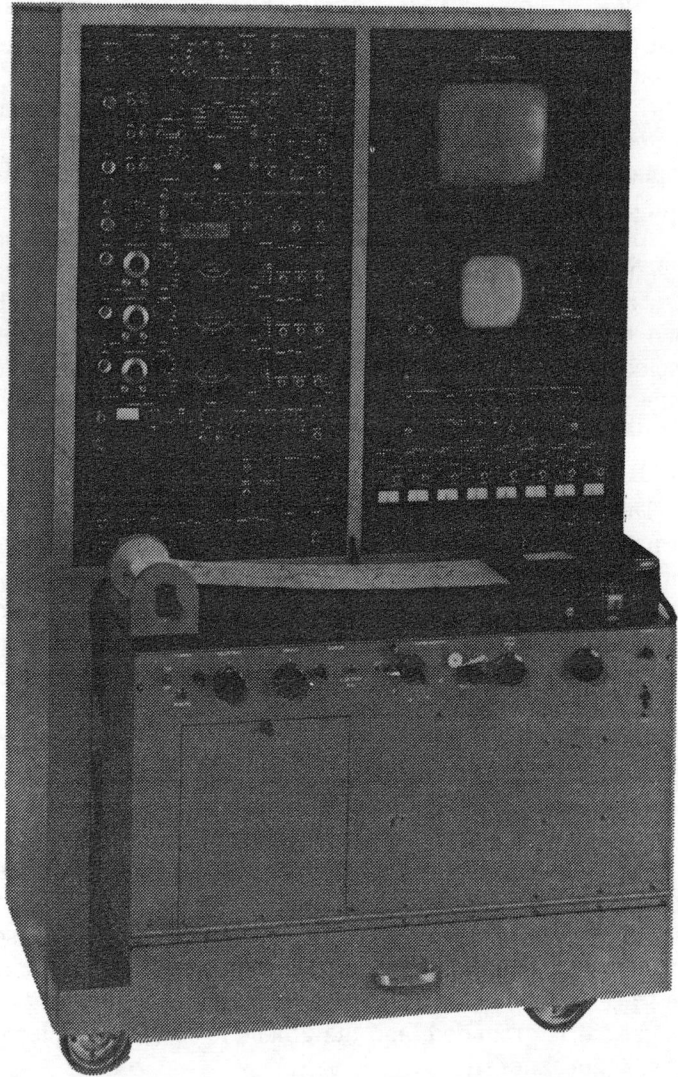

Fig. 10-3. An older version of the previous physiological monitoring system that is still very much in day-to-day use. (Courtesy E for M)

The galvanometer in pen-type recorders is limited to a frequency response of 100–200 Hz. If these are used, it is common practice to display frequencies below 75 Hz directly. Those of greater frequency are displayed after being integrated, which produces an envelope waveform representing the *time average* of the high frequencies in the entire band.

Other phonocardiographs use a high frequency recorder such as those using the light-beam or high-velocity ink-jet galvanometers.

A variation on the phonocardiograph theme is the *intracardiac* recording. A tiny piezoelectric crystal microphone on a special catheter tip is inserted into the chambers of the heart or into the great vessels near the heart.

An *apex* cardiograph is a special type of phono machine designed to record the low-frequency sounds generated by the apex of the heart as it beats or rubs against the chest wall Such measurements are often made in terms of force or displacement, but they use the same type of electronic equipment. The microphone, however, must be carefully selected for its ultralow frequency response.

EXERCISE ECG LABORATORIES

The exercise ECG or "stress test" is a somewhat new form of medical diagnostic test, though it uses some rather ordinary electrocardiograph equipment. The ECG preamplifiers are relatively simple one-lead or multilead versions. In fact, a common configuration is to use a three-lead ECG machine that is automatically switched through four groups of three leads each, until all twelve leads are run.

The main piece of unique equipment is a treadmill on which the patient is made to walk. This piece of equipment is a source of some trouble and may be the cause of noisy ECG recordings. The moving fabric or rubber tread acts much like a Van de Graff generator, producing static charges that are transferred to the patient. This creates some spike like baseline "grass" artifacts on the ECG recording. These artifacts can be quite high in amplitude, high enough to render the trace useless. But this should not be a problem so long as the patient is grounded, and the ground is usually completed through the handrail.

It is often the case, however, that the technicians who conduct the test will try to be helpful and tape the handrail or cover it with a nice soft cloth. This will substantially improve the patient's comfort, but at the expense of a severely deteriorated ECG tracing. If the towel or tape insulating the handrail is removed, the patient will naturally hold onto the rail for balance, and this effectively grounds his body.

An alternative to having the patient grip the cold, hard metal might be to wrap the rail in the conductive foam or velpack material used to store and ship CMOS ICs and CMOS circuit boards. CMOS integrated circuits are easily damaged by static discharges, so they are shipped in a special foam that is conductive. The finished printed circuit boards are shipped inside a special plastic bag made of a conductive material. Although I have not tried this technique, the same principle should work to discharge the artifact-causing static as easily as it does for CMOS circuits.

COMPUTER-BASED SYSTEMS

Many medical instrument manufacturers have produced instrument packages that are computer based. These either replace or supplement their regular line of analog instrumentation. Some have gone the route of the computerized central monitoring system, as was briefly discussed in Chapter 6. Others, such as the unit pictured in Fig. 10-4, are designed for a variety of tasks including use in the catheterization laboratory.

The E-for-M model shown in the picture is based on, and built around, the popular *PDP/11* minicomputer manufactured by the Digital Equipment Corporation (D.E.C.). Sizes range from the *PDP-11/05* with over 8000 words of memory to the *PDP-11/45* with one 124,000 words. The input to the computer is through specially designed E-for-M interface circuits, from the *VR-6* analog instrumentation system discussed previously, or a similar piece of equipment.

The oscilloscope shown in Fig. 10-4 is a non-fade memory type in which the analog trace can be frozen and held for comparison or examination. The instrument also includes a character generator for display of alphanumeric data on the CRT screen. Data input for this function can be from the *VR6* analog package, catheter position panel, oxygen panel, or a keyboard. Disc drives are available as an option so that memory size can be expanded considerably.

If you will allow me a momentary digression, please consider this trend as something that foretells the future. The minicomputer and micropressor are going to make computer-based instruments more common in all areas of electronic instrumentation, especially the medical in-

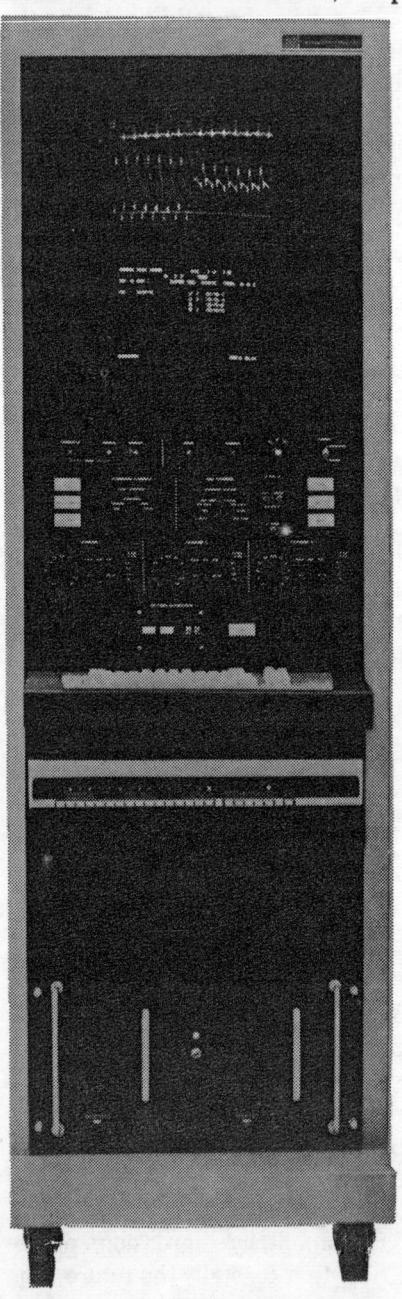

Fig. 10-4. Computer-based catherization laboratory instrumentation system. (Courtesy E for M)

struments field where electronic gadgets must sometimes make a computation based on several inputs. Your are then well advised to study the computer texts listed in the bibliography, which is by no means comprehensive; there are undoubtedly some very good books not listed. The list does, however, reflect those books which I have bought and read, and found to be useful.

HOLTER MONITORS

These instruments are protable ECG tape recorders that are worn by the patient on the pants belt or in the leather-like carrying case with a strap around the neck. Their purpose is to provide the physician with a 12-hour record of the patient's ECG signal. They use a three-inch open-reel tape that runs at approximately 0.152 in./sec. This requires only approximately 400 to 500 feet of tape to make up to 12 hours of recording.

The tape is recovered from the patient and played back at 7½ ips—almost 50 times faster than it was acquired. A special tape player fitted with a CRT display is used to spot anomalies such as PVCs and other arrhythmias, even though played back at high speed. When one of these anomalies is spotted, the tape is slowed down and played at the regular speed. A strip chart is then made for examination by the physician.

The recorder's slow motor is a sophisticated design using a 40 Hz synchronous hysteresis motor driven by a polyphase, digital logic controlled power supply. The main problems encountered with these instruments are broken patient cables and dirty tape heads (normally an operating technicians job, but occasionally seen in the repair shop). A few cases of abuse are also found because Murphy's Law requires that at least one patient a month drop the recorder!

CARDIAC OUTPUT COMPUTERS

A cardiac output computer might be a digital instrument based on a minicomputer or microprocessor, or it might be a simple analog computer designed to calculate only one function. Regardless of the system, though, most seem to use the *dilution technique*, responding to either temperature or dye-concentration changes in blood flow.

The *cardiac output* (C.O.) is a measure of blood flow volume. This will have a value between three and five liters of blood per minute for a healthy adult who is at rest. The *stroke volume* is the amount of blood ejected by the heart during each beat. The cardiac output is then equal to the stroke volume (in liters/minute) times the heart rate (in beats/minute).

The *mean circulation time* (M.C.T.) is a figure obtained by dividing the body's total blood volume by the cardiac output. Both C.O. and M.C.T. are available on some cardiac output computers.

Dilution Methods

Dilution methods for finding the cardiac output require an injectate to be added to the blood at a calibrated, known rate. The concentration is then measured downstream. The cardiac output (C.O.) is then equal to the injection rate (in milligrams/minute) divided by the concentration (in milligrams/liter). Once again, the C.O. result is in liters/minute.

Dye dilution uses a dye, such as cyanine-green, and measures the concentration using a densitometer or colorimeter. *Thermodilution*, on the other hand, uses cold saline (lower than body temperature but not chilled) as the indicator and a special thermistor transducer as the transduction element.

In the thermal method, the fast response time (0.1 seconds) balloon thermistor catheter is passed via a cut-down, usually in the right arm, through the patient's venous system to the heart. The tip of the catheter is passed through the heart via the right atrium and right ventricle to the pulmonary artery. Besides the thermistor in the tip, there is a balloon further back that causes occlusion and helps hold the position. A lumen located near the entrance to the right atrium is used to expel the chilled injectate. After the saline is injected, the transducer begins to record temperature changes. The graph at the transducer output has the high temperatures close to the origin, producing a curve like Fig. 10-5. This curve is then integrated electronically and plugged into the equation:

$$C.O. = \frac{G_B \, G_S \, K}{H_B \, H_S} \times \frac{V_S \, (T_{BI} - T_{SI})}{\int T_B \, dt}$$

where T_{BI} = initial blood temperature
T_{SI} = initial saline temperature
T_B = real-time blood temperature
G_B = specific gravity of human blood

G_S = specific gravity of the saline solution
H_B = heat content of blood
H_S = heat content of saline solution
V_S = volume of saline injected
K = a constant
dt = time differential

Under normal circumstances, with the usual solutions specified, a new constant (K') can be used to replace the factor $[G_B G_S K/H_B H_S]$. This constant takes the value of 0.054 or 0.065, depending upon usual catheter and solution types. This reduces the above equation to:

$$C.O. = \frac{V_S K' (T_{BI} - T_{SI})}{\int T_B \, dt}$$

Further simplification occurs if you can standardize the amount of injectate used (the V_S term) to, for example, 10 cc. This is done in some models of cardiac output computer. The area under the T_B-vs-t curve is calculated by an electronic integrator while T_{BI} and T_{SI} are either measured automatically or manually entered into the computer from front panel dials.

Analog C.O. Computer

The block diagram of one typical analog cardiac output computer is shown in Fig. 10-6. This is highly simplified so that

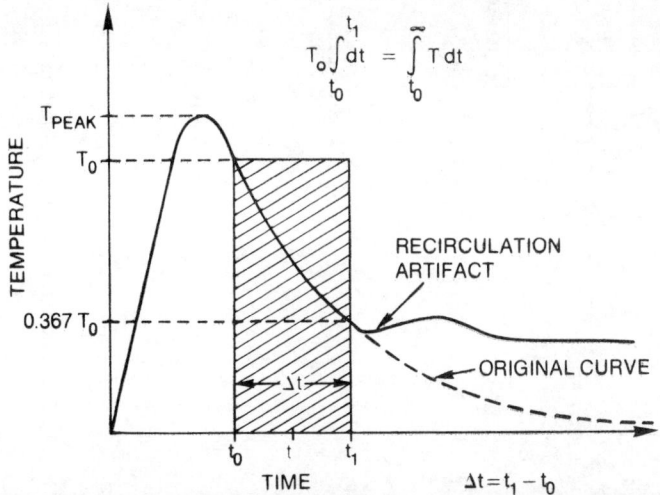

Fig. 10-5. Graph of temperature vs time in cardiac output measurement.

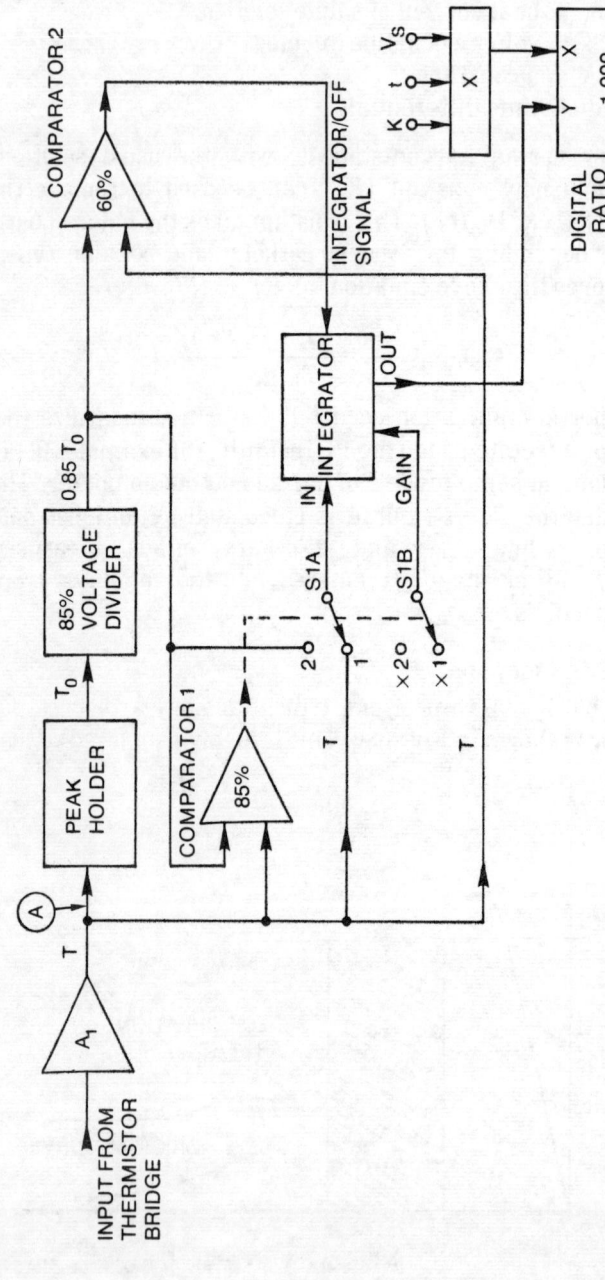

Fig. 10-6. Block diagram of the Columbus Instruments cardiac output computer.

the process can be explained more easily. This particular breed of cardiac output computer makes use of a well-known property of exponentially decaying curves to calculate the cardiac output, even though there might be significant artifacts present to cause errors. Such errors are caused by the recirculation of the injectate.

Refer to the graph in Fig. 10-5. This curve is an exponential decay function from point t_0 on. It approaches $T = 0$ as an asymptote at $t = \infty$. Unfortunately, the recirculation artifact will enter the picture before a proper integration of this last portion of the curve can be completed. But only a good approximation is actually needed, so we can use the rectangle method to find the area under the exponential portion of the curve.

We can assume that this curve becomes truly exponential when it has dropped to approximately 85% of peak value T_{PEAK}. This is designated T_0 on the graph of Fig. 10-5. We allow the T curve to continue falling until the value of T is equal to $0.367\ T_0$. This occurs at time designated T_1. The area of the rectangle formed by side $(T_0 - 0)$ and time $(t_1 - t_0)$ is nearly, to a very good approximation, equal to the area under the exponential portion of the curve from $t = t_0$ to $t = \infty$.

The Columbus Instruments cardiac output computer of Fig. 10-6 uses a modified version of this *geometric integration* scheme. The thermistor in the catheter tip is part of a Wheatstone bridge circuit that is balanced when in normal-temperature blood. This bridge circuit will produce the output waveform of Fig. 10-5 when the saline is injected. The output signal is then amplified by A1 in Fig. 10-6, and signal T appears at point A. This T signal is simultaneously fed to a *peak holder*, an *85% comparator*, a *60% comparator*, and an *electronic integrator* (through input selector switch, S1). At time $t = 0$, switch S1A is in the number 1 position, so the integrator will have a gain of unity (1) and will integrate signal T directly.

The peak holder also follows the T signal, but its output will always store a dc voltage that is equal to the highest previous amplitude on the T curve. Once the curve passes the point $T = T_{PEAK}$ the value of the peak-holder remains constant at the value attained by T at that point. A resistive voltage divider produces an output that is 85% of this value, or in other words, $E = 0.85\ T_{PEAK}$.

This 85% voltage is fed to the input of comparator number 1. The other input to this comparator is the analog output of amplifier A1, the signal T. The input to the integrator is connected to the output of amplifier A1 from $t = 0$ until $t = t_0$. At that point in time, the waveform T has dropped to the 85% trigger point that is supposed to signify the onset of the exponential decay portion of the curve. This causes the comparator to toggle, causing switch S1 to go into position number 2.

At this point, the integrator has performed the mathematical operation:

$$\int_{t=0}^{t=t_0} T \, dt$$

From now on, though, the integrator will integrate the constant $0.85 \, T_{\text{PEAK}}$. This potential is fed to both the integrator and to the 60% comparator. The integrator gain has also been increased to by a factor of two, to $\times 2$. This means the actual integration is:

$$2\int 0.85 \, T_{\text{PEAK}} \, dt = 2T_0 \int dt$$

Integration will now continue until T falls to 60% of T_0 (which is also 49.9% of T_{PEAK}). This occurs at a point approximately half way between T_0 and $0.36 \, T_0$ making the time interval equal to $\frac{1}{2}(t_1 - t_0)$. This is the reason why it was necessary to double the integrator gain.

At $t = t'$, the 60% comparator number toggles and shuts off the integrator input but holds its value at the integrator output. This voltage is the value plugged into the denominator of the cardiac output equation, which now becomes:

$$\text{C.O.} = \frac{K V_S (T_{\text{BI}} - T_{\text{SI}})}{\int_{t=0}^{t_0} T \, dt + 2 T_0 \int_{t_0}^{t'} dt}$$

The readout meter is special. This readout is actually part of the computation circuitry rather than being simply a readout device. Known as a *ratio digital voltmeter*, it is designed to read out a voltage equal to the *ratio* of two input voltages, X and Y. Its display, then, indicates $E_{\text{RO}} = X/Y$. The output of the integrator (the denominator of the equation) is fed to the Y input. Another voltage representing the numerator is fed to the X input, and the ratio computation is made.

This C.O. circuit is an analog computer using operational amplifiers to sum voltages from front panel controls. More recent computers use thermistors to find the initial blood temperature before injection is made, using the same thermistor as for T. A standard tactic used to simplify the design is to fix the temperature of the saline injectate at 25°C (room temperature). Many models will also specify either 5 or 10 cc for the volume of injectate, V_s.

A new type of cardiac output computer is made by AVCO and is to be used in conjunction with their intra-aortic balloon pump. Although it is too new at this writing for details to be presented here, I can offer a few conjectures based on having seen one under test in the manufacturer's service facility. The speculation is that its microprocessor (see!) is the Intel *8008*, and that the microprocessor is used to compute the cardiac output directly from an AVCO algorithm that makes use of the pressure, beats per minute, and balloon volume signals available on the service connector normally located on the rear panel of the balloon pump console.

Chapter 11
Cardiac Radio Telemetry

Many hospitals use radio telemetry links to monitor certain patients. This allows them to keep track of their ECG signals while simultaneously allowing the patients to be ambulatory. The patient wears a cigarett-pack size, VHF or UHF FM radio transmitter. The nurse's station, or a separate central monitoring console, is equipped with a set of single-channel receivers that match the number of transmitters in the system on a one-to-one basis. These stations are also equipped with oscilloscopes, alarms, strip chart recorders, and the other electronic equipment that is normally part of the ICU/CCU type of monitoring system.

Figure 11-1 shows a radio telemetry monitoring system with two channels. The patient wears the transmitter (Fig. 11-2) on his belt. This allows him to walk about the hospital, but only in a zone prescribed from considerations of signal coverage and the quick availability of medical assistance should an emergency develop.

Equipment at the central station includes receivers for two or more channels. (More channels are possible and more than two are usual.) Each channel has a companion heart-rate meter module. Each channel also has an oscilloscope, although in many cases a common multichannel instrument serves all patients. Also common to all patients in the system is a strip chart recorder. Patient selection and

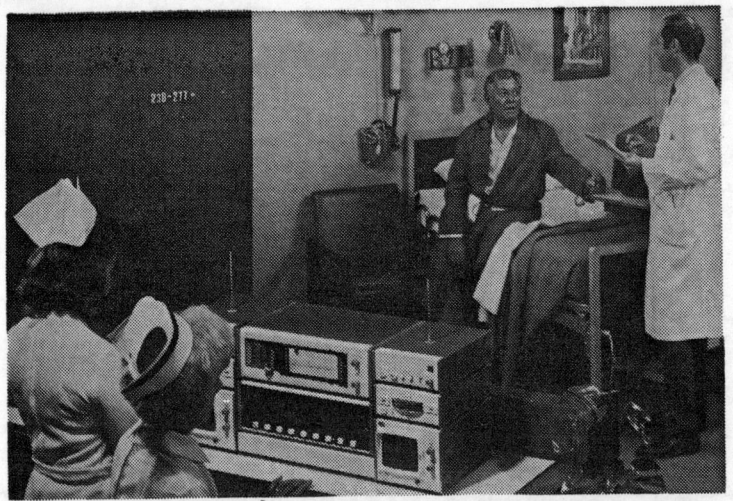

Fig. 11-1. Radio telemetry system is used to monitor a heart patient's ECG waveform at the nurses station while allowing the patient to be ambulatory. (Courtesy Hewlett-Packard)

various alarms can be provided through a suitable module designed for that purpose.

Bedside monitoring—not always provided in telemetry systems—can be provided by a slave or remote oscilloscope at bedside. In this system, the signals are picked up by the telemetry receivers and routed back to the patient's room via hard wires. (The techniques of hardwire distribution are discussed in the chapter on central monitoring systems, so they will not be repeated here.) Such a telemetry system allows the patient to easily exercise by walking about the corridors but without sacrificing the necessary ability of monitoring his electrocardiogram.

Examples of typical cardiac radio telemetry equipment are shown in Fig. 11-3 (transmitter) and 11-4 (receiver). Three wires from the transmitter serve both to acquire the ECG signal from surface electrodes on the patient's skin and as the radio antenna for the transmitter output circuitry.

Telemetry receivers, like much medical equipment of other types, tend to have a bare minimum of external controls. In Fig. 11-4, for example, the size of the displayed signal (amplitude of the oscilloscope or chart recorder) and has access to a 1.0 millivolt calibration signal. Two warning lights are also provided one indicating bad electrodes on the patient's body, the other for weak signal input to the receiver.

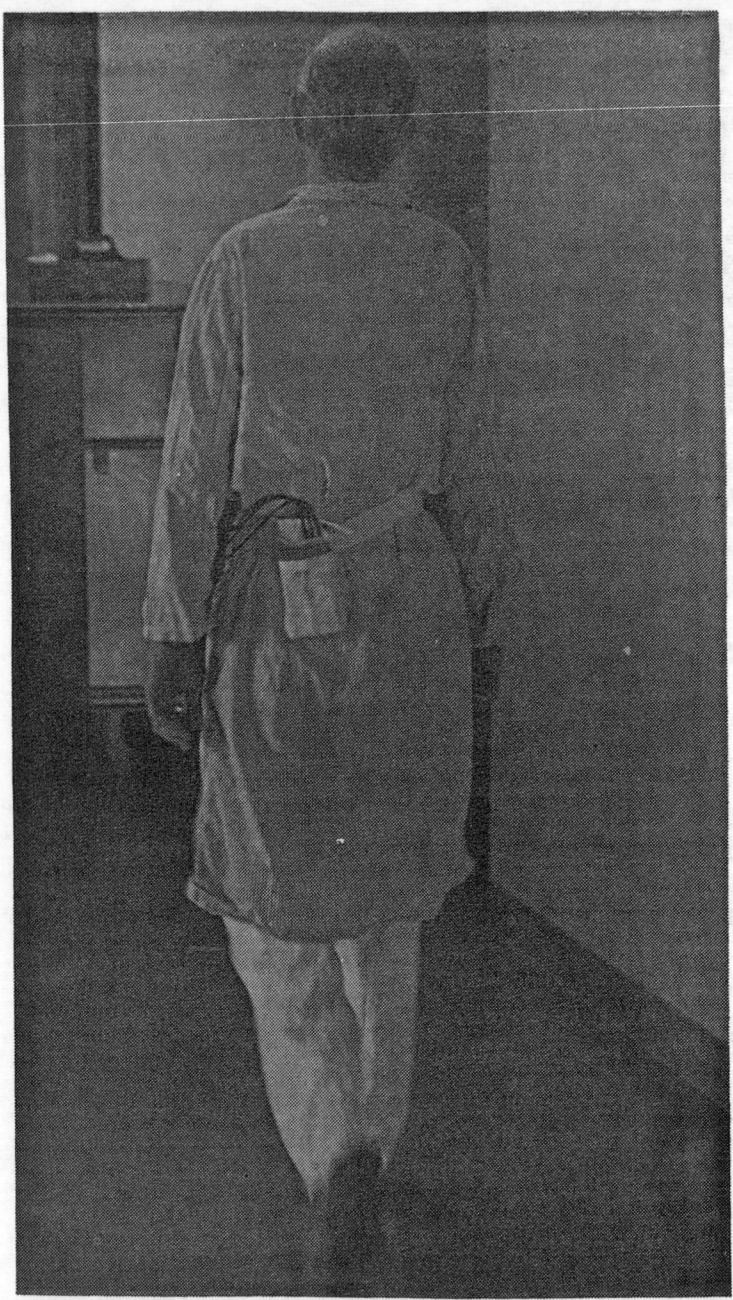

Fig. 11-2. The patient is allowed to walk around a certain specified area of the hospital that is well within the range of the telemetry system and emergency help should it be needed. (Courtesy Hewlett-Packard)

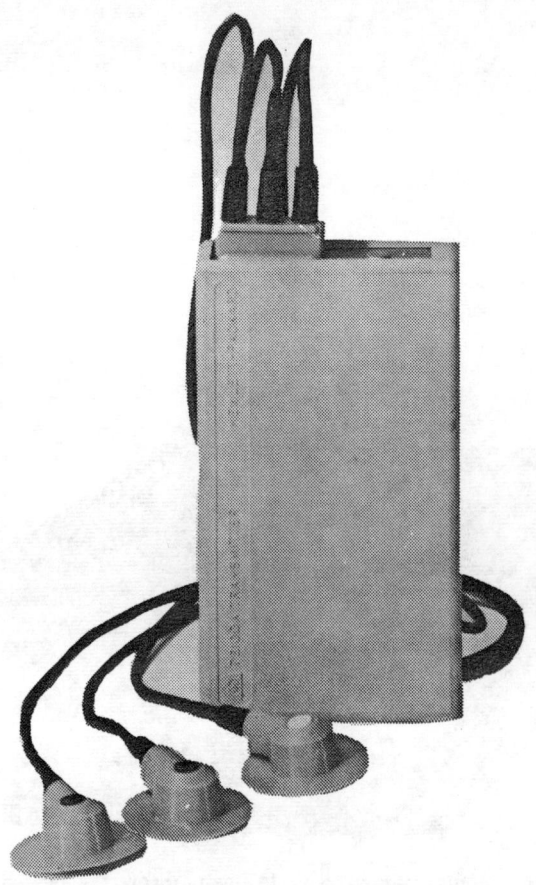

Fig. 11-3. This typical belt transmitter for cardiac telemetry uses the ECG pickup leads as the radio antenna. (Courtesy Hewlett-Packard)

The weak-signal lamp could be turned on by any factor that reduces signal amplitude, including a weak battery in the transmitter or a patient wandering into a zone where the signal pickup is poor. Since there might be several of these insufficient coverage zones, care must be exercised in selecting the area where the patient is allowed to wander. Hopefully, there will not be any areas close to the central monitoring console where the signal level drops too low for proper coverage. Even the high sensitivity of these receivers cannot totally make up for the extremely low power of the transmitters, so coverage is limited.

Two major design philosophies are found in single-channel, medical telemetry links. These can be designated

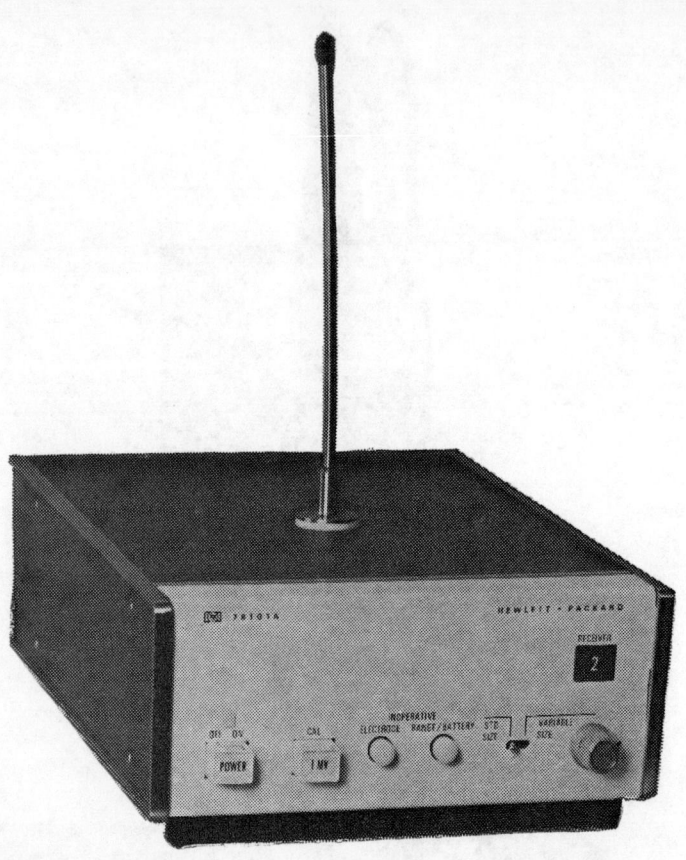

Fig. 11-4. This single-channel, radio telemetry receiver is located at the nurse's station and is connected to the regular monitoring equipment. (Courtesy Hewlett-Packard)

direct-FM (or simply *FM*) and *FM/FM*. Figure 11-5 is the block diagram of a direct-FM system. The patient's ECG signal is acquired by two or three chest electrodes. This signal is amplified by a preamplifier stage to about 0.5 to 3.0 volts (peak). This amplified signal is then applied to the transmitter's frequency modulator, then through the frequency multipliers, and finally power amplifier stages.

In communications equipment, we normally have a final amplifier that is not a frequency-multiplier stage, but in radio telemetry for medical purposes, the small power and size requirements permit many designers to combine functions. They may well "double in the final" as well as boost the power level to the specified output.

In FM/FM systems the same sort of thing occurs, except that the ECG signal is used to frequency-modulate an audio-range, voltage-controlled oscillator (VCO). This, in turn, is used to frequency-modulate the transmitter's main frequency control oscillator. The double modulation scheme wins the designation *FM/FM*. Obviously, the FM/FM receiver must also include a decoder for the audio FM, so the ECG wave-form can be recovered.

FM TERMS AND TECHNIQUES

Frequency modulation implies that the frequency of a radio carrier is changed or varied in a manner proportional to the amplitude of some lower frequency modulating signal. Let us assume that a positive-going amplitude on the modulating signal causes the carrier frequency to increase, and a negative-going modulating signal causes the carrier frequency to shift downwards. Also, let us further assume a notational system where F_0 is the unmodulated carrier frequency F_H is the minimum frequency of **the** carrier under modulation conditions.

On positive-going excursions of the modulating waveform, the carrier of the transmitter will shift frequency an amount ΔF (read *delta F*) to the frequency $F_0 + \Delta F = F_H$. The size of ΔF is proportional to the *amplitude* of the modulating signal, *not* its frequency. The speed with which the carrier shift is made is proportional to the frequency of the modulating

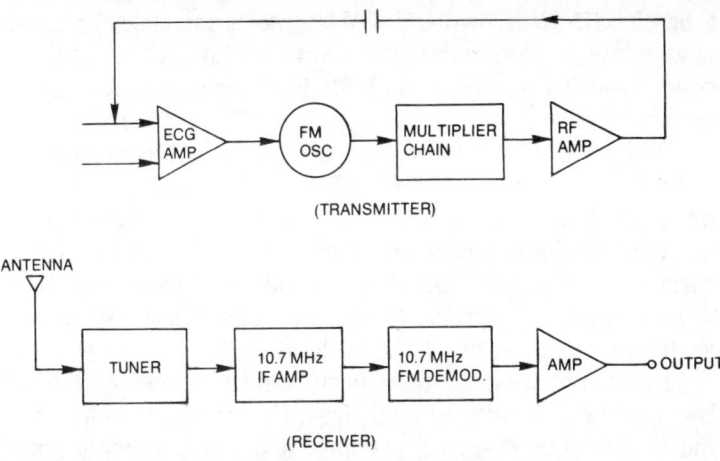

Fig. 11-5. Direct-FM telemetry system.

signal, but the maximum frequency shift of the radio carrier is proportional *only* to the amplitude of the modulating signal. Similarly, on negative swings of the modulating signal, the carrier shifts to a frequency $F_O - \Delta F' = F_L$. For a sine-wave modulating signal that is baseline symmetric (no dc component), we can state that

$$|\Delta F| = |\Delta F'|$$

The quantity ΔF is called the *deviation*, but it is often the case that the FM terms *deviation* and *frequency swing* are confused. Deviation (ΔF) is the amount of frequency shift during modulation from F_O to *either* F_H or F_L extremes. That is,

$$\Delta F = F_H - F_O$$
$$\Delta F' = F_O - F_L$$

If F and F' are not equal, then they are called *positive* and *negative* deviation, respectively.

Frequency swing, on the other hand, is the *total* shift from lower to upper extremes, or $F_H - F_L$. If the modulating signal is symmetrical about the baseline, then the frequency swing is equal to $2\Delta F$.

Frequency-modulated radio systems can generally be divided into *narrow* and *wideband* catagories. A narrow-band system is one where the deviation is small for a given amplitude-modulating signal. Most authorities agree that narrow-band systems have frequency deviation on the order of 5 or 10 kHz. Narrow-band FM is the usual case for most landmobile communications (commercial utility, safety, police, and fire) and for the VHF FM marine radiotelephone service.

Wideband FM systems have deviation specifications in the 10 to 80 kHz range. FM broadcasters, TV broadcasters, and most cardiac radio telemetry systems use this form of modulation. For example, the television-sound signal is an FM carrier with about 25 kHz deviation, while the FM broadcasters and cardiac telemetry transmitters use 75 kHz as the specification for "100% modulation."

Frequency modulation is preferred in telemetry systems because it can be almost noise free. Contrary to the claims of much hi-fi equipment advertising, it is not *absolutely* noise free. But FM gives superior performance under some rather trying conditions that would usually wipe out most amplitude-modulated systems. FM is also fairly easy to implement using solid-state technology; a statement that could not be made two decades ago. Modern solid-state devices can operate well into the UHF region, and special diodes can be used for actually modulating the carrier.

Noise, at least the impluse variety often called *static*, tends to amplitude-modulate radio signals. FM signals, though, use frequency variations to carry the modulation information. In some FM receivers, a limiter stage clips the amplitude of all signal levels greater than some minimum amplitude. This clipping is responsible for eliminating the amplitude spikes of any noise that is modulating the carrier. In other types of FM receivers, the detector/demodulator circuit is designed to have little sensitivity to amplitude variations, so it will not reproduce or pass amplitude variations in the input signal. In either event, if the radio signal is strong enough to reduce or *quiet* the receiver's background hiss, then the noise rejection of the system will be quite high. But signals too weak will still be subject to noise, and this can cause artifacts in the demodulated output signal.

TYPICAL ECG TELEMETRY TRANSMITTERS

For the time being, we shall limit our discussion of FM telemetry transmitters to those of the direct-FM variety. A typical block diagram is shown in Fig. 11-5. The ECG amplifier usually consists of a differential gain stage and sometimes a 60 Hz notch filter to eliminate interference from ac powerlines. Because of the compactness requirement, most ECG telemetry transmitters use one or two operational amplifiers to provide the needed high gain for this function.

In most cases the designers have been constrained to use a single, small battery for operation of the transmitter. Batteries between 5.6V and 12V are very much in evidence, while the standard 9V transistor radio battery is very common.

This power-supply constraint also makes the use of micropower operational amplifiers very attractive. Many designers choose such devices because of their low current drain in quiescence and their ability to operate from relatively low battery voltages. Several semiconductor manufacturers offer dual and even triple operational amplifiers in a single

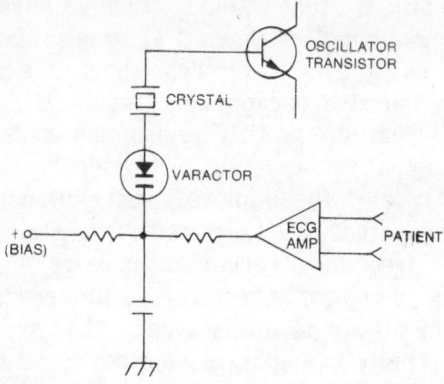

Fig. 11-6. A popular type of FM modulator uses a variable capacitance diode (varactor) to pull the frequency of an oscillating crystal an amount proportional to the amplitude of the modulating input voltage from the ECG preamplifier.

TO-5 type can, a 14-pin DIP, or a 14-pin flatpack, integrated circuit package.

The signal developed in the amplifier stage is fed to a crystal oscillator (Fig. 11-6) that is usually operated in the 10 to 50 MHz range, depending upon design choices. Contrary to popular belief, crystal frequencies are not absolute and can be changed quite a bit from that marked on the can or holder. One of the factors affecting the resonant frequency of a piezoelectric crystal is the capacitance it sees looking into the oscillator circuit. In the FM oscillator/modulator of Fig. 11-6, a special variable capacitance diode (called a *varactor*) is connected in series with the crystal. This type of semiconductor diode has the characteristic that its junction capacitance will vary in a predictable manner with changes in reverse bias potential. All diodes will exhibit this phenomenon to some degree, but the varactor is designed to enhance this feature and make it controllable. The ECG signal developed in amplifier A1 causes frequency deviations in the oscillator by varying the capacitance of varactor D1.

The stages following the oscillator are frequency multipliers as well as amplifiers. Such stages have an output frequency that is some integer multiple of the input frequency. This can actually be accomplished in any nonlinear circuit such as semiconductor diode, class-B amplifier, or class-C amplifier (class-A amplifiers cannot be used because they are linear). It is merely necessary to tune the output of such a circuit to an integer multiple of the input frequency. The output tank circuit is used to select one of the harmonics generated by the nonlinearity of the stage. Frequency deviation is also multiplied by there stages.

Let us assume that a transmitter for ECG telemetry is to operate on a frequency of 215.76 MHz with a symmetrical deviation of ± 75 kHz. The stage following the oscillator is a frequency doubler, and that feeds a tripler, which feeds another doubler. This makes a multiplication factor of $2 \times 3 \times 2 = 12$ times the oscillator frequency and the oscillator deviation.

A crystal for the oscillator that is suitable for this example would have a frequency $1/12$ of 215.76 MHz, or 17.98 MHz. The output of the first doubler would have a frequency of twice the crystal frequency, or 35.96 MHz. The tripler circuit takes this signal, feeds it through an additional nonlinear stage (the flywheel effect of the doubler tank tends to "re-linearize" the output signal) and picks off the third harmonic of the doubler stage, or 107.88 MHz. Similarly, the last doubler picks off the second harmonic of the tripler output, or 215.76 MHz.

Since we also multiply the oscillator deviation by the same factor, we must set the deviation control to produce at deviation at the oscillator that is also $1/12$ of 75 kHz, or 6.25 kHz. Of course, in the practical service of such instruments, we would simply adjust the *output* deviation even though we are actually adjusting a control located in the FM oscillator, three stages back.

Another modulator design is used in only a few ECG telemetry transmitters. But this circuit finds a lot of

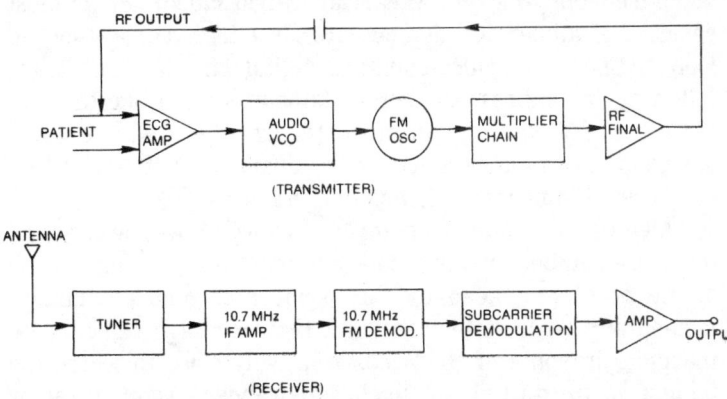

Fig. 11-7. FM/FM telemetry system.

205

application in other forms of radio communications transmitters. This is the *reactance* modulator, which receives a fixed frequency signal from the crystal oscillator and varies its *phase* in a manner proportional to the modulating signal. This version of angular modulation is often called *phase* modulation or simply *PM*. Actaully, we find phase-modulated transmitters in wide use (even though most are labelled "FM") in all fields of radio communication other than medical telemetry systems.

FREQUENCY MODULATION RECEIVERS

The demodulation of simple amplitude-modulated signals is relatively easy. All that is required is a simple envelope detector such as a diode rectifier. Frequency modulation and phase modulation, on the other hand, require a detector that is phase and frequency sensitive. Such circuits are the Foster-Seeley descriminator, ratio detector, quadrature detector (now available in integrated-circuit form), phase-locked loop, and even a digital or "pulse counting" version using a monostable multivibrator and an integrator.

In direct-FM systems, we need only a superhetrodyne receiver with an FM demodulator, such as one of the types discussed earlier, plus some sort of dc or low-frequency ac amplifier following the demodulator to build up the signal to a level that can be accommodated by a strip chart recorder or oscilloscope.

In FM/FM systems, on the other hand, the next stage following the demodulator is another demodulator for the audio-frequency-range FM carrier, called *subcarrier*. In most cases, the subcarrier demodulator is either a phase-locked loop (PLL) or a pulse-counting digital circuit. The stages following the subcarrier demodulator are much like those of the direct-FM variety. In most, though, there will be some low-pass filtering to remove the residual audio subcarrier that survives the subcarrier demodulation process.

Medical telemetry transmitters are very low powered and therefore can be expected to have a low coverage range. Some of the problems faced by the servicer of such equipment, incidentally, will reflect the fact that coverage tends to be marginal in some of the areas relatively close to where the patient is permitted, or likely, to wander. Another factor affecting FM ECG telemetry is the fact that many of the frequencies assigned for this use are shared with other services, so the telemetry systems must be able to tolerate interference from those transmitters. Fortunately, good receiver selectivity, low "audio" section bandwidths, and the well-known FM *capture effect* tend to reduce the severity of such problems.

Many of the FM telemetry channels coincide with VHF and UHF television broadcasting channels. In fact, many are in the actual guard bands that are part of each channel. Although this arrangement can produce obvious problems, it is a blessing in disguise in some cases because it allows us to use, where applicable, low-cost master antenna TV (MATV) system components such as preamplifiers and couplers. For example, you can use multi-set couplers to mix together, in one transmission line, signals from several remote antennas located both centrally and in various radio troublespots located at points in your unit. In a similar manner, multi-set distribution systems located at the central telemetry console can break out and distribute those signals to their respective receivers. This greatly simplifies and design of local systems since you can use off-the-shelf components, which eliminates the need for a high-level design capability. Such systems must be carefully balanced, however, or one source will dominate, creating a poor dynamic situation. Also, there is a limit to useful gain in the antenna system and amplifiers because of rf noise.

One interesting aspect to some ECG telemetry receivers is that their center of passband frequency is *not* the same as the transmitter frequency, as might be expected. The signal-loss lamp on the receiver's front panel is the reason. Most FM demodulators produce a zero output voltage at the center frequency. (This is especially true of the quadrature detector, integrated circuits popular in FM telemetry receivers.) The typical signal-loss light is triggered on by a comparator, such as the LM311 used in the American Optical equipment. To compensate for this effect, a 48 kHz offset in receiver frequency is provided. A carrier present in the passband will thus produce a dc offset voltage in the output, even if the signal is unmodulated.

SERVICING FM TELEMETRY

For simple, quick troubleshooting of medical radio telemetry transmitters, much can be said for the continuously variable type of television antenna, field strength meter (FSM). This is another example of the compatability of TV and telemetry components and equipment. The field strength meters are available at low clost, and they tune to the standard VHF and UHF television channels. Most FSM instruments have both a loudspeaker and meter for output indications. The meter is an S-meter or AGC voltmeter, and this is used to establish the strength of the TV stations being received. Such information is necessary for proper master antenna system design. Bioelectronics people can press these instruments into service because of the correspondence of frequencies—but only if the field strength meter is of the continously variable design; those with "click-stop" tuners in the front end are less useful for this application.

One of the tricks required when servicing any radio transmitter/receiver system is to determine whether the problem is due to the transmitter not sending or to the receiver not picking up and demodulating the signal. This is not as simple as it might sound where no test equipment is available. With the field strength meter, however, you can tell rapidly whether the transmitter is putting out rf power. That little bit of information will tell you whether to concentrate your efforts on the transmitter or the receiver.

More qualitative analysis—certainly desirable if you can afford the cost of test equipment—is made using a VHF/UHF frequency counter, low range rf power meter, FM deviation meter, and a spectrum analyzer. All of these are common items of test equipment used in professional communications shops. But it is not necessary to await the funding needed to acquire such prestigeous equipment before attempting telemetry repairs. You will find that most repairs involve the same sort of parts as in any other electronics: batteries, battery connectors, switches, pushbuttons, and input/output connectors of assorted types. These bad parts can be found using little more than a cheap voltohmeter (VOM) and a practiced, discerning eye.

Receiver servicing requires some sort of VHF or UHF (as the case may be) signal source. Of course, a laboratory-grade signal generator or synthesizer is desirable because it can synthesize all output frequencies from a single, internal, highly accurate and stable, crystal reference oscillator that can be frequency modulated to over 100 kHz deviation and amplitude modulated to over 120%. But unless you do an awfully lot of ECG telemetry work, this is not too practical. You can easily press a transmitter into service as an impromptu signal generator if the need arises. And again, the job reduces to the use of a VOM, oscilloscope, and a lot of communications and electronics horse sense. Your most important asset in servicing this equipment is a knowledge of how solid-state FM transmitters and receivers work.

Chapter 12
Scientific Instruments in Clinical Use

There are a number of scientific instruments used in the typical medical center that would seemingly be just as much at home in the research laboratory, chemistry laboratory, or other types of scientific facility. Some of these instruments are used in the same form as in the other areas, but others are adaptations of the more basic items used and found elsewhere.

PH METERS

The term *pH* is measurement describing the relative acid-base balance of a liquid. This figure is related to the concentration of the hydrogen plus (H^+) ion in the solution being tested. More specifically,

$$pH = -\log_{10}(H^+)$$

A neutral solution is one that is neither acid nor base, it has a pH of exactly 7.00. Acidic solutions have lower pH numbers while basic or alkaline solutions have higher pH numbers. The normal scale on modern pH meters covers the range from 1 to 14.

An electronic pH meter is little more than a millivoltmeter connected to a specialized electrode that can be immersed in the solution being examined. The electronics portion of the typical pH meter is millivoltmeter calibrated with a special readout scale. In fact, most meters have, in addition to the pH scale, a millivolts scale. The millivoltmeter function is selected by a front panel switch. A number of electronic millivoltmeter circuits are commonly used, but only one will be considered here as an example.

There are several electrode configurations in existence, but that shown in Fig. 12-1 is probably the most common in medical pH equipment. This system uses a *glass* electrode whose output voltage is measured relative to that of a *calomel* (mercurous chloride) reference electrode. Electrodes used to measure pH depend upon the development of electrical potentials across a barrier separating two materials of the same phase, or across the interface between materials of different phase (e.g., a metal-to-electrolyte interface). In the calomel reference electrode, this potential is generated by an interface of pure mercury (Hg) and a solution of potassium chloride (KCl) saturated with calomel.

One of the problems with some reference electrode designs is that a second potential might develop at the interface between the solution being tested and the KCl in the electrode. This problem is eliminated, or at least reduced, by the use of a salt bridge in the pipe from the calomel reference electrode. The calomel reference electrode is preferred because it possesses a reasonable long-term stability. That is to say, its half-cell potential does not deteriorate markedly over long periods of time.

The second electrode used in the pH configuration is the glass electrode, also shown in Fig. 12-1. This electrode produces a potential across a thin membrane, in this case a special glass. The glass bulb shown in Fig. 12-1 is the membrane, and it is immersed in the solution being tested. The solution on the inside of the glass membrane is usually a chloride with pH = 1. A silver-silver chloride (Ag-AgCl) electrode connected to the output wire is immersed in the solution inside the glass bulb. The electrical potential developed across the glass membrane is approximately 60 millivolts per pH unit at 30°C, but it will vary from approximately 50 mV to around 70 mV per pH unit over the range of 0°C to 100°C. One manufacturer presents a graph of the pH meter's output (Fig. 12-1B) showing it to have a negative slope. The glass electrode is preferred over some of its competitors because it will work consistently, with little fuss and care, under a variety of really trying conditions.

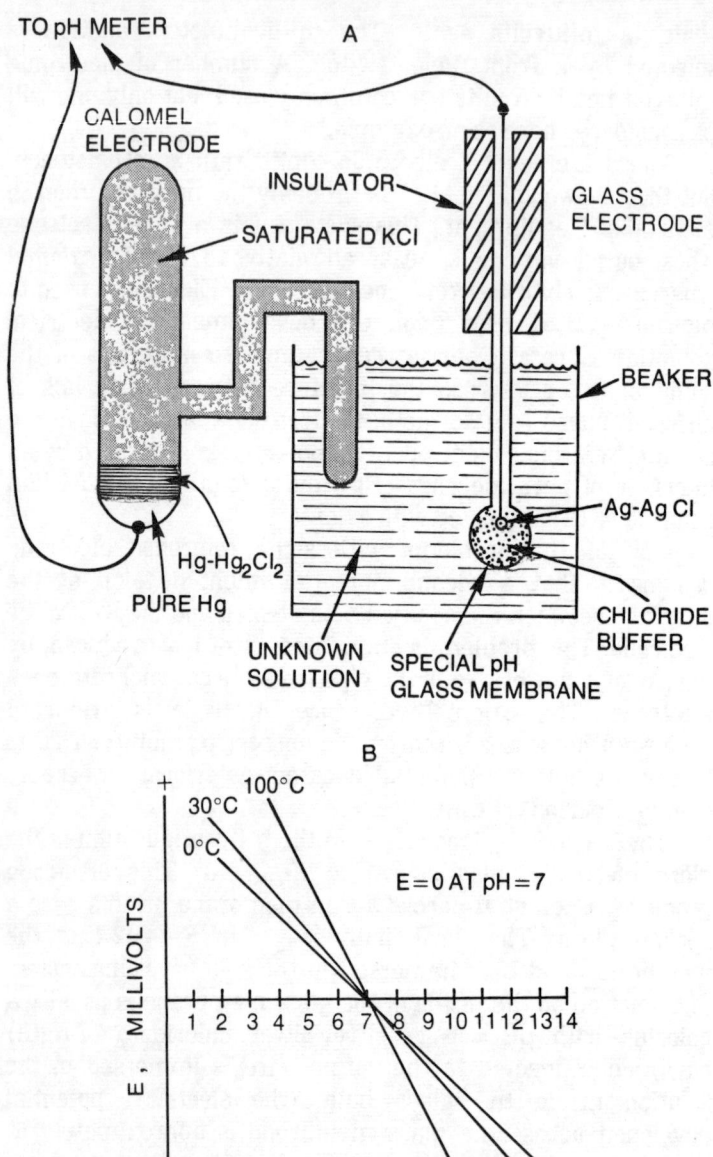

Fig. 12-1. (A) construction of calomel and glass electrodes used in the electronic measurement of pH. (B) output curve of the pH electrode set. Temperature affects the slope, but it is a nominal 57 mV/pH in most common probes.

Medical pH meters come in several configurations that can be classified most easily by electrode construction. *In vitro* instruments for measuring fluids are similar to that of Fig. 12-1. In caridac cath and gastroenterology applications, however, this design is unsuitable, so another mechanical design is required for *in vivo* studies inside the patient's body.

In the blood gas laboratory, they use a combination housing with both reference and glass electrodes (and possibly another type of electrode to be discussed shortly) in one common housing made of glass. This is water filled and uses a pump to pull blood from the syringe in which it was taken from the patient and deliver it to the measuring site. Circulating water cleans and flushes the system after use.

The cell potential across the glass electrode's membrane is produced through the migration of a tiny number of ions across the barrier. Therefore, the glass electrodes have a very high impedance, normally between 200 and 300 mehgohms. In order to prevent loading of the electrode by the amplifier input, it becomes necessary for pH meter input amplifiers to have an extremely high input impedance. This figure should not be less than about 1000 megohms (10^9 ohms), and many are able to boast input impedances up to 10^{12} ohms.

A TYPICAL PH METER

Figure 12-2 shows a partial schematic of a typical pH meter. I have selected an operational amplifier model because this choice makes the description simpler. The input stage, amplifier A1, must be a low-drift high-input-impedance design. This almost requires the use of a special FET operational amplifier for A1, but a few designs use 741-type op-amps preceded by a discrete JFET or MOSFET stage. Many pH meter input amplifiers are "chopper" desgins that preserve the low baseline drift requirement.

At pH values close to seven, only a very small voltage appears across the input terminals. This is especially true of medical pH meters where the normal range for human blood pH is close to seven all of the time. These instruments will rarely see an input voltage over 50 or 60 millivolts. Under these conditions, it is quite possible for the drift of the input amplifier to contribute significantly to overall error.

A chopper input circuit helps to eliminate some of these drift problems. In a few modern designs, amplifier A1 will be

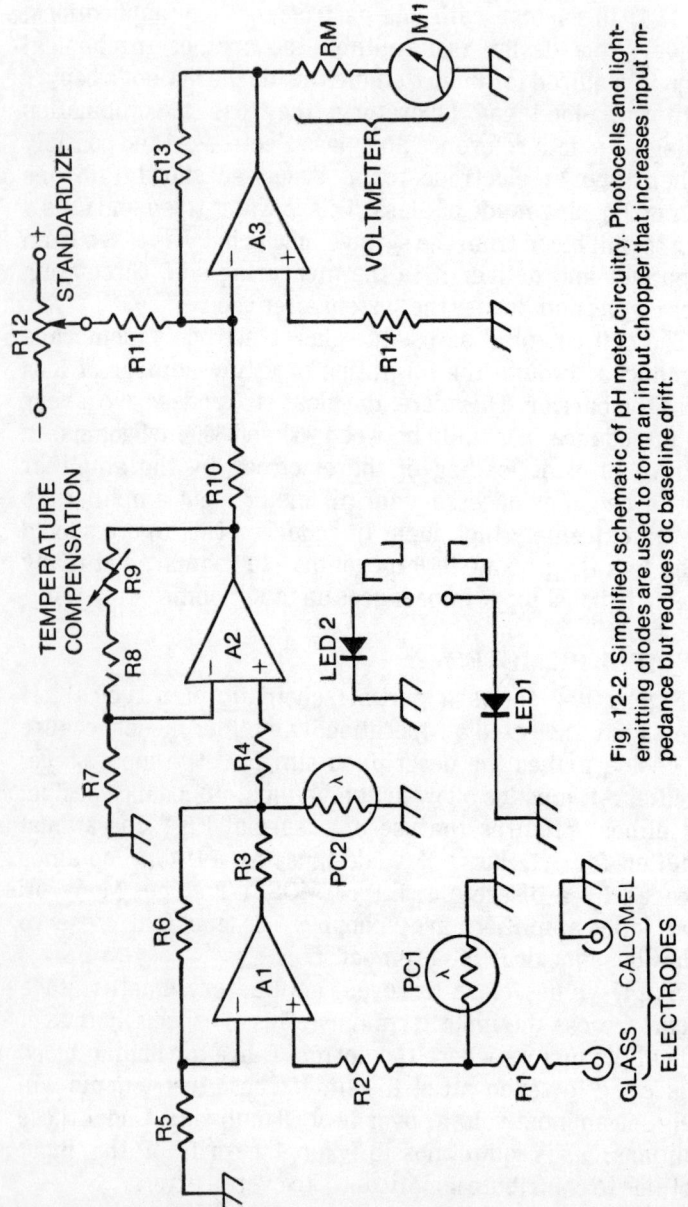

Fig. 12-2. Simplified schematic of pH meter circuitry. Photocells and light-emitting diodes are used to form an input chopper that increases input impedance but reduces dc baseline drift.

an integrated circuit or "module" type with JFET or varactor choppers built in. In others—and that includes most in actual use—amplifier A1 will be one of the conventional chopper designs.

In this example version, a pair of light-emitting diodes (LEDs) are driven in push-pull such that one will be dark while the other is lighted. Each LED is coupled to a photocell (photoresistor) that has an extremely high resistance when dark and an extremely low resistance when illuminated. Resistors R1/R2 and R3/R4 have a very high resistance relative to the illuminated resistances of PC1 and PC2. When PC1 is lighted, the junction of R1/R2 sees a very low resistance to ground, and this effectively shunts the signal to ground by the familiar voltage-divider action. Similarly, when PC2 is lighted, the junction of R3/R4 is effectively shunted to ground.

Amplifier A1 could be a chopped type, and it probably would be. Its ac coupling would thus take advantage of the low drift inherent to such circuits because of their feedback action.

Amplifier A2 provides additional amplification and temperature compensation. The output slope of the pH electrode curve (see Fig. 12-1B) varies with temperature over a voltage range of approximately 20 millivolts with changes in temperature of 0°C to 100°C. Potentiometer R9 sets the gain of amplifier A2, and hence the system gain, to compensate for differences in pH sensitivity.

The final amplifier in the cascade, A3, is also used to provide dc offset to calibrate the system. There are several ways of doing this calibration. One is to short the input terminals together and adjust potentiometer R12 until output voltmeter M1 reads a pH of exactly seven.

Another, and more accurate, calibration technique is to use a standard buffer solution of known pH to adjust the instrument. The operator dips the electrodes in the solution and then adjusts potentiometer R12 until meter M1 reads the same pH as the calibrated buffer solution. This is a more accurate technique, but only if the user follows good laboratory practices to avoid contaminating the buffer solution.

In most older instruments the readout device is an analog panel meter. Such panel meters are quite often very large in size to increase resolution. Newer instruments, however, use digital readouts.

BLOOD GAS ANALYZERS

Medical pH meters are usually part of a somewhat more sophisticated instrument package known as a *blood gases machine*. These instruments measure the pH and the partial pressures of carbon dioxide (pCO_2) the oxygen (pO_2). The standard pCO_2 electrode is actually a modified pH electrode. This is usually called a *Severinghaus* electrode after one of the principle inventors. This electrode has a thin membrane over the glass bulb of the pH electrode, and this new membrane is semi-permeable to carbon dioxide. The internal solution is also modified to add a little sodium chloride. The normal technique is to measure the pH of the blood and compare it, on a nomograph, with the pH values of standardized calibration solutions with partial pressures of 60 and 30 torr (mmHg). This is sometimes referred to as the *Astrup* method.

Oxygen concentration is measured using a thin platinum wire, called the oxygen electrode, and a silver-silver chloride (Ag-AgCl) reference electrode. A tiny current is made to flow between these two points; the magnitude of this current is proportional to the oxygen concentration of the solution in which both are immersed. Most pO_2 meters use a small battery to energize the electrode. You will find that a large number of instruments use a popular, small mercury battery, the RM-1 or HG-1, depending upon the manufacturer.

The Clark pO_2 electrode is an improved version and is the type most often encountered in medical gas measuring equipment. In Fig. 12-3 the Clark pO_2 electrode, the Ag-AgCl reference electrode, and the platinum cathodic surface are both mounted inside of a glass housing and are bathed in a saturated potassium chloride (KCl) solution. Across the opening is a polythene membrane that is semi-permeable to oxygen molecules. The current, set up by battery RM-1 and potentiometer R1, flows between the two electrodes. This instrument is used to drive a current amplifier.

Most of the blood gas analyzing instruments used in the hospital will use a combination electrode. The blood gas analyzer manufactured by Radiometer (Copenhagen, Denmark), for example, features such an electrode. By judiciously mounting the two types of electrode so that they do not mutually degrade each other's performance, it is possible to make a Clark-Severinghaus electrode assembly. This is the type most often seen on clinical blood gases machines.

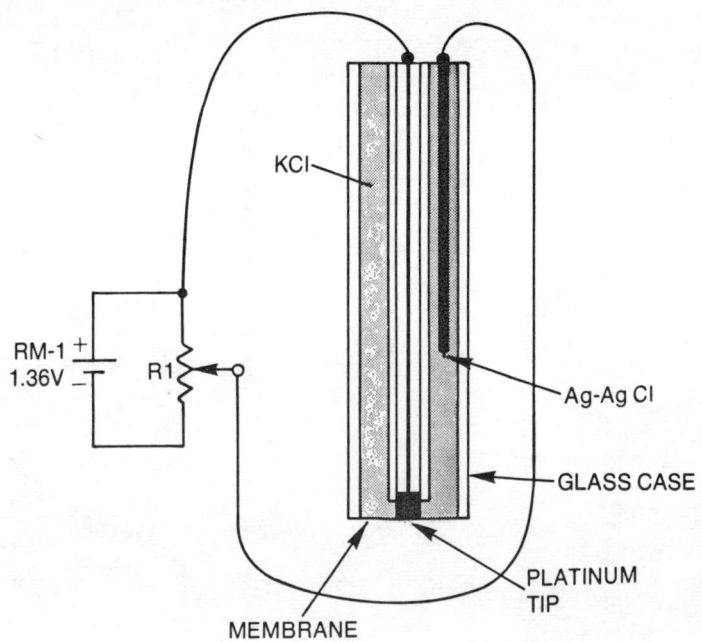

Fig. 12-3. Typical construction of a Clark gas electrode.

RADIATION DETECTORS

The gas-filled tube is probably the most popular type of radiation detector. Such tubes can be operated in any of three modes: ionization chamber, proportional counter, and Geiger counter. The main difference between these three is the voltage level applied to the gas-filled tube. A schematic of a typical gas-filled tube is shown in Fig. 12-4 with its operating curve.

Regardless of the mode, the operation of this tube is dependent upon an internal electric field set up through the application of a high potential difference across the two electrodes. Radiation particles, which enter mostly through the thin window on the end of the tube, ionize some of the gas molecules. The electric field can then operate on these particles and pull some of them toward the inner electrode, where they form a current that flows out through the external resistance. This current has an impulse character and so produces a spike-like pulse across the resistor. This pulse is the signal fed to the counter.

The gas-filled radiation detector is most popularly associated with the hand-held Geiger counter. In some

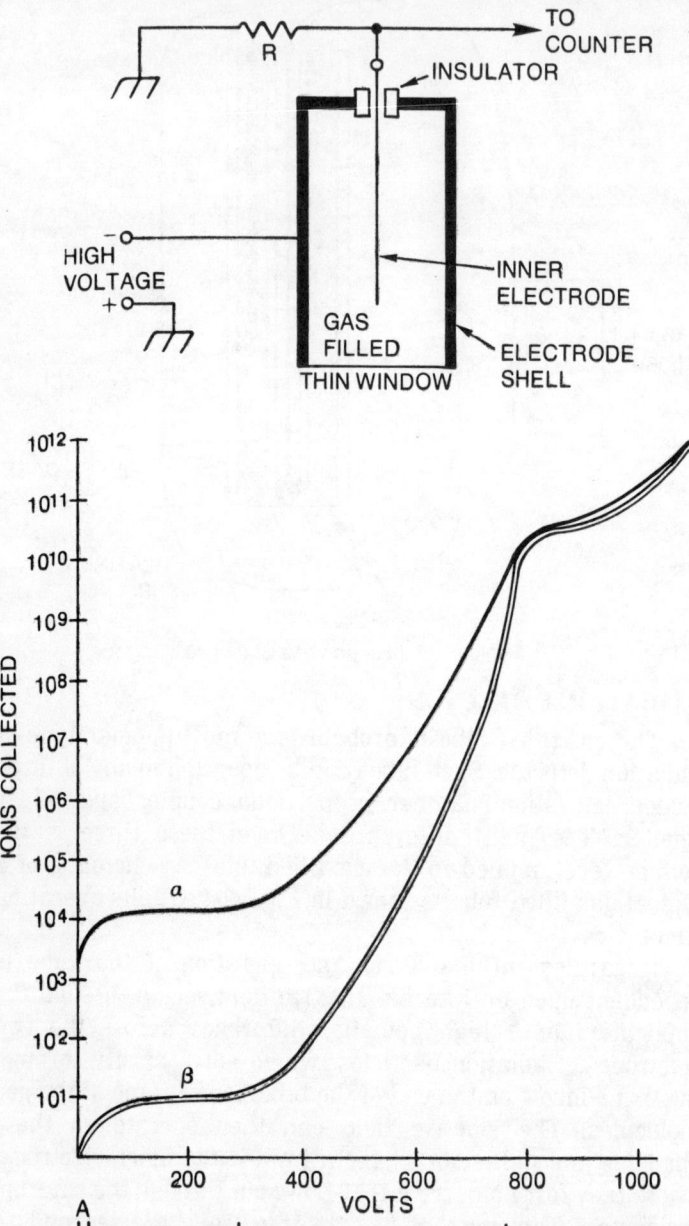

Fig. 12-4. The mechanical construction of a gas-filled radiation detector. The characteristic curve shows the properties and operating conditions of the gas-filled tube.

laboratory instruments, on the other hand, the gas-filled "tube" is actually a dome, and the inner electrode is a small loop of wire. In these instruments there is a little compartment, accessible through a trap door, that accepts samples for radioactive testing.

Figure 12-4 shows the operating curve of a typical gas-filled tube. Two curves are given here, one for alpha (α) particles and the other for beta (β) particles (high-speed electrons). A low-voltage bias (region A of the graph) creates only a weak electric field inside the tube. This field is too weak to attract many of the particles formed when radiation ionizes the gas.

The second zone, however, presents a somewhat different situation. In region B, which extends from approximately 100 to 240 volts, the tube operates as an ionization chamber. Nearly all of the ions produced in this region of operation appear as a current flow in external resistance R. The voltage drop across R is proportional to the level of radiation intensity. We can, therefore, use a gas-filled tube as an ionization chamber to measure the intensity of gamma-ray sources such as X-ray generators.

The third region on the characteristic curve, region C, extends from around 240 volts up to just under 800 volts. In this part of its curve, the gas-filled tube operates as a proportional counter. In this type of operation it is found that the electric field is strong enough to impart sufficient kinetic energy to the ionized gas particles that they create additional ions through the mechanism of collision. Because of this, the ionic current in the external resistor producing the voltage spike is magnified proportionally to the applied voltage. The proportional counter is thus capable of counting ions in the chamber on a one-by-one basis.

The name *proporitonal counter* is derived from the fact that the amplitude of the output pulse is proportional to the kinetic energy of the incident ionizing radiation particle. A particle with higher levels of energy will ionize more gas molecules than low-energy particles. This current can be multiplies by as much as a million times through the creation of new ions by the collision of the original ions with un-ionized gas particles.

The last region of the curve, region D, is where the gas-filled tube becomes a Geiger counter—the name erroneously applied to instruments of all three classes. At voltage levels from around 800 to well over 2000 volts, the gas-filled tube operates in a somewhat different manner than described previously. The ion multiplication effect of the proportional counter becomes so intense in this region that the tube can be said to abruptly discharge or *avalanche*. This produces as single pulse across the external resistor with pretty much the same amplitude every time it occurs, which implies that Geiger counter output pulses are totally independent of the kinetic energy of the impinging radiation.

Gas-filled tube specifications very somewhat from one manufacturer to another. Most tubes use argon, at a gauge pressure of approximately 100 torr, as the internal gas. A small amount of impurity (usually bromine) is added to quench the discharge; otherwise, the tube would remain ionized and would behave more like an argon glow lamp than a radiation detector. Typical output pulses from these tubes are on the order of a few microseconds, so the amplifier circuitry must be able to follow moderate to fast rise-time pulses.

SCINTILLATION COUNTERS

Scintillation is a word used to denote a process similar to that which generates light on the screen of a cathode ray tube. When a radiation particle strikes an atom of certain phosphorous materials, its kinetic energy may be added to the energy of the orbital electrons. When an electron is thus excited, it jumps to a higher energy level. It is, however, unstable in this high-energy state and will soon fall back to its normal, or ground, state. But energy must be conserved, and just as it attained extra energy from the radiation, it must lose energy as it returns to its normal state. This energy is released in the form of light energy called *photons*. Quite simply then, a scintillator is a device that allows the counting of the light flashes produced by scintillation.

A stylized scintillator tube is shown in Fig. 12-5. In this instrument, the scintillation crystal is attached to a *photomultiplier* tube—a specialized vacuum tube capable of making a very large output current for even very dim light inputs. The cathode of the photomultiplier is a photoemitter material that produces an electron for every impinging photon. (For more information on the photoelectric effect, see the chapter on X-rays.)

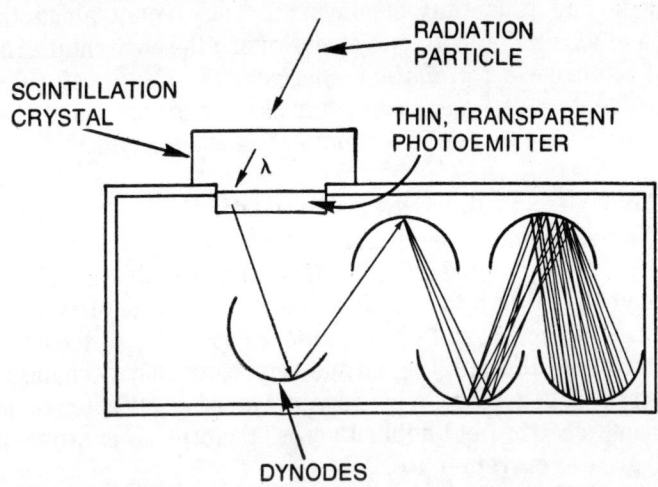

Fig. 12-5. A scintillation radiation detector uses a photomultiplier tube to increase its output current levels.

The typical photomultipler tube has 10 anodes or *dynodes* arranged so that electrons reflected from the first will strike the second, those from the second strike the third, and so forth. Each dynode has a potential with respect to the cathode that is approximately 100 volts higher than that of the preceding dynode. This is usually implemented by connecting each successive dynode to an appropriate tap on a resistive voltage divider.

Each electron emitted by the cathode surface is therefore accelerated by a potential of approximately 100 electron volts (eV). This means that each electron will have a 100 eV kinetic energy when it strikes the next dynode. And when it does strike the next dynode, its kinetic energy will knock loose several more electrons from the metallic dynode material; these are sometimes called *secondary* electrons. This process continues, the electron count increasing at each dynode, until the tenth dynode, where it is collected and delivered to the external circuit.

The scintillator/photomultiplier produces a current that is proportional to the kinetic energy of the indicent radiation. Such tubes, then, are used to measure the energy of the radiation. Most of the better scintillation assemblies can generate nanosecond duration pulses up to a very high counting rate, making them more sensitive than the gas-filled tubes. The scintillation assembly is often associated with a

221

cathode ray tube that displays the pulse count along the vertical axis and the kinetic energy along the horizontal axis; this comprises a *radiation spectrometer*. Many of these instruments use a computer-like memory and an add-to-memory circuit for accumulating pulse counts.

SEMICONDUCTOR RADIATION DETECTORS

The elements of semiconductor theory form the basis for the operation of diodes and transistors, and this should be somewhat familiar to you. If a radiation particle strikes the semiconductor crystal, its kinetic energy can dislodge an electron, and through the normal semiconductor mechanism, a current is generated. This current can be accelerated by an external electric field applied across the crystal, creating an even greater current pulse.

The pulse amplitude from this type of detector is substantial, and it is nearly linear for a wide range of particle kinetic energy (usually 20 keV to 200 MeV). Pulse durations down to the nanosecond range can be achieved.

TYPICAL GEIGER COUNTER CIRCUITS

The block diagram of a typical Geiger counter survey meter is shown in Fig. 12-6. Most of these instruments are intended for portable operation and so will be battery powered. Typically, two or four size D dry cells are used. High-voltage bias for the gas-filled tube is developed in a special power supply in which an oscillator drives the primary of a high-voltage transformer. The ac voltage on the secondary of this transformer is rectified and then applied to an RC filter network consisting of a string of one-megohm resistors and 0.01 μF filter capacitors. There might also be a special high-voltage neon regulator in the circuit.

Pulses from the gas-filled tube are coupled through capacitor C1 to an input amplifier. The pulses from this stage are used to trigger a monostable multivibrator (one-shot) to produce one constant-amplitude, constant-duration pulse for every trigger pulse received from the amplifier output. These pulses are time averaged in the integrator following the one-shot to produce a dc level that can be read on the output meter. This meter might be calibrated in units of *events per unit time* (EPUT) or in units of radiation.

Many meters have a calibration point marked on their scales. The idea here is to feed a precise 3600 Hz pulse train

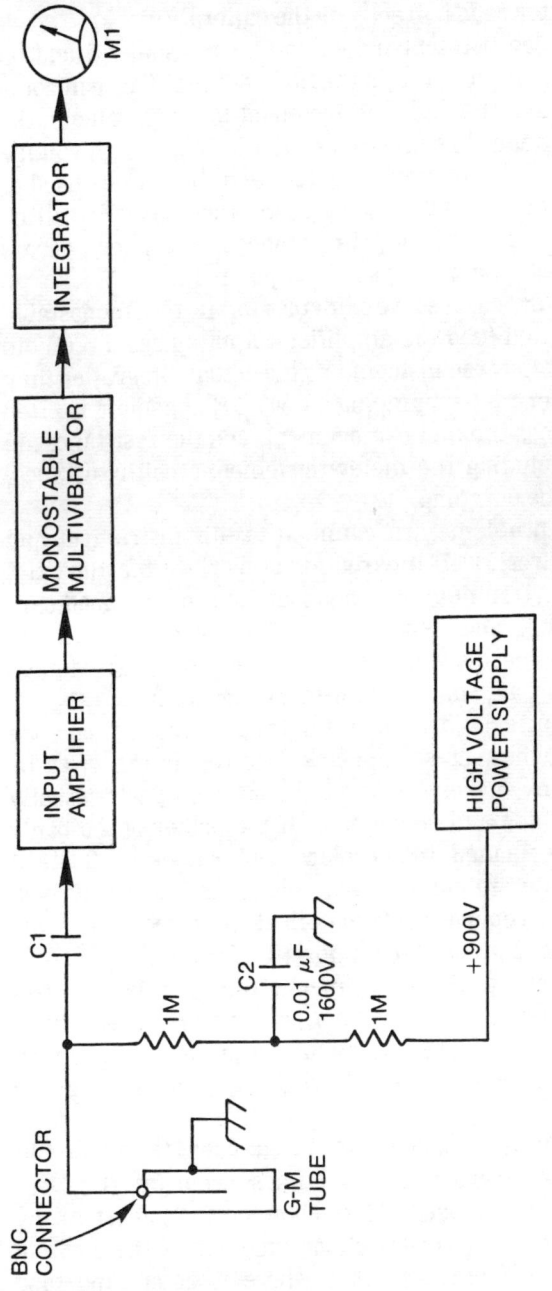

Fig. 12-6. Block diagram of a radiation survey meter. Pulses developed when the gas-filled Geiger-Muller (G-M) tube fires and discharges C1 are coupled to a one-shot multivibrator and an integrator.

into the amplifier input and adjust the calibrated so that the meter reads directly on the calibrate mark.

One other adjustment potentiometer is usually found on these instruments. It controls the high voltage. This control is adjusted to make the high voltage equal to some value in the 800–900 volt range. In some cases there will be a high-voltage position of the function/range switch, and this can be used to set the high-voltage potentiometer. In other cases it will be necessary to use a high-impedance voltmeter across appropriate test points to make the adjustment.

Many lower cost survey meters omit the monostable multivibrator and feed the amplifier output pulses directly to the integrator. In these instruments the actual integration may be a function of meter damping. A 500 μF capacitor is often connected across the meter movement, and the resistances in the circuit, including the meter movement's coil resistance, contribute to the damping.

Very few problems are common to this instrument and most seem to work well if cared for properly. Unfortunately, the hospital environment does not seem to promote good care for instruments, and some types of problems do pop up occasionally. There seem to be two main problems: damage from the battery acid and intermittent connectors.

Dry cell batteries leak electrolyte, and this will corrode anything it touches, or so it seems. The repair can often be accomplished by merely cleaning the affected parts, usually the battery holder and connectors. If the holder is too badly damaged to be cleaned, then replacement is in order. Some of the survey meter manufacturers charge an extremely high price for these replacement holders. I once received a $45 quote on a cheap nylon holder for two D cells! Give some thought to making a replacement from similar holders available through any consumer electronics or hobbyist electronics supply house. Many of these can be adapted, although the best choice usually requires some shopping to locate.

The other problem is an intermittent connection with the Geiger tube. A break will sometimes occur at the BNC connector, if such is used. Most commonly, at least in my experience, the break occurs at the tube end of the cable, a couple of inches from the point where it enters the tube housing. The repair is easily accomplished by cutting the cable a few inches back from the tube and reconnecting it in the proper manner. Since this will usually require disassembly of a tube housing, do this carefully! If this attempt does not cure the problem, try replacing the BNC connector. A special high-voltage BNC connector is sometimes used, and this may not be readily available. In this case you might try wiring the cable directly to the instrument. A black nylon strain relief will keep the cable intact and keep it from damage.

Most survey meters have a radioactive test strip on the case for testing of the instrument. If this is missing or seems to be dead, you can purchase test discs.

DENSITOMETERS

A basic densitometer is shown in Fig. 12-7. A lamp is powered from a highly regulated source and positioned so that its light can fall on a photoresistor. This resistor is connected into an electronic circuit similar to the plethysmograph in the chapter on transducers. A sample being tested is then placed in the light transmission path, and its effect on the photocell output is noted. A filter is often provided because the parameter being measured may be sensitive to wavelength. A popular application of this principle is used in blood analyzers, which use photometers.

FILTER AND FLAME PHOTOMETERS

A photometer is a specilized densitometer used to determine the concentration of certain solutions. An example of a simple photometer is shown in Fig. 12-8. This is basically a voltage bridge circuit in which a pair of matched photovoltaic

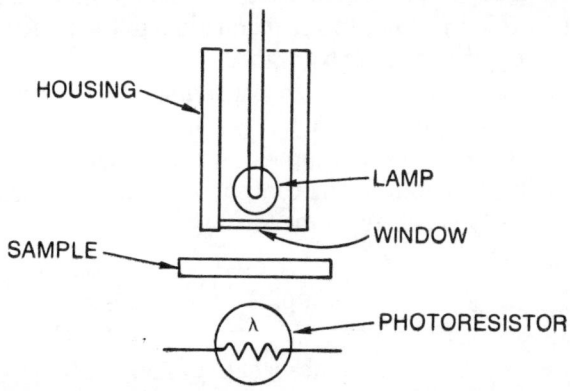

Fig. 12-7. Basic configuration of a simple densitometer.

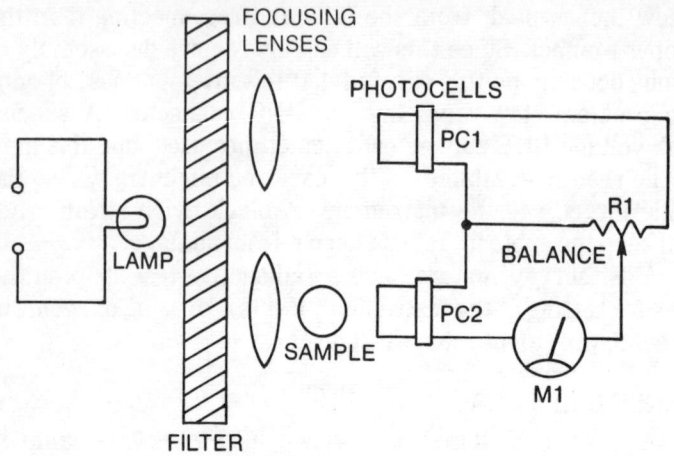

Fig. 12-8. The basic photometer consists of a pair of densitometers. Their relative outputs are compared to analyze the concentration of a sample.

selenium cells are connected in a circuit with a galvanometer and a balancing potentiometer. Potentiometer R1 is adjusted with the sample removed until the circuit is balanced. The sample is then inserted into the light transmission path of one photocell. This unbalances the circuit, thereby deflecting the meter. Potentiometer R1 is then adjusted until the meter is again centered. If the potentiometer is fitted with a calibrated dial, it is possible to tell something about the relative transmissibility or absorbancy of the sample.

A filter is used to select the most appropriate light wavelength from the white-light lamp source. The absorptivity of the sample is dependent upon the light's path length, the nature of the material, the concentration of the material, and the wavelength (color) of the light used.

It is usually necessary to use a sample cell to calibrate the system. What you are actually doing is comparing the absorptivity of a sample supplied by the manufacturer to that of the unknown sample. The concentration of the standard will be known, so you can apply the formula:

$$\text{Concentration of sample} = \frac{\begin{pmatrix}\text{absorbancy}\\\text{of sample}\end{pmatrix} \times \begin{pmatrix}\text{concentration}\\\text{of standard}\end{pmatrix}}{(\text{absorbancy of standard})}$$

This equation can be worked mechanically. The standard cell is often labeled with a calibration figure that represents the simulated concentration. Adjustment of the potentiometer then gives you the ratio of absorbancies in the equation from the result read out on a dial.

Most of these instruments are relatively simple, yet they can produce a high degree of accuracy. Problems requiring service are mostly mechanical and include lamp replacement.

A popular modification of this basic photometer system is called the *flame* photometer and is used to measure the concentration of sodium (Na) and potassium (K) in the blood. In this instrument, the light source is replaced by a flame that is adjusted to burn colorless. A specially designed flame nozzle, with air and gas intakes, plus an aspiration tube to suck blood into the flame, is located in a chimney. This nozzle is positioned so that the flame burns opposite the photocells. A calibrated amount of lithium salt is added to the sample to create a red flame. Filters separate the various colors (sodium creates a yellow flame and potassium a violet flame) so that the photocells can respond to an appropriate input. Modern flame photometers commonly used in hospitals to measure the concentration of blood sodium and potassium usually have a digital readout.

Chapter 13

Ultrasonic Instruments

Medical ultrasonics is a field that, by all accounts, is expected to expand by a large margin over the next few years. It encompasses a large number of different instruments or devices that are diagnostic or therapeutic. In most electronic specialties, the words *ultrasonic* and *ultrasound* usually denote a signal that has a frequency above the range of human hearing but below something loosely termed *radio* frequency. For most applications, this will mean 20,000 to 150,000 Hz, the exact limits being dependent upon who is setting them and for what purpose they are needed. Medical ultrasound, however, usually involves frequencies ranging from approximately 20 kHz to well over 10 MHz.

Some physical therapy "ultrasound" is actually radio-frequency waves well into the UHF region. This latter, though, is more properly relegated to the field of *diathermy*. The use of frequencies to 10 MHz under the heading "ultrasound" is not really a contradiction because it assumes another factor, and that is the *nature* of the physical wave generated. To be sure, a 2500 kHz or 10 MHz *electrical* signal would generate an electromagnetic radio wave that would propagate into space if the signal source was coupled to a radio antenna of appropriate dimensions. This is not, however, the case in medical ultrasonics. In this class of instruments, the generated wave is purely *sonic*, and any sonic wave, ultra-

or otherwise, is a mechanical disturbance in some medium such as air, water, or human tissue.

ULTRASONIC TRANSDUCERS

As an example of how an electrical signal can generate a mechanical wave, consider first the operation of an ordinary permanent-magnet loudspeaker. This device is familiar to most readers. The main components of the loudspeaker are the voice coil, permanent magnet, and a paper or fiber cone. The main purpose of any loudspeaker is to function as a highly specialized air pump. The cone is the part that actually moves the air, and it is usually conical in shape (hence the name), but has a planar surface. The voice coil is a small cylindrical coil of wire placed concentric to the cone at its center. The voice coil surrounds the permanent magnet in such a way that the magnetic field generated by electrical currents flowing in the voice coil interacts with the magnetic field of the permanent magnet.

When you connect a loudspeaker to a signal source, its voice coil becomes a miniature electromagnet. On one half of each cycle of the input waveform, the small magnetic field generated by the voice coil has a polarity opposite that of the permanent magnet, so it is attracted to the magnet. Since the voice coil is attached to the cone, and both are reasonably free to move, the cone pulls in toward the magnet. This creates an air void in the space immediately in front of the cone's former position, so air rushes in to cancel the void under the force of atmospheric pressure. This creates one half of the acoustical (mechanical) wave. On the alternate half of the input waveform, the magnetic field around the coil reverses, and this causes the two magnetic fields to repel each other. The cone is thus driven outward, toward the listener, creating a compression wave in the air. In other words, the loudspeaker creates a compression wave on one half of the signal and a rarification wave on the alternate half.

The loudspeaker is considered an ultrasonic transducer, but only in the lowest ultrasonic regions. It is limited in its frequency range because of its own inertia. Because the cone is relatively massive, the cone can only respond linearly to the input signal to about 15 or 20 kHz. Even when the cone is replaced by a low mass, very thin metallic diaphram, the frequency response is still limited to perhaps 100 kHz or so.

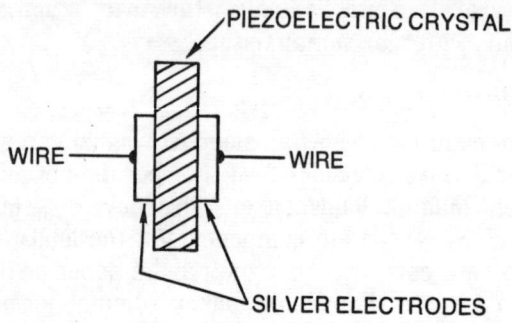

Fig. 13-1. A piezoelectric crystal element mounted between electrodes forms a basic ultrasonic transducer.

Thin piezoelectric crystal elements, however, are able to vibrate at rates up to millions of times per second.

Piezoelectricity is a property of certain naturally occuring and synthetic crystals, such as quartz. If a properly cut slab of such a material is mounted with electrodes as in Fig. 13-1, a voltage is generated across those electrodes whenever the crystal slab is mechanically deformed. If the slab is squeezed, for example, a voltage of one polarity will appear across the electrodes. Deformation in the opposite direction creates a similar voltage level but of opposite polarity. The piezoelectric element will also demonstrate resonance. If it is subjected to a mechanical wave from the surrounding medium that has a frequency close to the mechanical resonant frequency of the slab, as determined by its physical size and other factors, it will commence vibrating. This causes an ac voltage to appear across the electrodes that has the same frequency and shape as the impinging mechanical wave. The piezoelectric element can therefore be employed as a receiver transducer in an ultrasonic system. It is a device that can perform as a mechanical-to-electrical transducer.

But there is also a reciprocal function noted in piezoelectric transducers. If a voltage is applied across the electrodes, the voltage causes the crystal to deform. If the applied voltage is alternating, the piezoelectric crystal will vibrate back and forth, describing simple harmonic motion between limits imposed by the amplitude of the applied voltage. This is a highly interesting phenomenon because the same element can respond to both mechanical and electrical input stimulus.

Although any electrical or mechanical stimulus can make a crystal deform to some extent, only frequencies close to the natural resonant frequency of the element can cause an oscillatory vibration of long duration. Frequencies off resonance are soon damped, so only signals close to the natural resonant frequency of the slab are capable of sustaining oscillation and therefore producing a significant response.

Because of the dual mechanical/electrical nature of the piezoelectric phenomenon, we are free to use any particular crystal as either transmitter or receiver. In one case, it will be a sonic-to-electrical transducer, while in the other it is an electrical-to-sonic transducer. In some instruments you can easily see the dual personality of these transducers because they have a single piezoelectric crystal used as both transmitter and receiver transducers.

In most cases, an ultrasound instrument first transmits a sonic wave, then examines it at some remote point or at the same point as it originated. In the latter case, you are actually looking at a reflected wave. Medical ultrasound might use either pulses or continous wave (CW) modes, depending upon the application. Almost all are low powered; the exceptions are some instruments used in physical therapy. In the usual diagnostic instrument, it is necessary to impose a low-power constraint both for reasons related to patient safety and to crystal transducer life expectancy.

A CW diagnostic instrument uses two transducers, one for receive and one for transmit. The two transducers may, however, be totally interchangeable.

Pulsed systems fire timed bursts of ultrasound energy, so they are capable of receiving the reflection echoes with the same transducer during the quiet period between bursts. The designer is then free to use a single transducer for both functions, much like radar systems that use a single antenna system.

PROPERTIES OF SOUND WAVES

Before proceeding with typical ultrasound instruments used in medicine, first consider the physics associated with all waves in general, and ultrasonic waves in particular. First, let's examine electromagnetic wave propagation through any medium, and that includes a vacuum. The velocity, frequency, and wavelength of any propagating wave are related by:

$$V = F\lambda$$

where V = velocity of propagation
F = frequency in events per unit of time, usually cycles per second (hertz)
λ = wavelength

A well known example of this, taken from radio theory, is the relationship:

$$F = 3 \times 10^8/\lambda$$

Where λ is the wavelength (in meters) and the constant, 3×10^8, is the approximate velocity of light (in meters per second) or any other electromagnetic wave.

In keeping with standard practice in the physical sciences, we shall use international metric units. Where MKS (meter-kilogram-second) units are used, velocity will be expressed in meters per second, wavelength in meters, and frequency in hertz (cycles per second). If, one the other hand, CGS (centimeter-gram-second) units are used, as they often are in medical instrumentation, simply replace meters with centimeters in both velocity and wavelength specifications. (Note, however, that the velocity of light in the CGS system becomes 3×10^{10} cm/sec.)

Example. Ultrasonic energy is known to travel with a velocity of 1000 m/sec in a certain type of human tissue. If a 10 MHz signal is applied, what is its wavelength?

If $V = F\lambda$, then $\lambda = V/F$, so

$$\lambda = (10^3 \text{ m/sec})/(10^7 \text{ Hz})$$
$$= 10^{-4} \text{ meters, or } 10^{-2} \text{ centimeters}$$

Time and Distance

Timing the interval between when a burst of energy originates and when it is received can give us the distance traveled. In cases where transmitting and receiving transducers are on opposite sides of the path to be determined, we use the formula:

$$L = VT$$

where L = *path length*
V = velocity of propagation
T = time in seconds

Again, either MKS or CGS units may be used, but it is important that you keep both velocity and length in terms of the same system of measurement if you want to wind up with a correct answer.

In medical ultrasound, the second signal used to trigger the timer circuitry may well be a *reflected* echo. In fact, reflected-signal designs are probably the most common. If the receiver transducer is located coincident with the transmitter transducer, then a modified formula is necessary because the signal path is actually twice as long as was true in the previous case, so:

$$L = \tfrac{1}{2} VT$$

Example. An ultrasound pulse burst is applied to a type of tissue in which the velocity of propagation is 1200 m/sec. The reflection echo is observed to return to the point of origin in 50 μsec. What is the thickness of the structure in which the wave has traveled?

First, we must do a little units conversion. Microseconds is not a usable unit in our system, so we must express this information in seconds:

$$50 \,\mu\text{sec} = 50 \times 10^{-6} \text{ sec} = 5 \times 10^{-5} \text{ sec}$$

Now, let us solve the actual problem at hand.

$$\begin{aligned} L &= \tfrac{1}{2}VT \\ &= \tfrac{1}{2}(1200 \text{ m/sec}) \, (5 \times 10^{-5} \text{ sec}) \\ &= 3 \times 10^{-2} \text{ meter} \end{aligned}$$

But in most medical settings, it is more appropriate to use centimeters because they result in more convenient sized numbers. The proper conversion is:

$$(3 \times 10^{-2} \text{ m}) \, (100 \text{ cm/m}) = 3 \text{ cm}$$

Reflected Waves

Figure 13-2 illustrates the phenomenon of reflection. You may easily recognize this situation and the relationships presented if you have ever studied optics in high school, technical school, or a college physics course. The principle is the same, even though the medium and type of wave are different.

When a wave strikes a surface that has sufficient density compared with the medium in which the wave travels, some or all of the energy is reflected. We have all seen this phenomenon because it is the way an ordinary mirror works. In medical ultrasonics, the "mirror" may be bone or other dense tissue. A line *normal* to the surface is one that is perpendicular to that surface. That is to say, the normal line and a tangent line to the surface form mutual right angles. All angles in this type of problem are, by convention, only the acute angles (less than 90 degrees) of the pair formed. In Fig. 13-2, angle θ_1 is the angle between the normal and the incoming or *incident* wave, and θ_2 is the angle between the normal and the *reflected* wave.

If the surface is of irregular shape, the normal is just a line drawn at right angles to the point on the surface where reflection actually occurs. This simplifies the problem without deteriorating our understanding of the process. In all cases, however, the angle of the incident wave is equal to the angle of the reflected wave: that is $\theta_1 = \theta_2$.

Refracted Waves

A total or 100% reflection only occurs if the surface material is totally opaque to the incident wave. If it is not, another phenomenon, known as *refraction*, occurs. In this phenomenon, the wave energy is split, with some wave energy being reflected at the surface interface, and some wave energy being refracted and passing through. The effect is similar to the reflections seen on a window pane while at the same time looking through the pane.

The angular relationships are somewhat different with refracted waves than with reflected waves (Fig. 13-3). According to Snell's law, the angles of the incident wave and the refracted wave also depend upon the velocity of the wave, whether it be sound or light wave. This is expressed by the formula:

$$\frac{\sin \theta_1}{\sin \theta_2} = \frac{V_1}{V_2}$$

Where V_1 and V_2 are the velocities of the waves in the two materials, and θ_1 and θ_2 are the angles of the waves with respect to the normal in each material.

Since the density of the materials affects the velocity of the waves passing through them, you will find that the densest

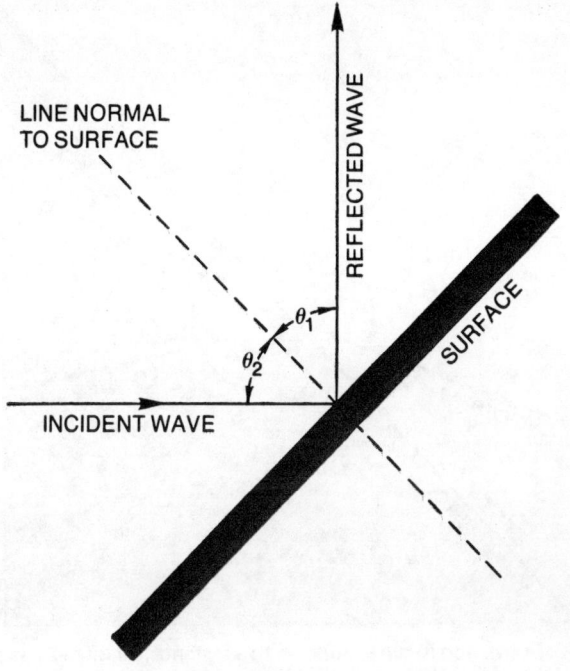

Fig. 13-2. Reflection is a phenomenon encountered in ultransonics.

materials have the slowest wave velocities. You will also find that two homogeneous materials having equal wave velocities will neither reflect nor refract the wave; the wave will pass through the materials unchanged. But in general this is not the case, so it can be said that ultrasonic waves will change direction as they strike the interface between different body tissues, producing varying amounts of reflected and refracted wave energy. For example, when an ultrasound wave is transmitted into the abdomen, it will pass through various interfaces formed by muscles, intestines, and other tissues having differing densities. In most medical ultrasound applications, both reflection and refraction take place at the same interfaces, giving rise to a variety of signals (including secondary reflections) that must be carefully processed and interpreted before any meaningful information can be deduced.

Doppler Shift

Several classes of medical ultrasonic instruments operate on a principle known as *Doppler shift*. Perhaps the best way to

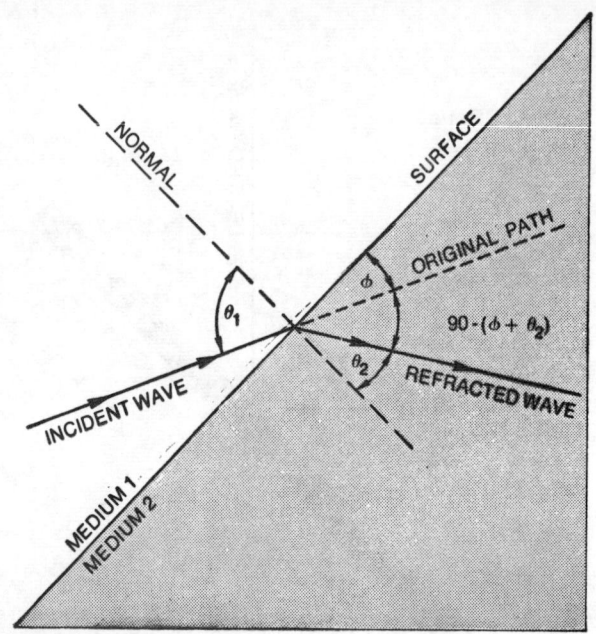

Fig. 13-3. Refraction in ultrasound. In this instance, medium 2 has a higher density than medium 1. A wave originating in medium 2 would follow the same path, but in the opposite direction.

present this phenomenon is to discuss the most classic example of Doppler shift, the train whistle. The only time you hear a train's whistle at its normal or natural frequency is when it is at rest relative to your own motion. If the train is in motion, however, a change in frequency will be noted by an observer who is not in motion with the train. Such an observer could be located in a stationary position along the tracks someplace, perhaps at the train station platform.

As the train approaches the station, the pitch of its whistle increases because the velocity of the train compresses the sound waves emitted by the whistle. This causes a rise in pitch as the train approaches. This can be explained in terms of the equation $V = F\lambda$. The velocity term is now a composite of the sound wave's velocity *plus* the train's velocity. The increase in pitch is greater for trains approaching with the fastest speeds.

As the train passes the observer, the apparent pitch changes, and the whistle appears to drop in pitch. The motion of the train away from the observer now subtracts from the actual sound velocity, lowering the pitch.

It is the *motion* of the train that creates Doppler shift. If the train is at rest relative to the observer, no Doppler shift can occur.

In another application of the Doppler principle, the wave source is stationary and the waves are reflected off a moving object or target. The amount of Doppler shift is also proportional to the velocity of the moving object. This is the same principle used by policemen operating a radar trap.

Doppler shift is also the basic principle of operation underlying a whole class of medical electronic instruments.

ULTRASONIC DOPPLER FLOW DETECTOR

Figure 13-4 shows an example of a typical Doppler flow meter. This is a continuous-wave instrument and uses two

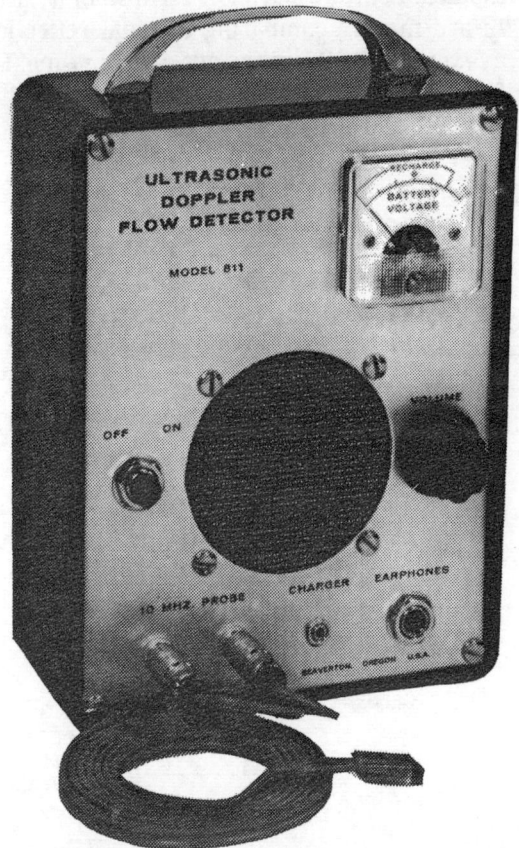

Fig. 13-4. An ultransonic blood flow detector. (Courtesy Parks Electronic Laboratories.)

transducers installed in a common transducer head assembly. The head is placed on the patient's skin surface immediately over a vessel to determine if blood is actually flowing. This particular model operates at a frequency close to 10 MHz. The ultrasonic wave is reflected back toward the receiving transducer by the moving blood and vessel walls. The return signal, though, will have undergone a slight Doppler shift and will therefore have a frequency that is slightly different from the transmitted signal. It is the shift in frequency that is of interest here because the frequency change follows the pulsing pressures of the blood in the vessel.

A simple diagram of such an instrument is shown in Fig. 13-5. The 10 MHz signal originates in the transmit oscillator. In most designs, this stage will be a self-excited oscillator because absolute accuracy and short-term stability are not too critical. We are merely comparing a signal reflection to its original wave, only a few milliseconds apart in time. Even if a severe drift is present, the oscillator frequency would not shift too much in this short time span.

The signal from the transmit oscillator receives further amplification before being applied to the transducer head, where it is converted into a sonic wave by the transmit

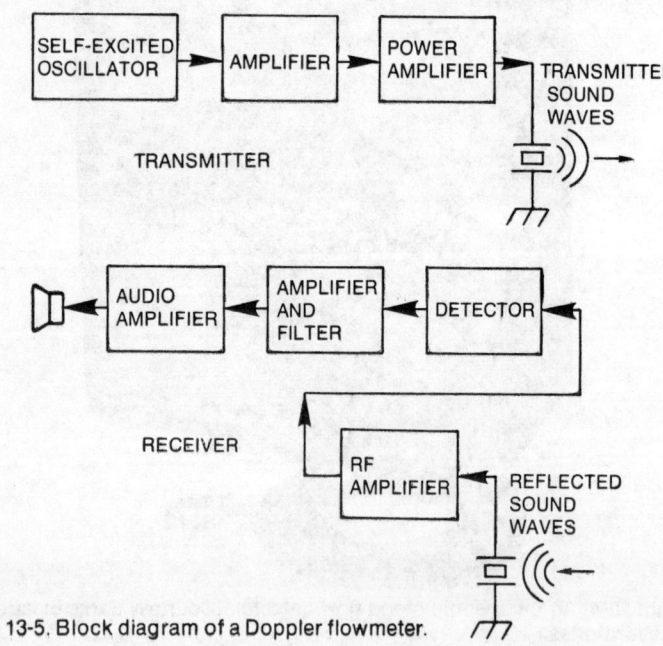

Fig. 13-5. Block diagram of a Doppler flowmeter.

piezoelectric transducer. In many instruments of this class, the interchangeability of the two transducers is emphasized by the fact that two connectors are supplied, but they are not marked as to which is for transmit and which is for receive.

The reflected ultrasonic wave excites the receive transducer, and this generates the receiver input signal through the piezoelectric phenomenon discussed earlier. If the reflected signal is from a non-moving object, it will have the same frequency as the transmitted signal. That is to say, there will be no Doppler component. But if the reflecting surface was not stationary, there will be a measurable Doppler shift. This shift is detected and then processed in an audio amplifier. Most flowmeters of this class, incidentally, use a loudspeaker or earphone as the output, but a few also have a meter.

Most service problems associated with this type of instrument are due to a dirty or abused transducer assembly. You will often be able to clear up the problem by simply cleaning the transducer face and checking the electrical connections.

Sonic waves do not couple efficiently to the skin or any other tissue across a low-density air barrier, so some form of direct coupling medium must be used. This is actually a jelly-like paste that must be cleaned off the transducer after each use. In many instances, though, it is found that users have not followed instructions too well. The old dried paste interferes with the proper operation of the instrument.

Another frequently encountered service problem is battery failure. Almost all ultrasonic Doppler instruments are portable and battery operated. Invariably, or so it seems to this jaded servicer, somebody leaves the instrument turned on, which soon discharges the nickel-cadmium batteries. Some of the Parks models (as in Fig. 13-4) incorporate an automatic turnoff circuit on the power supply that automatically turns off the instrument after a few minutes of usage, thus preserving the battery. This also saves the battery from damage caused by completely discharging.

FETAL HEART DETECTORS

Doppler shift of the ultrasonic wave forms the basis of operation for a class of instruments called *fetal heart detectors*. Such instruments are manufactured by a number of companies, including Roche Medical Electronics and

Hewlett-Packard. Some relatively simple instruments in this class are the electronic stethoscopes; others are more elaborate and resemble cardiac bedside monitors. All of them, however, operate on the same Doppler shift principle.

In trying to hear fetal heart sounds using a regular acoustical stethoscope, it is sometimes found that the normal abdominal sounds of the mother mask the sounds of interest. This can make the fetal heart sounds very difficult to hear using traditional methods. But in the ultrasonic version, most acoustrical sounds cannot pass through the piezoelectric transducer because it responds to only a narrow band of frequencies.

Fetal heart-sound monitors operate at frequencies around 2.5 MHz. They usually have both receive and transmit crystals housed in a single transducer assembly, which is placed on the abdomen above the uterus. Ultrasonic waves strike the beating fetal heart, reflecting a Doppler shifted wave that is picked up by the receive crystal element and processed in a manner like the flowmeter discussed earlier. Also present in the input signal are some artifact components created by the moving abdominal wall and other internal structures. Fortunately, these artifacts have frequencies different from those of the fetal heart sounds, so some judicious filtering serves nicely to clean up the signal heard at the output.

SERVICING DOPPLER EQUIPMENT

Servicing an ultrasonic instrument, such as the flowmeter and fetal heart sound detector discussed earlier, is complicated by the same problem existing in all transmitter/receiver systems—determining which half of the system is at fault. If you have an oscilloscope that will display the output signal of the transmitter, it will be quite useful for checking this type of system. (Incidentally, this is one powerful reason why you should lobby to purchase an oscilloscope with a vertical frequency out to at least 15 MHz.) Once it has been determined which half of the system is at fault, common service techniques will soon find the bad part.

Microphonics

One of the more common problems associated with ultrasonic instruments is an effect resembling microphonics, a term that originated back in the vacuum tube days. If a vacuum tube audio stage is subjected to vibration with one of the internal tube elements loose, the vibration would modulate the electron stream and thereby appear in the output signal. This is not quite the mechanism as in the ultrasonic version of microphonics, but the results in the audio output have a similar sound.

If the ultrasonic instrument is microphonic, or if it appears to break into oscillation at the slightest provocation, look first to the transmit oscillator. Such problems are generally caused by a mechanical or acoustical frequency-modulation of the oscillator. Most of these circuits employ either a Hartley or Colpitts self-excited design. It is the coil in the LC resonant tank circuit that is most commonly at fault. These coild are generally tuned by an adjustable ferrite core; that is, they are slug tuned.

Loose cores are a very common cause of microphonics and audio oscillation symptoms. At the frequencies commonly used in ultrasonic instruments, there might actually be two cores. One core is fixed and forms a cup around the outside of the coil; the other core is an adjustable slug inside the coil body. Both cores, however, are inside of a metal shield can.

Although it may be easier to simply replace the shielded coil assembly, it may prove quicker (especially if replacements are not readily at hand) to repair the defective assembly. All you need to do is carefully disassemble the shielded coil to a point where you can cement the cup core and slug core. For the fixed cup core, you can use almost any handy adhesive substance. I have successfully used Elmer's white glue, various epoxy products, the cyanoacrylic "super glues," and good old rubber cement.

The slug core, however, is supposed to be adjustable. A hard-setting glue will set you up for a coil replacement, and possibly weeks of down time while a part is obtained, should additional repairs or subsequent transducer replacement necessitate returning the transmit oscillator. For the tuning slug, it is recommended that you use a product such as Glyptal, a thick fingernail polish, or even hot-dripped wax from an ordinary candle. These products will all hold the slug firmly in place, yet allow for future adjustment. While this may not be exactly easy, it will still be possible without undue effort.

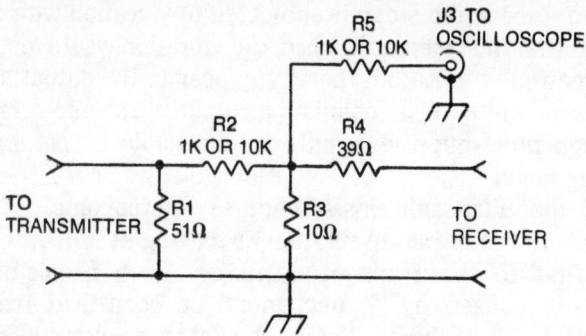

Fig. 13-6. This resistor attenuation pad uses the transmitter signal for receiver alignment and a troubleshooting signal generator.

Transducer Tests

A test jig is useful for servicing and adjusting ultrasonic Doppler instruments. The transmitter is often tuned to the transducer, first by connecting the transducer, then by immersing it in water. If mechanical vibration from the environment is kept to a minimum, you should be able to spot a slight disturbance at the water's surface due to ultrasonic wave action. Tune the transmitter adjustments inside of the instrument for maximum disturbance of the water. This phenomenon is a little hard to see, but it is easier and cheaper than some of the alternatives. While you have the transducer in the water bath, try moving it back and forth while listening to the output. This will create a swish-swish sound in the output, which is a relatively good indicator of instrument performance.

The attenuation pad of Fig. 13-6 is now connected between the transmitter and receiver. This pad provides a signal of proper amplitude for troubleshooting or alignment of the receiver circuits. If the instrument uses a common input/output jack for the transducer assembly, jacks J1 and J2 will be part of that connector. If these jacks are separate, as in Fig. 13-4, separate connectors are required. J3 is a semi-isolated output to an oscilloscope, voltmeter, or dc voltmeter equipped with a demodulator probe. The dc voltmeter may not be useful in all situations and should be regarded only as an option.

The pad is designed to present a constant impedance in the neighborhood of 50 ohms to both the transmitter and the receiver. R1 was selected because it is the nearest carbon resistor value to the nominal fifty ohms specification. R3 and R4 sum to 49 ohms, allowing R3 to be part of a voltage-divider network. R2 is selected according to the desired amount of attenuation: 10,000 ohms for 60 dB and 1000 ohms for 40 dB. All resistors can be quarter or half-watt carbon-composition types and should be mounted inside a small shielded container. This last precaution is a good reason to opt for the smaller quarter-watt types. Of course, a rather bewildering variety of connectors may prove necessary if more than one brand or model of Doppler instrument is to be serviced. Alternatively, if numbers are few and service rare, the connectors can be jury rigged for each use.

If past experience is a valid teacher, you can well expect that most service problems in Doppler equipment will involve the transducer, mechanical damage to the instrument, or worn-out parts such as switches, jacks, and so forth. This leads me to caution you to look for the obvious before attempting any time-consuming or detailed troubleshooting procedures. And leave all tuning adjustments alone—they rarely shift that much by themselves. Disturbing such adjustments will only compound your problems. In all likelihood, it will prove impossible to realign the set until after the real problem has been located and corrected. Never troubleshoot with a diddlestick (alignment tool).

ECHOENCEPHALOGRAPHS

This class of diagnostic instrument uses ultrasonic waves in a radar-like manner to locate certain features inside the patient's head and to measure their distance from the skull wall. In the basic echo system there will be a transducer assembly containing both transmit and receive crystals. An ultrasound pulse is fired and its return echo received. These pulses are displayed against a timebase on an A-scan oscilloscope, which shows amplitude vs time. An example is shown in Fig. 13-7.

Oscilloscope sweep is initiated from the left side of the cathode ray tube screen when the ultrasonic pulse is fired from the transmitter. This pulse shows up as the first spike on the CRT trace. A midline structure, dividing the left and right halves of the brain, creates a weak return echo shown here as the second spike. A stronger reflection off of the far wall of the skull creates the third spike. Incidentally, it is not necessary to

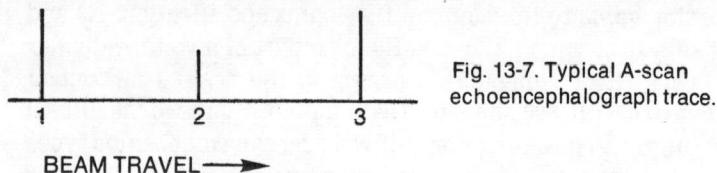

Fig. 13-7. Typical A-scan echoencephalograph trace.

use any special CRT marker circuitry to create the first spike because the reflection from the near wall of the skull will be quite large, and this also eliminates a potential calibration error in marker timing.

Normally, the second spike is equidistant between the first and third spikes. If a tumor or other defect displaces the midline structure, this relationship is destroyed and the second spike will appear offset, either the left or right side. Sometimes cell or fluid masses will create a fourth spike with an amplitude proportional to the object's size. The distance from the skull wall at the transducer's point of contact is given by the $L = \frac{1}{2}VT$ equation given earlier. Velocity V of 2.5 MHz ultrasonic waves in brain tissue is approximately 1500 m/sec, and time T can be easily measured from the calibrated oscilloscope time base and the graticule on the CRT screen.

The technique of echo ranging finds use in other than the simple A-scan mode discussed here. You can define sizes, for example, by taking a number of readings at different points and computing distance L from the equation. You can get a good idea of size, providing the object is large enough to render negligible errors in L due to errors in oscilloscope time-base calibration. Some sophisticated instruments do this calculation automatically by firing pulses from numerous angles then displaying the processed signals on a CRT screen to be viewed and photographed if a permanent record is required.

Analysis of the oscilloscope trace can provide further information regarding the nature of the object. If it is primarily fluid-filled, reflections will be created only at the interfaces, so there will be two additional spikes. Solid objects, on the other hand, produce noisy traces consisting of multitudinous spikes, sometimes enough to actually give the illusion of solidness.

Chapter 14
Balloon Pumps, Pneumotachometers, and Cardiomemories

This chapter is included to catch some of the special medical instruments that do not fit nicely into other subject chapters. The special items here are intra-aortic balloon pumps, pneumotachometers, and ECG memory recorders.

INTRA-AORTIC BALLOON PUMPS

An AVCO intra-aortic balloon pump is shown in Fig. 14-1 and 14-2. This machine provides temporary cardiac assistance to the patient's left ventricle using a technique known as *counterpulsation*. This technique operates by decreasing the aortic pressure (see Fig. 14-3) immediately prior to the ejection of blood from the left ventricle of the heart. Counterpulsation theoretically accomplishes two purposes: a reduction of the work done by the left ventricle and an improved perfusion of the heart muscle.

For discussion of balloon pump operation, assume a deflated balloon located as shown in the aorta (Fig. 14-3). The pump inflates the balloon, which distends the aortic wall just prior to the time when the spaces around the balloon fill up with blood. The action of the inflating balloon causes an increase in aortic pressure. When the balloon is deflated just prior to ventricular contraction, the aorta resumes its former shape and size, and the aortic pressure decreases.

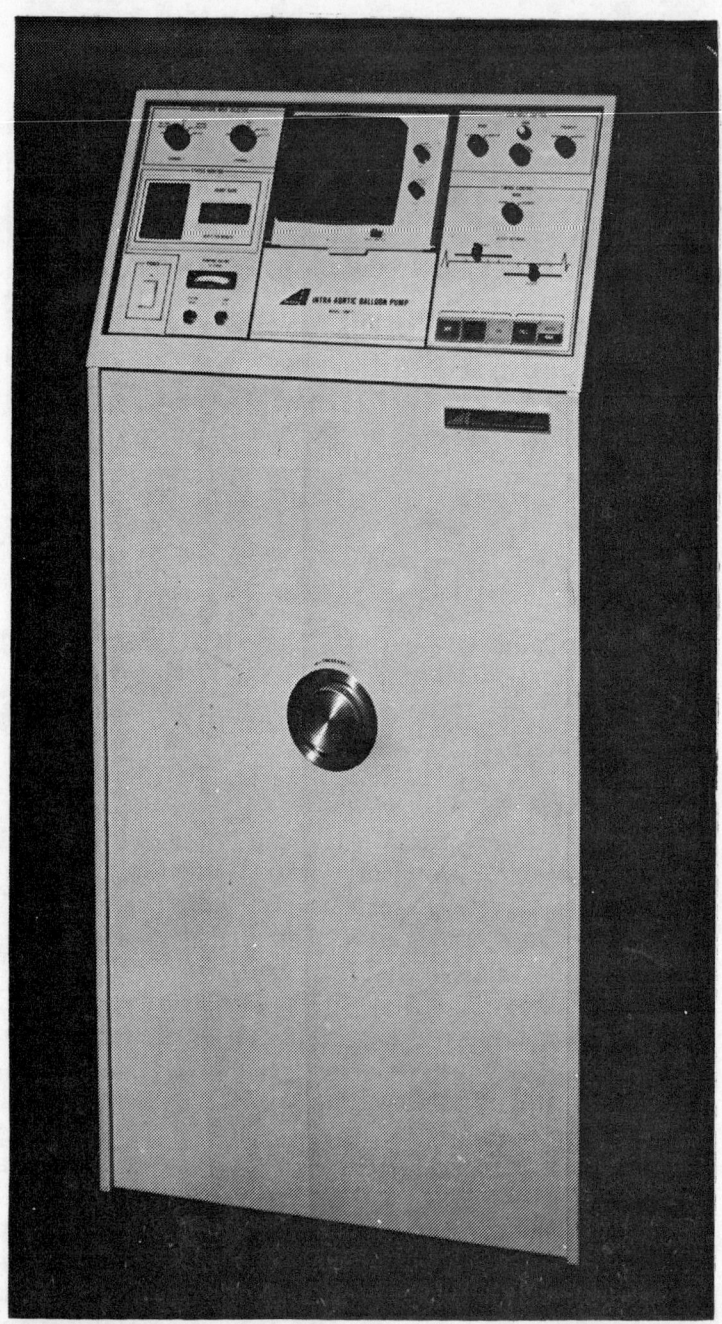

Fig. 14-1. AVCO intra-aortic ballon pump, model IABP-8, sold and serviced by Roche Medical Electronics.

Basic Pump Mechanism

A block diagram of the balloon pump mechanism is shown in Fig. 14-4. The balloon inflation and deflation is caused by an isolating piston operating with helium gas. Helium is used because it is a very lightweight gas, which is an important requirement because the balloon must be capable of changing volume rapidly. Hydrogen, of course, is even lighter than helium, but it must be disqualified for use in the balloon pump because of its high inflammability.

A size-D tank of medical-grade helium is located just inside of the rear door of the balloon pump housing. Its job is to supply the helium gas used on the balloon side of the isolating piston. The system can be loaded with helium by either manual or automatic operation of the pump cycle.

A gas surveillance system is incorporated into the pump and is used as a safety precaution. Should something go amiss with the pump, the surveillance system operates a *vent* relay, which opens the patient side of the piston to the atmosphere.

A high pressure against the machine side of the isolation piston causes the inflate cycle while a sudden vacuum generates the deflate action. These pressure levels are supplied by a compressor/vacuum-pump assembly located in the bottom portion of the pump housing. The vacuum and drive pressure is controlled by an electrically operated pulse valve. The coil of this valve is connected to an electronic drive circuit that is triggered by the patient's ECG waveform. The ECG signal can be acquired from either a bedside monitor connected through a phone-plug patch cord to a jack on the rear panel of the pump, or through direct pickup through the pump's own internal isolated ECG preamplifier. A connector for a standard five-pin ECG patient cable is provided on the rear panel of the pump.

Besides the vent (to atmosphere) valve, there are several other helium valves, controls, and monitors to be considered. On top of the helium bottle is a preadjusted regulator that is used to limit pressure supplied to the system to a range of 20–25 psi. There is also a pressure-sensitive switch that turns on a *helium low* lamp on the alarm panel of the front console. Following the pressure switch there is another regulator that is designed to limit line pressure to a level of 15 torr (mmHg). Controlling the gas system are four valves in a manifold. The manual and auto-fill valves control the flow of helium into the

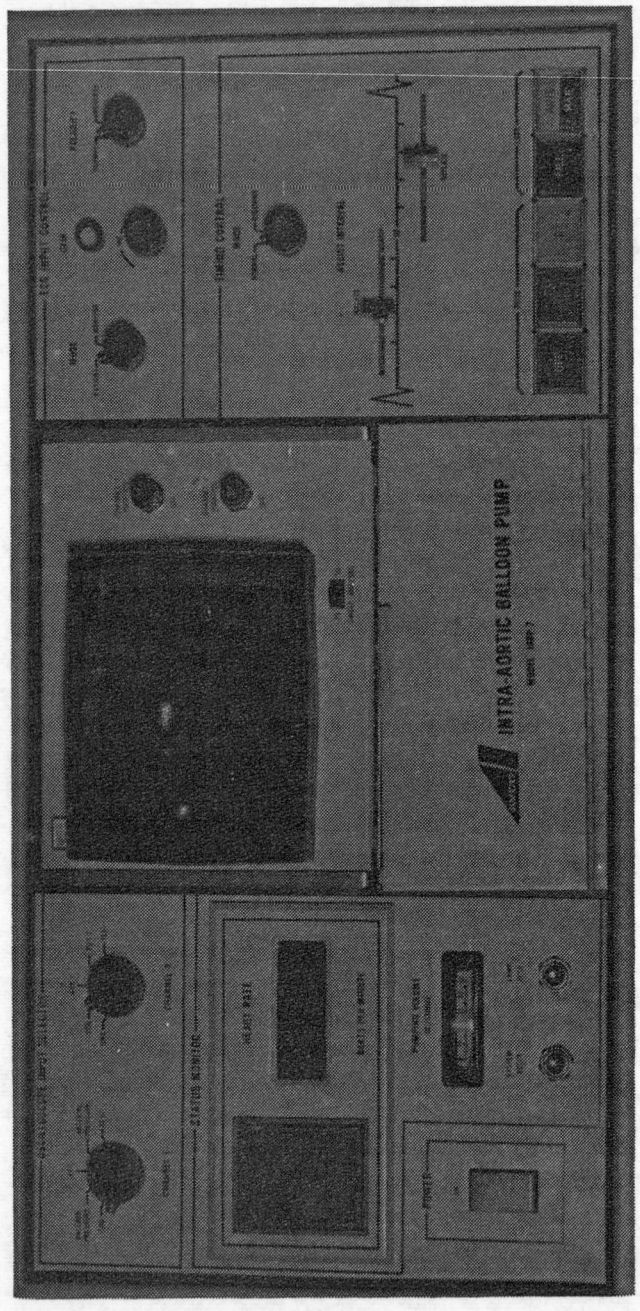

Fig. 14-2. Operator's console on the AVCO balloon pump.

manifold. Both *vent* and *slow-release* valves go directly to atmosphere.

The output port of the manifold goes to the drive side of the isolation piston. A pressure transducer in this line keeps track of balloon pressure and its amplified output waveform is displayed on the console oscilloscope. A mechanical control on the piston sets the pumping volume and a resistor ganged to this control is used to derive the stroke-volume signal used by the surveillance system. The volume control knob, incidentally, is the knob shown on the lower portion of the pump housing in Fig. 14-1.

There are three different balloon sizes differentiated by their respective volumes: 20 cc, 30 cc, and 40 cc. Each balloon is equipped with a resistor molded into the plastic gas connector that attached the balloon hoase to the pump assembly. This resistor is needed so that the gas surveillance system knows which size balloon is being used without the necessity of depending upon the operator to set a special switch. These values are: 270Ω for the 40 cc balloon, 510Ω for the 30 cc, and 1000Ω for the 20 cc.

Console Controls and Features

The console of the pump (Fig. 14-2) is the upper section and contains the bulk of the electronics. The top cover shroud must be taken off before the electronics can be serviced. The design of this particular instrument is good from the servicer's point of view, which leads me to suspect either that good human engineering was at hand or that the guy who designed it had a service and troubleshooting background. All that is required to remove the shroud is to take out two small screws at the corners along the rear lip of the top cover. The cover can then be gently lifted off and be set aside.

The oscilloscope shown in Fig. 14-2 is a specially constructed version of the Hewlett-Packard model *7803B*. On the upper left-hand side of the console is an oscilloscope input selector switch bank. One position of each switch connects its respective channel to ground so that the position controls can be adjusted to place the baselines at appropriate points on the CRT screen. The patient's ECG may be displayed on either channel, but channel 1 can also accommodate the patient's arterial-pressure waveform and the balloon-pressure waveform generated by the pump's internal pressure transducer.

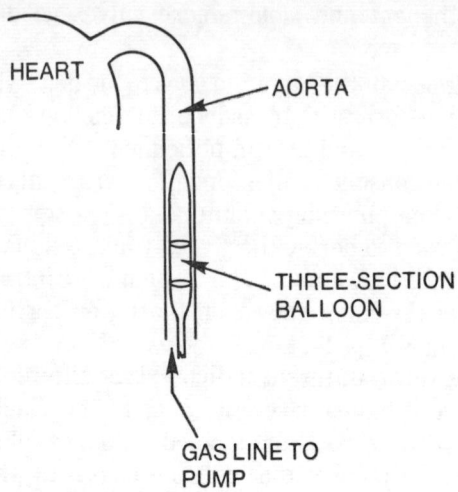

Fig. 14-3. Placement of the three chamber AVCO balloon in the patients aorta.

Controls for the ECG preamplifier are in the upper right-hand corner of the console. The *mode* switch selects the input from either the patient cable or the patch-cord input from a regular bedside monitor. The polarity switch is needed because the circuits following the preamplifier want to see only positive-going R waves. An amplifier gain control adjusts the ECG amplitude to a point where each R wave causes flashing of the systole lamp. This should occur with a deflection on the oscilloscope screen of 1.5 to 2.0 centimeters.

Located below the ECG preamplifier are the inflate/deflate timing controls and the drive-control switches. The controls are adjusted so that the inflate occurs at the top of the t wave and deflate between p and R waves. The controls are calibrated in terms of percentage of the patient's R-to-R interval, but it is best to examine the ECG signal on the oscilloscope for the exact placement of marker flags, generated by the timing circuit, on the ECG waveform. The inflate marker is positive-going while the deflate marker is negative-going.

These flags, incidentally, can be a good troubleshooting indicator in some cases. The flags are mixed with the ECG signal at the input of a summing amplifier that drives the oscilloscope. If the pump is not driving but the flags are present, you may feel safe in exonerating the logic circuitry up to the input of the *weaning* control. This circuit, which has its

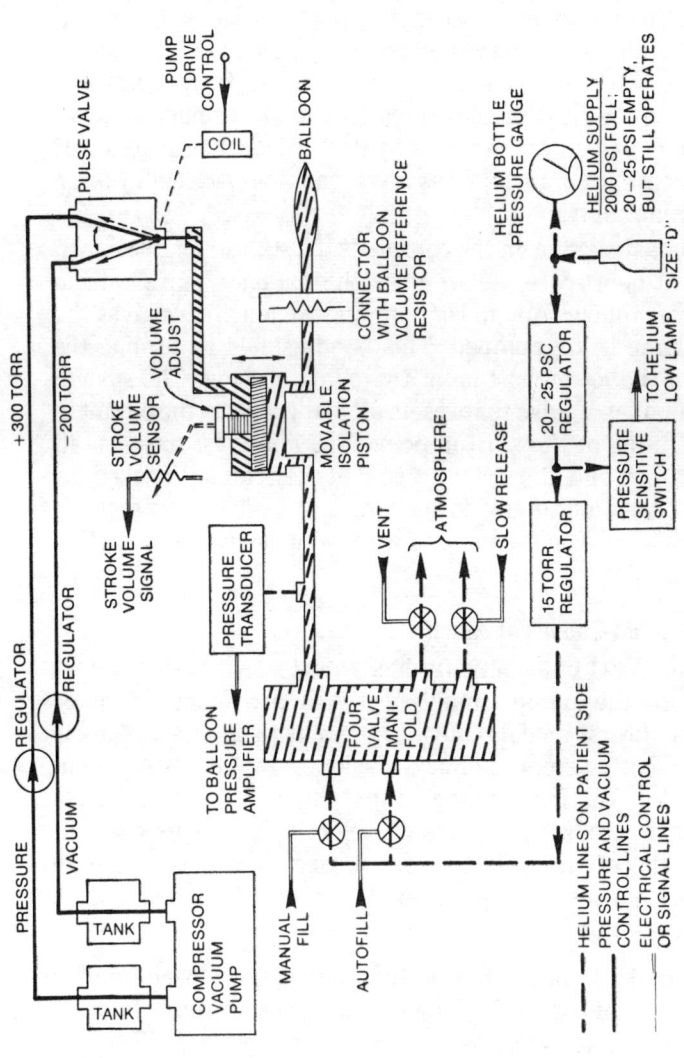

Fig. 14-4. Block diagram of the IABP-7 and IABP-8 pneumatic and electronic control systems.

control knobs located just inside the small trap door beneath the oscilloscope, is used to ease the patient off of the pump. The wean circuit contains a 3-bit digital counter and appropriate logic gates that are used to decode the counter output according to commands from the selector switch. This causes the pump-drive solenoid on the pulse valve to be energized either on every R wave, every second R wave, every fourth R wave, or on every eight R wave. If the flags are present on the ECG display, then look to the weaning control, the pulse valve, or the pulse-valve driver transistors. Of course, absence of the marker flags leads to the circuitry prior to the wean control.

The last section on the console is the status monitor panel. A digital heart-rate meter gives the patient's pulse rate in beats per minute. An analog pumping-volume meter gives the gas volume being pumped. This is adjustable by turning the knob on the lower portion of the pump housing. The *system reset* supplies a pulse that resets all of the logic in the circuit to the condition at the startup point. The *lamp test* turns on all panel lamps and alarm lamps so that they can be checked for proper operation; if any do not come on, it will be necessary to replace them. The meaning of each lamp is given in a section to follow.

Meaning and Causes of Alarms

The AVCO balloon pump has an extensive alarm system built into the pump, many of which are found on other manufacturers' models. Most of the alarms are part of a gas surveillance system and are designed to improve patient safety by venting to the atmosphere if certain alarm conditions are present. Besides electronic and mechanical faults, there are several user-caused problems that can generate alarms. The following is a short description of each alarm condition:

Vent. This lamp tells you that pumping has been forcibly terminated by the safety surveillance system built into the pump, the pump cycle has been turned off, and the balloon side of the isolating piston has been vented to atmosphere.

Pump Inop. This alarm will occur with a *vent* alarm and indicates either that no pumping has occurred for 12 seconds or that the balloon remained inflated for longer than 1.5 seconds. Check to be sure that gas volume is properly adjusted

(10 cc or higher) and troubleshoot any additional alarm lamps. Turn the power off, wait at least two seconds, then turn power back on to resume pumping. If pump fails again, another fault must be assumed.

High Gas Volume. This alarm will occur with a *vent* alarm and indicates the amount of gas being pumped is too great for balloon size. Check the *pumping volume* meter on front console to see that the volume is the same as the balloon size. If the reading is greater than balloon size, readjust the volume knob for the correct reading. Also check the balloon connector, rear connector, and purge hole cover for slow leaks.

High Leak Rate. This alarm will occur with a *vent* alarm and may indicate that gas is escaping, which is probably the most common fault. Other causes include: several ectopic ECG beats in succession and improper deflate timing. (See *troubleshooting high-leak situations*.)

High PVC Rate. This alarm does not vent the system, but serves to warn the operator that more than 19 PVC (in normal) or 9 PVCs (in bigeminy) occurred in a 60-second period.

ECG. Indicates that the ECG signal is either missing, too low in amplitude (1.5 to 2.0 cm deflection on scope), or is of too poor a quality to be used for triggering. This alarm will be followed by a *pump inop* and vent condition in 12 seconds. Causes include: bad ECG electrodes on patient, broken monitor, and gain control set too low. Check the ECG amplitude and quality and adjust or make repairs as needed. There are two methods for acquiring the ECG; if one is of too poor a quality, try the other.

Push System Reset or **Low Heart Rate**. These alarms tell you that the patient's heart rate is less than 30 beats per minute, and it may also be accompanied by an *ECG* alarm. Check the patient's pulse rate, and if greater than 30 BPM, check the ECG electrodes. If the problem is only a low heart rate, try pumping in the manual mode. This does, however, defeat the automatic fill feature, so an operator must remain with the pump to keep a check on balloon pressure and to refill manually every few minutes.

High Press. This alarm causes the system to vent if balloon pressure exceeds 27 torr. This alarm can be triggered by attempting to adjust the volume-control knob while pumping, by a volume that is too high initially, and by a drifting pressure regulator. If the volume is amiss, go to the standby mode, adjust the volume to the correct value, and then press the system reset to resume pumping. A drifting regulator, however, cannot be easily corrected since it is a function of warm-up. If time allows, warm the machine up for two hours before intended use. If there is no time available, disregard the fill instructions (fill for 1 sec) and hit the fill button very quickly. Resume pumping. After one or two hours of pumping, you can follow normal fill procedures.

Low Press. This alarm will be accompanied by a *vent* alarm and sometimes a *high leak* alarm. It always indicates a sudden loss of pressure, which can be caused by a kink in balloon line, an explosive leak (which can be dangerous if occurring in the balloon), certain ECG arrthythmias or a run of ectopics, an improper manual fill technique (if the alarm occurs shortly after going to the auto mode, suspect this as a cause), and an atrial pacing signal interfering with the timing. The best troubleshooting procedure is to discontinue pumping, place the pump in standby mode, and observe the balloon pressure on the oscilloscope. If it is ±5 torr, resume pumping; but if it is −20 torr, discontinue pumping, search for obvious leaks, and if none are found, notify the surgeon for balloon removal. If the alarm is a result of atrial pacing signals, try relocating the ECG leads or go to manual pumping.

Troubleshooting High Leak Situations

The balloon pump is equipped with an automatic gas surveillance system, as was mentioned earlier. *High leak* or *low press* alarms can occur erroneously with either a string of ectopic beats in the patient's ECG or with improper filling of the balloon. The system will vent soon after being placed in the auto mode if the balloon is improperly filled.

Make one—and only one—attempt to resume pumping. This is done by going through the regular startup procedure. If the pump again vents within 60 seconds, another fault must be assumed. Turn the balloon drive controls to off. Examine the status monitor alarm lights for a *helium low* indicator. If this alarm lamp is on, replace the helium cylinder and resume pumping. Inspect the plastic tubing at the balloon catheter and at the connector on the back of the pump for a secure fit. Check the O-ring seal on the balloon connector. Check the assist interval on the oscilloscope presentation of the balloon pressure waveform; this interval (Fig. 14-5) should have a 0.5

cm duration. Resume pumping, but if venting occurs again, turn the pump drive off the initiate troubleshooting to find an internal leak.

To isolate the leak, switch the pump drive off and the auto/manual switch to manual. Cross-clamp the plastic tubing a few inches from the back of the pump (Ask the medical people for a hemostat or similar clamp; they are seemingly made just for this purpose.) Turn the channel-1 selector to the *balloon pressure* position.

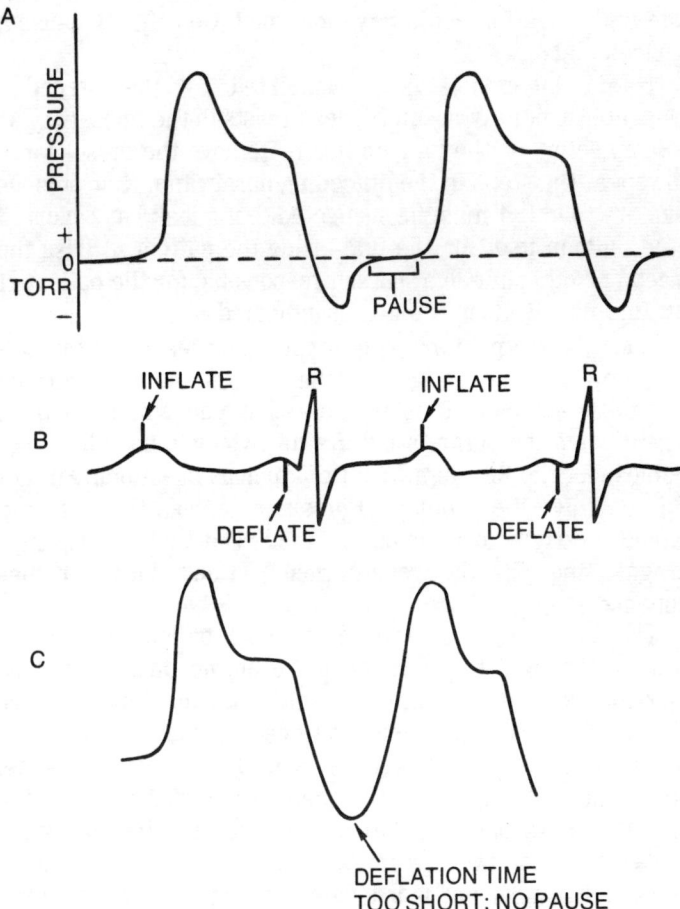

Fig. 14-5. Waveforms associated with the aortic balloon pump. (A) normal balloon pressure waveform. (B) patient's ECG waveform showing inflate and deflate timing markers. (C) improperly adjusted deflation timing control eliminates the pause or "rear porch" of the balloon pressure waveform, which may cause an alarm and vent-to-atmosphere condition.

Depress the fill button and hold for two or three seconds and then observe the pressure line on the oscilloscope screen for two minutes. If pressure drops more than 10 torr (one small CRT screen division) during this time, then there is an internal leak. If this is the case, look first to fittings, the plastic bowl of the cold trap, and the Teflon lines. I have seen several leaks in the cold trap (the O-ring gasket was defective) and in the Teflon lines from the compressor chassis to the pneumatic controls chassis. Also check the drain cock on the cold-trap assembly. It may not have been properly closed after the last drain and vibration could have loosened it enough to cause a high leak alarm.

If no internal leak is indicated by the preceding paragraph, you may assume a leak exists in the lines, the gas line connector, or the balloon itself. Remove the cross-clamp and repeat the steps in the preceding paragraph. If no obvious leaks are found, it must be suspected that a leak has occurred in the balloon itself or the line inside the patient. Advise the surgeon or other medical person responsible for the patient of your findings. Balloon removal is indicated.

There is one primary rule for locating leakes in the balloon pump and that is: suspect the obvious! As an electronic equipment servicer, it is unlikely that you will have been present when the pump failed. Rather, you will be called in to troubleshoot the problem. A little judicious questioning might help you solve the problem. For example, was the cold trap drained shortly before the pump failed? Did anybody trip over the gas lines in the recent past? (Don't laugh, it has happened.)

The electronics of the intra-aortic balloon pump are complex enough to warrant a recommendation that no adjustments be made without consulting the machine's service manual. The test equipment you need includes a dual-trace oscilloscope, voltmeter or VOM, a pressure/vacuum gauge, and a test load cell from the manufacturer. Also available from AVCO (through Roche) is a test set that interfaces the oscilloscope to the pump circuitry through a rather comprehensive service jack located on the pump's rear panel.

PNEUMOTACHOMETERS

The pneumotachometer is a device used primarily to tell if the patient is still breathing and to supply the breathing rate. The simplest type of pneumotachometer uses a bead thermistor placed just inside the patient's nostril. A constant current source (CCS) must be used to power the thermistor, and this supply must create enough current for the thermistor to just begin self-heating. One specification often made in this area is that thermistor temperature should increase approximately 1°C above ambient. This requires a current great enough to cause between 5 and 25 milliwatts of thermistor dissipation. Besides their use in some of the simpler pneumotachometers, the thermistor transducer is also seen in certain types of apnea alarms.

An example of a thermistor pneumotachometer circuit is shown in Fig. 14-6. Since the current remains very nearly constant, you can expect the voltage drop appearing across the thermistor to vary as the resistance varies, since Ohm's law must be obeyed. The resistance changes because the air breathed in and out by the patient cools the thermistor. It is important to design the constant current source so that current is limited to the amount required to provide self-heating, but no more. If the self-heating was more than minimal, the air coming through the nostril might not be capable of producing the cooling required to allow measurable resistance changes.

A similar device is shown in Fig. 14-7. This tranducer uses a very thin piece of platinum wire, which stretches across the inside of a piece of hollow tubing that also serves as a mouthpiece. The platinum wire is heated to a point barely above ambient and also operates through the mechanism of having the patient's breath cool the resistance element. Most of the instruments using the platinum wire transucer, though,

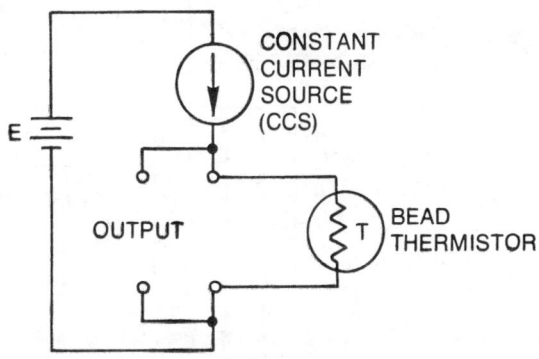

Fig. 14-6. Pneumotach transducer using a heated bead thermistor.

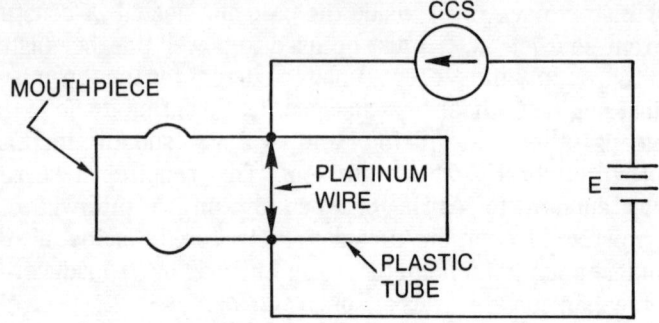

Fig. 14-7. Pneumotach transducer using a heated platinum wire.

place the resistance element in one leg of a Wheatstone bridge circuit.

Neither of the two types of transducer discussed so far are *directional*—that is to say, they are not able to distinguish between inhaled and exhaled air flow. Both flows can and do affect the thermistor in exactly the same manner. In fact, the waveform produced by these instruments exhibit a periodicity, but the frequency is exactly twice the actual respiration rate of the patient. By properly designing the logic circuit that drives the readout meter (using circuits similar to the heart-rate meter logic), it is possible to account for this fact, so everything is fine. Just do not take the actual waveform too seriously.

Figure 14-8 shows a type of respiratory transducer designed for use on a new type of respiratory alarm circuit. In

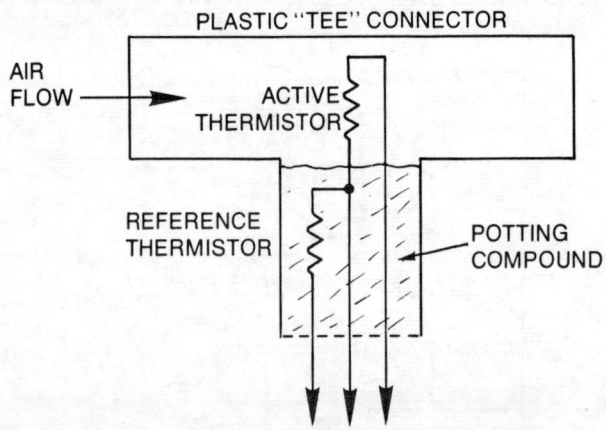

Fig. 14-8. The McCullough flowmeter transducer.

this design, which is a modification of an older principle, there are two thermistors built into one of the plastic tee connectors normally used in respirator systems. This transducer is placed in the expiration line of the respirator. Two thermistors are used, but only one is actively in the gas flow path. The other thermistor is used as a reference and is dead-ended in a potting compound made from a silicon preparation. In the original version, the thermistors were mounted to a stereo phone plug. (It seems that the larger size variety of these connectors has a thread diameter just about correct to fit inside one of the standard tee-fittings.) The thermistors are electrically placed in opposite legs of a Wheatstone bridge, and once again, they have a power dissipation just sufficient to cause mild self-heating.

In all of the transduction schemes of Figs. 14-6, 7, and 8, it is necessary to select the thermistors carefully. One factor that has proven very critical is the *thermal* time constant of the components. If a type with a long time constant is selected, it will respond with a highly damped waveform that is not very useful.

Air Flow Transducers

One fault found with the types of transducers discussed thus far is that they cannot be easily calibrated to derive any information other than the respiration rate. The transducer type shown in Fig. 14-9, however, can be used to quantify the process.

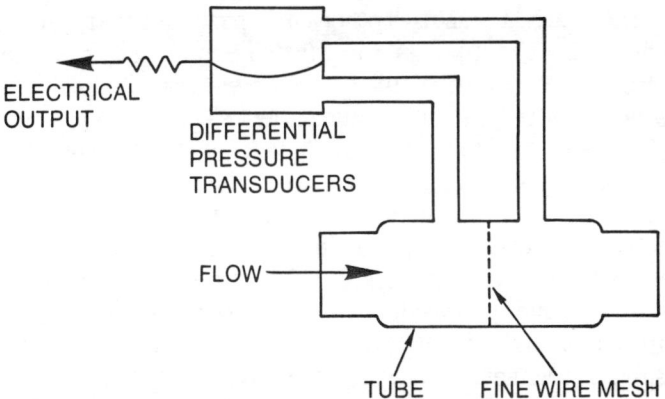

Fig. 14-9. A calibratable pneumotach transducer operates from the differential pressure created when the patient breathes into a tube obstructed by a fine wire-mesh gauze.

The *air flow* transducer consists of a fine wire gauze stretched across the airway. This transducer is used to drive a differential pressures transducer similar to those discussed in Chapter 2. Although physical dimensions vary somewhat from model to model, a relatively standard size is 5 centimeters diameter with a mesh density of 400 wires to the inch. The purpose of the gauze mesh is to offer enough airway resistance to create a pressure difference between the two sides, but not enough to restrict or interfere with the patient's breathing. If that were allowed, it would generate a tremendous error factor. In any event, the differential pressure should be no greater than about 0.75 torr.

Air flow transducers create a tiny differential signal proportional to approximately 7 millitorr per 10 liters per minute of airflow. The electrical signal developed by the differential pressures transducers is then proportional to the flow rate.

It is also a simple matter to derive a volume signal from this transducer, since volume is the integral of the flow rate. If we follow the pressure amplifier used to build up the flow signal with an electronic integrator, we will generate a volume signal. One parameter of interest here is the *minute volume*. To obtain that bit of data, it is common practice to use logic circuits that allow charging of the integrator for precisely one minute.

Other Pneumotachometers

There are at least two other basic pneumotach transducer techniques. The first is the *stretch strain gauge*. In this system, a rubber tube filled with an electrically conductive material is stretched across the patient's chest. This tube may be filled with mercury, copper sulphate, or electrode paste. As the chest expands during inspiration, the tube stretches, and that reduces its diameter. A reduced diameter in most electrical conductor increases its resistance. Similarly, when the chest relaxes as breath is exhaled, the diameter of the tube increases, and this reduces its electrical resistance. If a constant excitation current is fed through the resistance, a respiratory waveform is generated, much in the manner of the thermistor systems discussed earlier. However, the waveform generated by the strain gauge follows the same frequency as the breathing patient, not double the frequency as in the earlier systems.

The last type of pneumotachometer uses the *impedance pneumograph* technique for transduction. Here, changes in electrical impedance are picked up by electrodes on opposite sides of the patient's chest during respiration. A low-level current from an ac carrier oscillator is passed between the electrodes positioned on the subject's chest. Sometimes it is also possible to use these same electrodes for monitoring the ECG waveform, since the required placement for respiration monitoring is similar to that usually provided for a lead-I ECG.

An example of an impedance instrument designed along this line is the KDC neonate monitors often found in intensive care nursery facilities. Although this carrier technique appears similar to other carrier applications, it must be recognized that the signal amplitude must be kept very low. A demodulator in the monitor circuitry detects the amplitude shifts in the carrier that accompany respiration. Although this type of monitor cannot be easily calibrated for volume or flow rate, it can be used to derive the respiration rate and is also found in apnea monitors. That fact, coupled with the ease of operation, has made this a relatively popular approach.

ECG MEMORY RECORDERS

Some coronary care unit central monitoring systems incorporate a memory system in their design, as was mentioned in Chapter 6. These are made to store up to approximately one minute of the patient's ECG waveform; at least one system stores to 15 minutes. If one of the bedside monitors sounds an alarm, the central console alarm module freezes the recording presently on that patient's recorder channel. Two examples of such equipment are the Hewlett-Packard model *7805* and the American Optical Cardiomemory. Both record on quarter-inch magnetic tape and both use cartridges for ease of operation. The Hewlett-Packard model uses the Orrtronics Echomatic II cartridge, while the American Optical machine is designed around the popular Fidelipac cartridge (medium-size version) used in broadcasting. These are both very much like the old four-track tape cartridges that were popular in consumer tape players before the eight-track Learjet pack became almost universal in that market.

The Cardiomemory mechanism is an OEM drop-in version of the well-known Telex model 37 family of decks. In this type of mechanism, the pinch roller is part of the deck and is inserted into the cartridge, through a hole in the plastic case, by operation of the control arm. This arm also operates the ac power on/off switch.

The Telex deck is installed in a cabinet that also contains the American Optical electronics. Three printed circuit boards are used in this instrument and they also divide the separate functions required to make it all work: power supply, record modulators, and playback demodulators. Alarms are part of the power supply card.

Each Cardiomemory records up to four channels simultaneously and so can keep track of the ECG waveforms of four separate patients. If any of them generates an alarm situation, a 30-second alarm timer will initiate a countdown. When the 30 seconds have expired, this timer flags the control circuitry on the appropriate channel to cease recording on that channel until a manual reset button is pressed by the operator. This feature allows the machine to store the ECG waveforms from 30 seconds before to 30 seconds after the occurrence of the alarm.

Recorder Operation

ECG signals are too low in fundamental frequency for direct recording onto magnetic tape, so an FM recording technique must be adopted. Figure 14-10 shows a partial schematic of the input circuit used by American Optical. The input amplifier receives the ECG signal from the bedside monitor's remote output line. Transistors Q1 and Q2 form an audio-range voltage-controlled oscillator (VCO) operating with an unmodulated carrier center frequency of approximately 6760 Hz. This frequency varies in a manner proportional to the ECG waveform voltage amplitude, thus producing an FM signal. The output of the VCO is fed to a pair of digital logic gates that drive the record head. Notice that no high-frequency bias is used in this circuit as in audio tape recorders. Since this is an FM recording system, it is merely necessary to produce a spot on the tape for each cycle.

The playback demodulator in Fig. 14-11 sees a poor rendition of the square wave produced by the record process due to the filtering effects inherent in the system. Following the input amplifier, there is a Schmitt trigger stage that

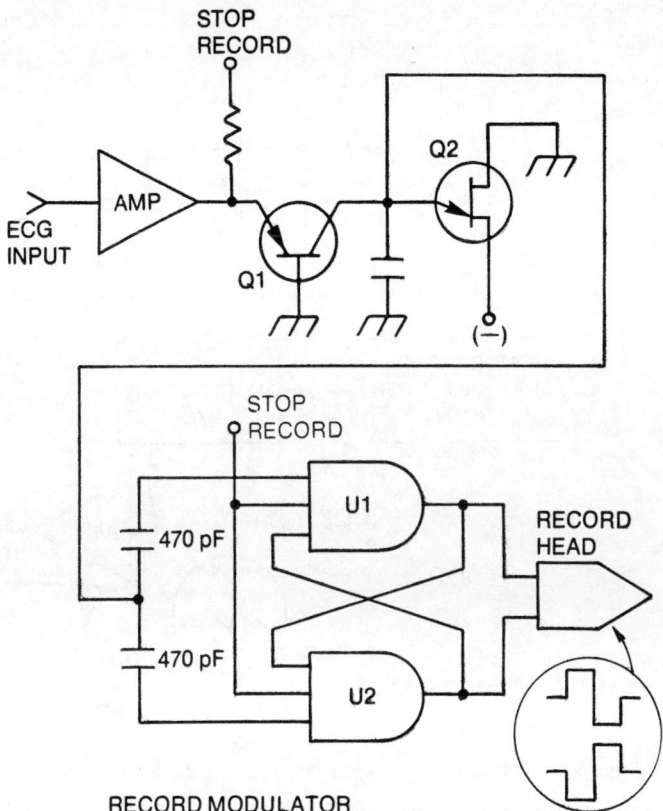

Fig. 14-10. Cardiomemory tape system, record modulator.

squares off the input signal and differentiates it to produce the spike-like pulses needed to trigger a monostable multivibrator (one-shot). The output of the monostable stage is a chain of well-defined pulses having equal amplitude and duration. These pulses are then integrated to recover the ECG waveform.

Servicing the Memory Tape Machine

Troubles with instruments such as the Cardiomemory can be either mechanical or electrical. These machines are operated up to 24 hours a day, every day of the year, which means that certain components will wear out predictably fast. Tape memory equipment use a classic capstan/pinch-roller system, and these rubber rollers wear out, as might be expected. Their replacement at specified intervals should be a

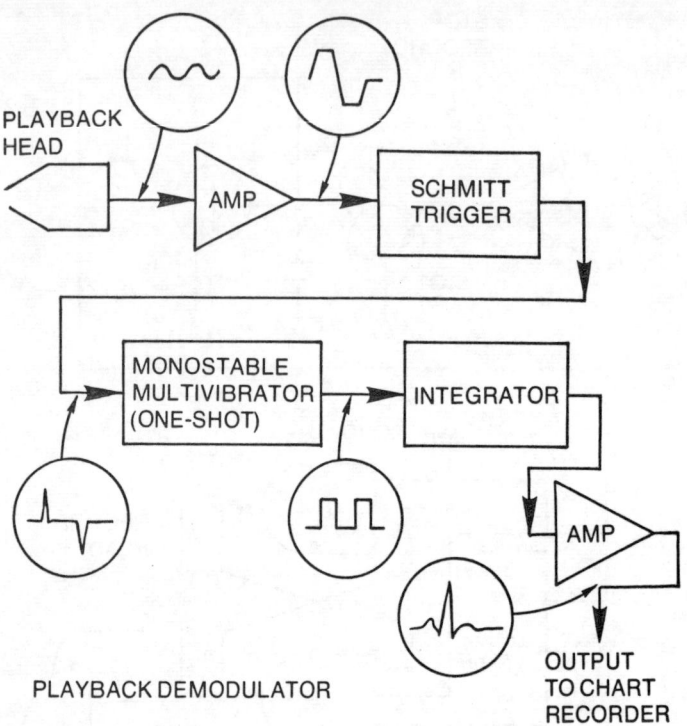

Fig. 14-11. Cardiomemory tape system, playback demodulator.

matter for your preventive maintenance (PM) program. (The choice of letters here is very fitting because it keeps you in bed at night, assuming that you are the one who has to provide the hospital with the p.m. emergency electronic service.)

There are several other parts that should be part of the PM program. The drive belts between the motor pulley and the flywheel and capstan assembly should be replaced occasionally, as should the nylon tip bearing on which the bottom bearing surface of the capstan shaft must ride. The capstan shaft and flywheel assembly should be removed and cleaned with alcohol or one of the other solvents used in the cleaning of electromechanical equipment. I would also recommend that the capstan be replaced at intervals of one or two years, unless trouble develops sooner. Memory equipment should be mounted horizontally (less than 20 degrees of incline) lest the capstan wear against the bronze bearings in the capstan housing.

Electrical problems in these machines mostly involve the heads and associated wiring. Some manufacturers provide helpful test features. For example, on the A.O. machines there is a *system test* position of the function switch that bypasses the heads, connecting together the demodulator input and modulator output. This can be used to help isolate many electrical problems.

Chapter 15
Test Instruments
and Repair Facilities

The exact nature of the tool and test-equipment inventory that is required varies markedly from place to place and situation to situation. But it is still possible to make some valid generalizations based on commonalities between all electronics servicers and medical electronics servicers in particular. In equipping any specific facility, however, some thought must be given to your own situation, so that needs can be assessed accordingly.

FACILITIES

Hospitals and service contractors usually share a common problem—limited space. Both find that the cost of commercial or light industrial square footage, and the pressures of numerous equal claims for that space, limits the amount of space available for an electronics service laboratory. You will, though, require enough floor space for a workbench, desk, a couple of file cabinets, and some parts storage space. These are actually bare essentials and should not be compromised. You may find that hospitals want to shunt their in-house electronics laboratories off to either the second basement (below the boiler room) or to the plant utilities penthouse (on the roof with the air-conditioning compressor).

Before accepting any quarters, you must be absolutely certain that adequate electrical power exists and that the space is accessible by elevator. Since most hospitals tend to grow in a poorly planned manner, reflecting the availability of money or the growth of the surrounding community, they tend to be a crazy quiltwork of different wings, where not all floors or locations can be reached by elevator. Even a short flight of stairs is totally unacceptable when you have to carry a couple hundred pounds of bulky equipment.

Workbenches

Workbenches can be made of wood or metal, as you please. If made of wood, of course, they can be easily custom designed by you, for your specific needs. Such a bench can be constructed either by you or by the hospital carpentry shop. If you opt to build it yourself, watch out for any union agreements, lest you upset some people.

In choosing or designing a workbench, make certain that you make it wide enough. There will be plenty of occasions to service some large and awfully bulky equipment. You will soon tire of being overcrowded on your own bench. Install a shelf along the back of the bench that is at least 12 inches wide; this can be used for test equipment.

Power to the bench can be provided at convenient points by using utility outlet strips. Be sure to check with the house electrician, however, to ascertain acceptable types. Many local electrical codes have rather strict requirements concerning this type of outlet system, and almost all require that only those types with a built-in circuit breaker or fuse be used. But this is a good idea regardless of the local codes. This is also an another area where the hospital union agreements can limit your freedom to install your own wiring.

At least one of the outlet strips, and preferably all of them if you can afford it, should be powered from an approved isolation transformer. This will prevent injury to personnel and damage to equipment from certain types of hazard that are known to exist. Also, rig a master power switch and circuit breaker that can cut all power to the bench in case of a catastrophic accident. This switch box should be located such that another person can turn off the power if the worker at the bench is being shocked. If the switch is inconveniently located, the rescuer would have to put himself in as much physical danger as the victim—and that isn't too smart.

Keep in mind, when designing your laboratory for safety, that most of the equipment sent up for repair is abnormal and defective, otherwise it would not be there in the first place. Never, never assume that the safety features work on any of the equipment sent to you for repair!

Service Manuals and Records

Your office equipment should include at least one desk, one chair, and one file cabinet. The files are to house both your library of service manuals and to keep your records of repairs and inspections. The records may be required by one or the other accrediting or licensing agency and to disprove any charges of neglect or incompetence in a malpractice suit against the hospital.

That library is your "ace in the hole" when servicing strange equipment, so stock your library with service manuals on all equipment in the hospital. Make an inventory of equipment in your facility and contact the manufacturers about a manual. In some cases, you will find that the users of the equipment have a service manual in their files, or more likely, stuffed in a box someplace. Ferret out these manuals and coerce, plead with, or threaten the users into giving them to you. Such manuals are usually more accurate than what might be sent to you by the manufacturer. Models do change, and the service manual supplied with the equipment when it was new should, hopefully, most nearly reflect the construction of that equipment.

In other cases, the manufacturer is your only source of manuals, and their policies will vary widely. Some will give you all the manuals you request for free, or for a ridiculously low price. Others will either deny your request altogether or set such an outrageously high fee that it is impossible for anybody to justify purchase. Many manufacturers, especially in the medical equipment market, have been known to become downright nasty at the very suggestion that they should actually supply a service manual. One manufacturer told me that his product was "high, space-age, technology and could not be serviced by *untrained* hospital personnel." (It had less complexity than a Japanese transistor radio!)

Do anything honorable—and whatever things dishonorable that you can tolerate—to obtain the service manuals needed to do your job. Beg, plead, implore, and coerce. Even try to convince the local salesman that his company's policies render the product totally unsafe and therefore unsuited to use in the hospital. And don't be afraid to ask the hospital administration to ban further purchases from an uncooperative company. You will soon find out that salesmen are sensitive to such "logical" persuasion.

SPECIAL TEST EQUIPMENT

Most test equipment common to all electronic service may be used to service medical electronics equipment. There are, however, a few special items that are required.

For ECG Machines

One such item is an *electrocardiograph waveform simulator*, usually dubbed a "chicken heart" in the trade. This device is a highly specialized signal generator that produces a voltage waveform closely resembling the human ECG waveform pattern. Chicken hearts are available in both portable and workbench models. I prefer the Parke-Davis model *3150* shown in Fig. 15-1 for at least two reasons. First, it

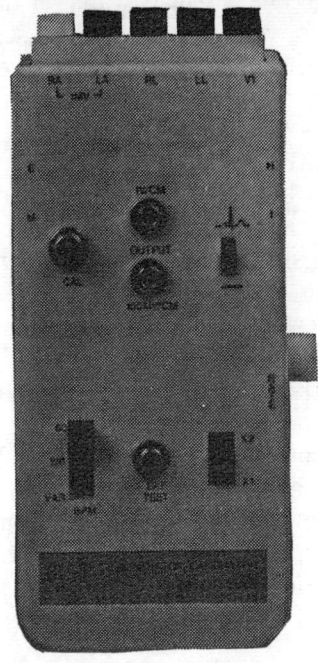

Fig. 15-1. ECG waveform simulation signal generator. Slang term for this instrument is "chicken heart." (Courtesy Parke-Davis)

produces all twelve leads—not just lead I. And second, it is slim enough to fit nicely into a tool case or labcoat pocket. Although not all of the features of the *3150* are desirable or necessary, you will find them helpful on occasion.

Portability is a requirement even for hospital-based technicians because much of your work will be on site. The equipment you work on will be either too much in use or too bulky to allow its removal to the lab for repair or inspection.

The availability of all twelve standard ECG leads will allow you to troubleshoot problems in the lead selector switch of the ECG preamplifier and in the patient cables. Those cables, by the way, fail frequently and are costly enough to have the medical people who use them interested in a repair, however temporary, rather than a replacement.

Electrosurgical Machines

Electrosurgical machines are little more than obsolete radio transmitters adapted to a special application. Of course, this little analogy doesn't hold water in the case of newer solid-state models, but it is valid for some of the older machines that are still in service and still very much alive. A few months prior to this writing, I found a machine that was still in daily use, still healthy and producing good output, and which has been purchased 23 years ago.

The similarity between the electrosurgical generator and a medium-wave radio transmitter is marked enough that procedures and instruments used in communications service are also usable in electrosurgery machine service. Because the typical electrosurgery generator operates in the 500–2500 kHz range, you are dealing with a relatively simple and well-behaved instrument, so can use some relatively simple test equipment.

Figure 15-2 shows a minimum, bare bones, electrosurgical tester that can be easily home-brewed from readily available components. This tester features two ranges in order to accommodate a wide range of rf power levels. Also provided are two different load impedances so that machines can be tested at either of the two commonly specified impedances, 250 and 500 ohms.

Resistors R1 through R4 are non-inductive types capable of dissipating at least 100 watts of rf power. If carbon resistors are available at reasonable cost, by all means use them. At these low frequencies, however, you can get away with using wire-wound resistors, provided that they are listed as *non-inductive*. These differ from regular power resistors in that the wire is wound in two bifilar coils connected such that their respective currents flow in opposite directions. This causes their magnetic fields to cancel each other.

Five-way banana binding posts are probably the most practical and universal connectors in this application. J1 and J2 are heavy-duty binding posts and are used to connect the tester to the output of the electrosurgical machine. J3 and J4, on the other hand, can be any convenient size binding post and are used for observing the electrosurgical output waveform on an oscilloscope (a desirable capability with modern chopped solid-state models).

Resistors R5 and R6 are selected to provide an attenuation suitable for the oscilloscope you are using. A ratio of 10,000:100 ohms is a good starting point usable by most people.

Meters M1 and M2 are thermocouple rf ammeters. M1 is selected to have a range of either 0–1.5 or 0–2 amperes and is used with higher powered machines. Meter M2, on the other hand, has a range of 0–500 milliamperes and is therefore useful on lower powered machines and on big machines set at lower power settings. Most rf ammeters are notoriously inaccurate on the lower ends of their scales, so M2 and M1 complement each other nicely.

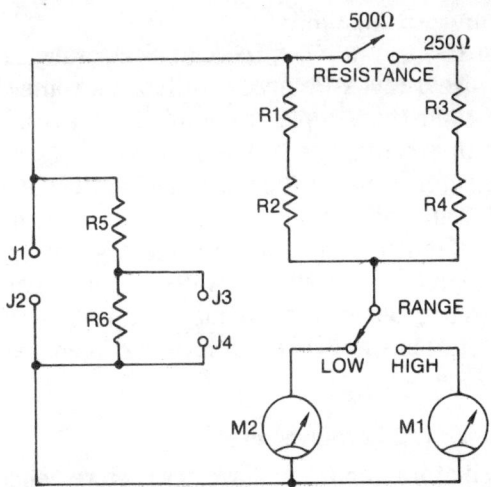

Fig. 15-2. Circuit diagram of an electrosurgery machine tester that can be built by the user.

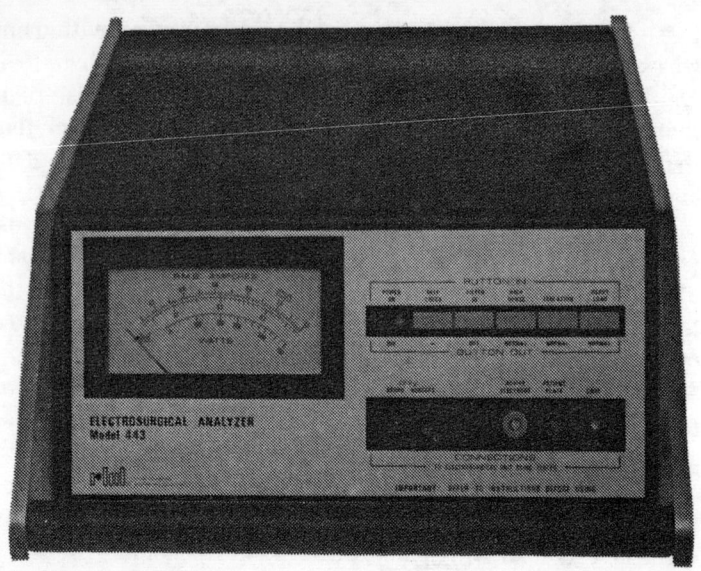

Fig. 15-3. Commercial electrosurgery machine analyzer. (Courtesy Neurodyne-Dempsey)

If you must ground one side of the the tester, then ground J2. This is not, however, recommended because grounded testers can prove dangerous to the servicer when the electrosurgery machine is improperly connected. Since the only reason to require a grounded tester is to interface with an oscilloscope, it might be better to only use an oscilloscope that has an A-minus-B capability.

Figure 15-3 shows a commercial electrosurgical analyzer made by Neurodyne-Dempsey. Although somewhat more expensive than the simple tester of the previous figure, it provides a more complete test of modern machines. Note that the manufacturer has calibrated the meter not only in rf amperes but in watts of power. This is advantageous because some manufacturers of electrosurgical generators specify their equipment's output in watts rather than current. Although you could easily calculate output power from the formula $I^2 R$, it is simpler to just have the figures available on the meter face.

Defibrillators and Cardioverters

Defibrillators and cardioverters store energy in a capacitor so that it can be discharged into the body of certain heart attack victims. The equipment you need to service and inspect defibrillators includes an oscilloscope (either storage type or with a Polaroid camera) and a defibrillator tester such as that shown in Fig. 15-4. These testers are actually little more than highly specialized integrating voltmeters that compute the energy in watt-seconds (joules) from the input voltage waveform.

The defibrillator is discharged through a dummy load resistor (50 ohms) located on top of the unit in the picture. The analyzer integrates the transient defibrillator voltage waveform, which is directly proportional to the energy delivered by the capacitor.

If your analyzer lacks an oscilloscope output jack, make one similar to that of Fig. 15-5. This is placed across the load resistor so its output is an attenuated version of the voltage

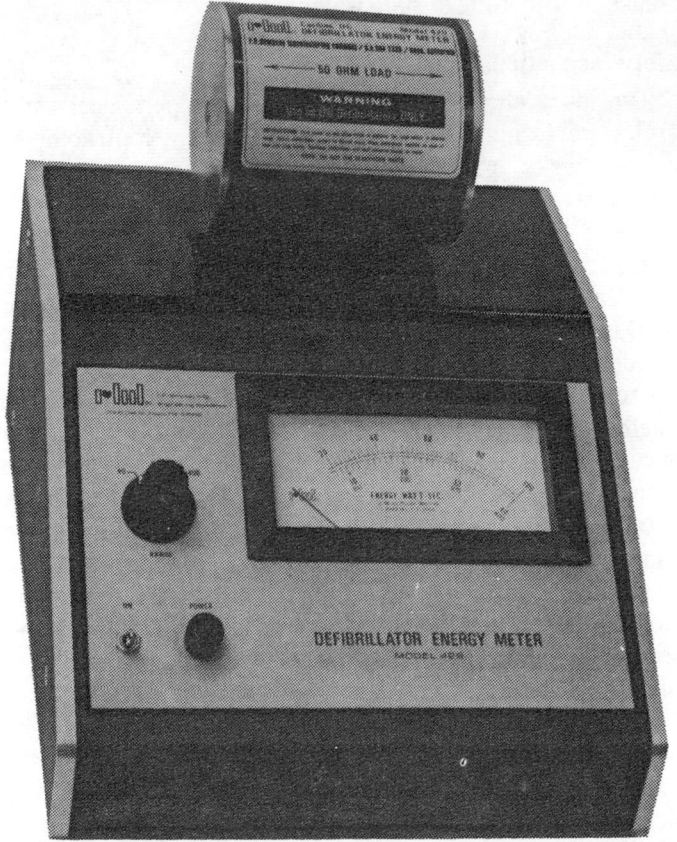

Fig. 15-4. Energy meter used to measure delivered output from a defibrillator. (Courtesy Neurodyne-Dempsey)

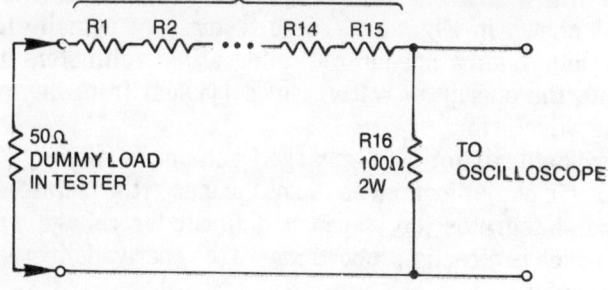

Fig. 15-5. Voltage divider across 50 ohm dummy load is used to adapt the defibrillator tester for oscilloscope viewing of the waveform.

applied to the dummy load. In Chapter 8 on defibrillators, we discuss the meaning of such waveforms.

Safety Inspections

One duty of many hospital electronics personnel (and a service performed on a fee basis by many contractors) is safety checks on equipment in patient areas, especially critical care areas. Details of certain classes of special safety problems are discussed in Chapter 16 and so will not be covered here. In order to perform the safety inspections, however, you will need certain special instruments and tools.

Dangerous current levels—in the medical context—are way down in the microampere range. You must therefore be able to test for leakage currents of less than 10 microamperes, which is the most often quoted specification. Similarly, you must be able to test for voltage drops on the order of a few millivolts between pieces of equipment. Figure 15-6 is a small, portable, combination microammeter and millivoltmeter made by Neurodyne-Dempsey.

Another portable instrument, also by the same manufacturer, is the Cordohmeter of Fig. 15-7. This is basically an ohmmeter adapted for use in medical electrical safety applications. On one range of the meter, you can check to see if ground leads have a truly low resistance, preferably in the milliohms range. In the other mode, this tester will check to see if there is more than one megohm between the powerline wires and ground.

Many areas of the hospital environment are "wet" zones—we find electrical cords and components soaking wet.

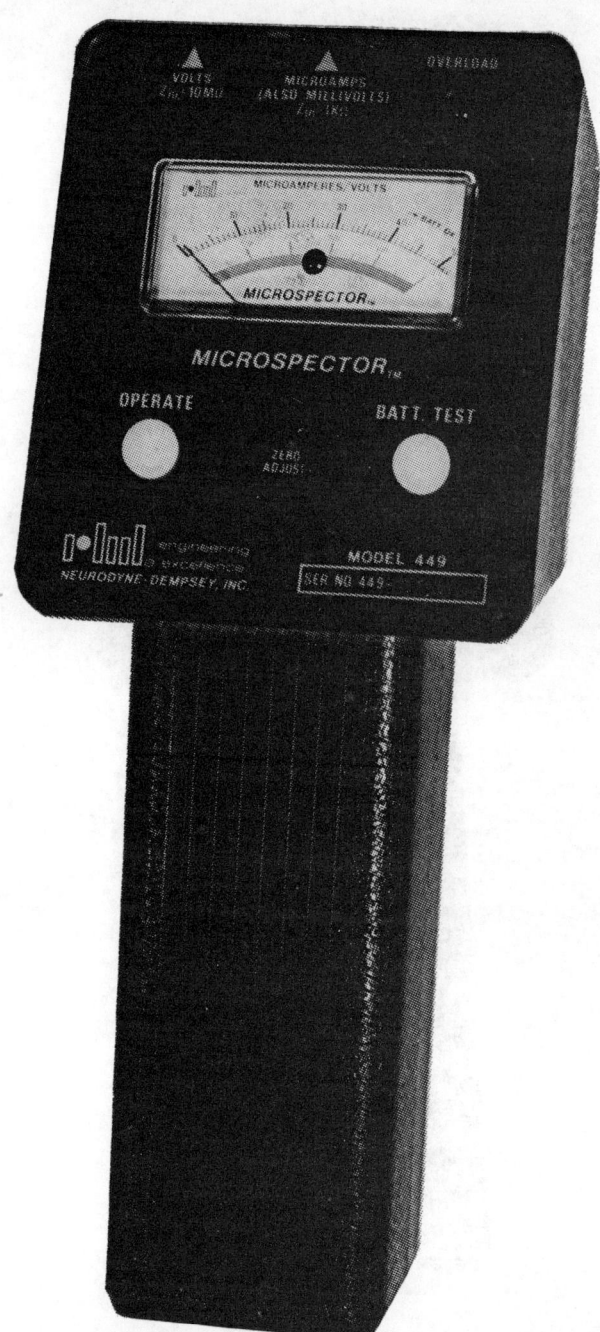

Fig. 15-6. Microammeter used to make ac leakage current survey inspections (Courtesy Neurodyne-Dempsey)

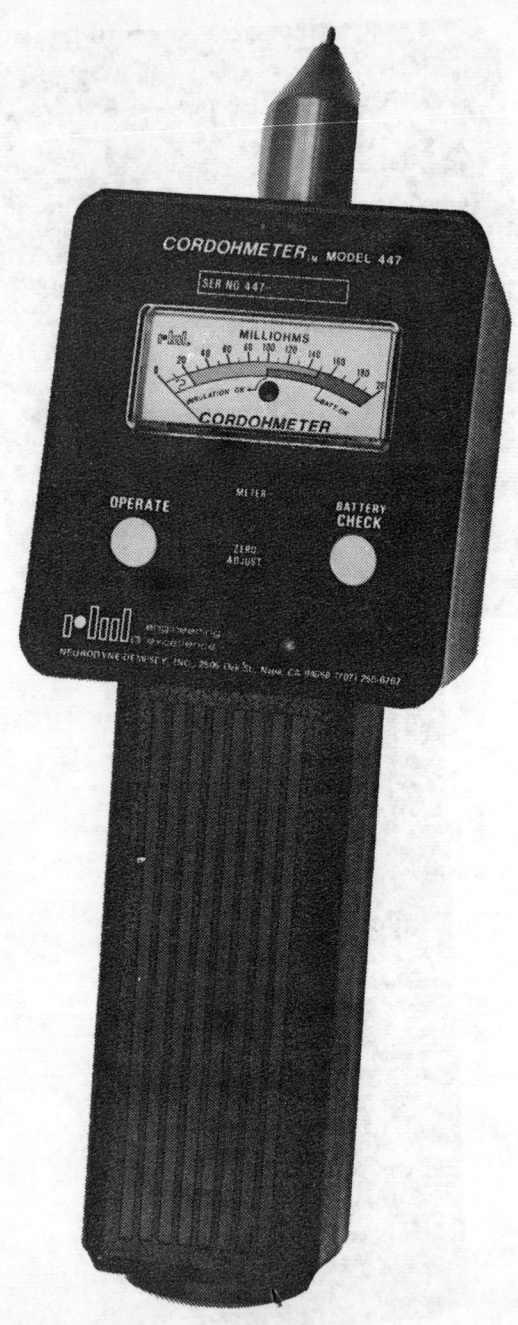

Fig. 15-7. Megohmmeter used to inspect electrical power cables. (Courtesy Neurodyne-Dempsey)

This lowers their resistance to ground and shunts some of the ac power to the chassis. Such a situation is a hazard, especially in kidney dialysis areas where some of the liquids are very conductive electrically relative to tap water. Distilled water, incidentally, is a poor electrical conductor, but impurities markedly reverse this situation and can make waterlogged equipment very dangerous.

Figure 15-8 shows a somewhat more comprehensive electrical safety analyzer that can be used to evaluate both the equipment and the electrical power distribution system. Besides having features found in other testers of a similar concept, this model also has the ability to check input-connector leakage currents in electrocardiograph machines.

Many areas of the hospital (especially those wet zones) must be protected by ground-fault interrupters (GFIs) in the electrical power system. If current down the ground wire (*not the neutral*) exceeds a certain allowable value, usually 5 mA, the GFI trips and removes power from the equipment served by that line.

The homebrew tester in Fig. 15-9 can be used to find the trip point of individual GFI devices. R1 and R2 are selected so

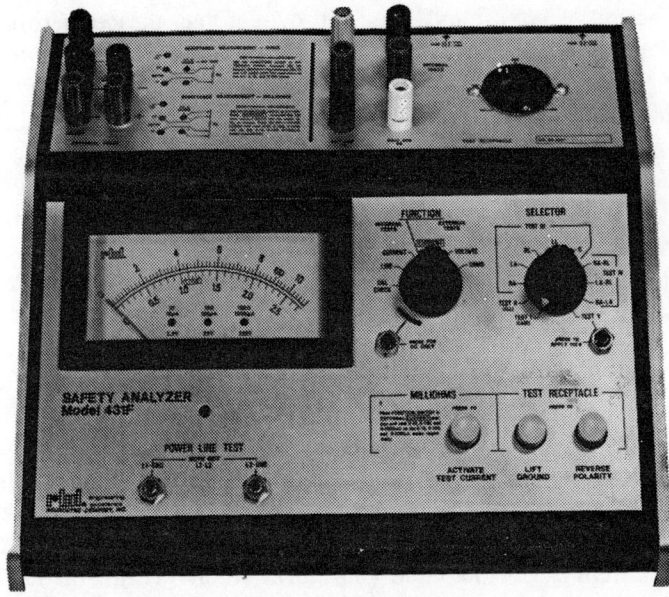

Fig. 15-8. Comprehensive electrical safety analyzer designed especially for hospital application. (Courtesy Neurodyne-Dempsey)

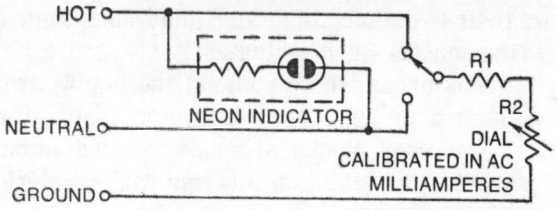

Fig. 15-9. Simple test circuit for inspecting ground-fault interrupters. Designed by C. McCullough, Bioelectronic Engineer at the George Washington University Medical Center.

that a current of 10 mA flows when the resistance of R2 is equal to zero ohms. R2 can be connected to a dial and calibrated in milliamperes. Initially, when making a test, set R2 to its maximum resistance value. Reduce the resistance slowly until the lamp goes out, indicating that the GFI has tripped.

MEDICAL INSTRUMENTATION CALIBRATION SYSTEM

One of the difficulties and frustrations of medical instrument service involves the test equipment. Test equipment of sufficient quality, yet highly portable, is often hard to locate. Many laboratories wind up with a hodgepodge collection of equipment acquired over a long period of time. Unfortunately, this can introduce compatibility problems, not to mention the motley appearance. Although it may take a bit of money and talk, there are now some new systems available to solve this age-old problem.

Figures 15-10 and 15-11, for example, illustrate a medical instrumentation calibration system (MICS) put together by Tektronix, Inc. This sytem is made up from its series *TM500* test equipment modules. While not a complete solution, this system is at least a partial answer to the test equipment integration problems of the medical electronics servicer. Two general configurations are recommended. A roll-around system can be built on a standard Tektronix Scopemobile cart, while a luggage-like portable system can be built in the power-supply mainframes. The Scopemobile system has an oscilloscope and two tiers of in-use instruments, plus a locked compartment in the lower tier for storage of unused instruments. The portable configuration shown in Fig. 15-11 has an oscilloscope module, a digital multimeter, and a digital frequency/period counter.

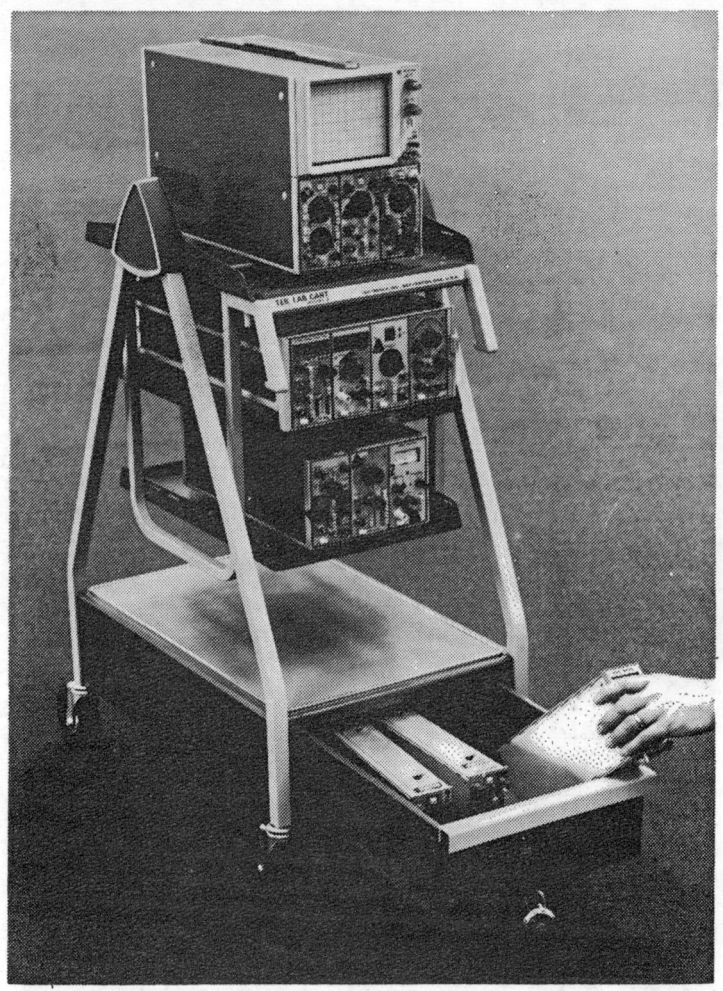

Fig. 15-10. Medical instrument calibration system (MICS) places all test equipment normally needed by the hospital electronics personnel on one cart. (Courtesy Tektronix, Inc.)

The *TM500* series includes a wide variety of test and measuring-equipment modules, but I would recommend only a few for an MICS cart. The standard MICS rack-up offered by Tektronix, incidentally, is a good compromise but there is no reason why you cannot mix 'em and match 'em to suit your own needs, prejudices, and budget. I suggest the following modules for medical work; you can select from them according to your own needs.

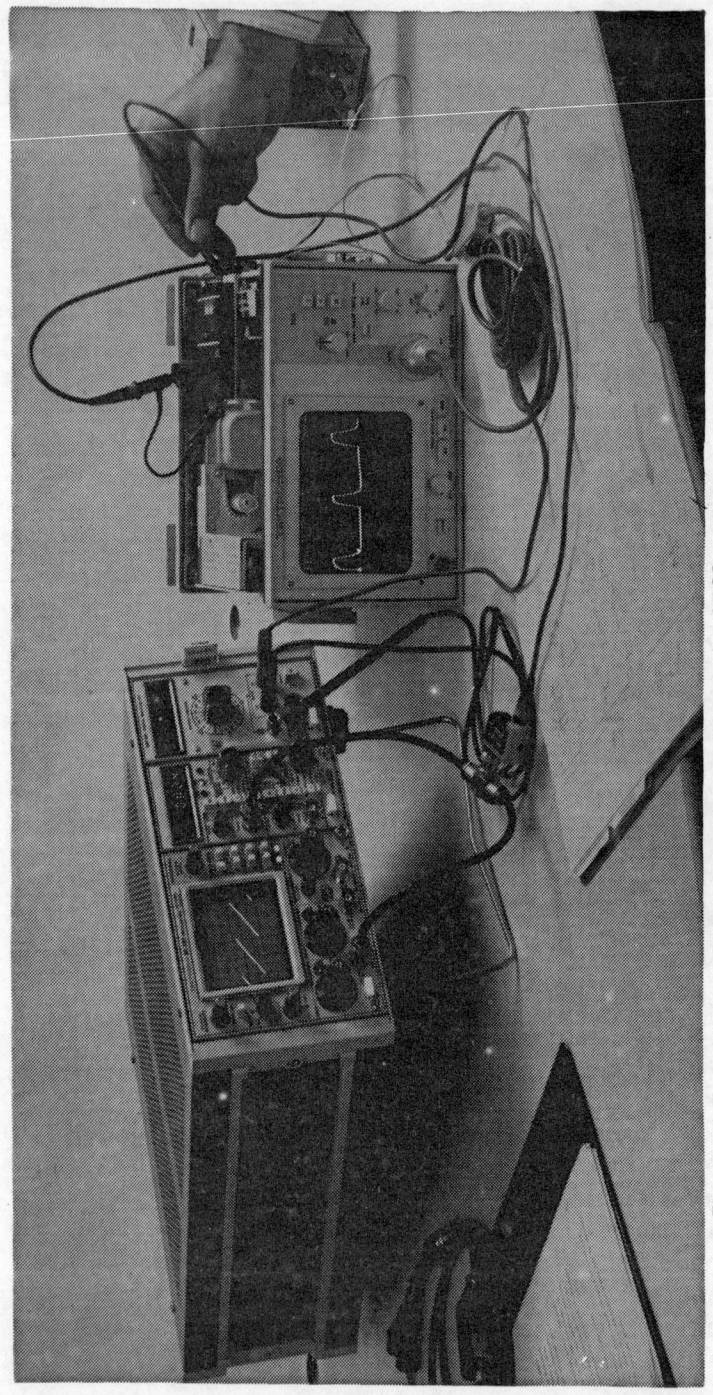

Fig. 15-11. Portable test-equipment system made up using MICS modules and a luggage-type power supply and housing. (Courtesy Tektronix, Inc.)

Counters:
- DC501—to 110 MHz
- DC502—to 550 MHz
- DC503—to 100 MHz, plus period
- DC504—to 80 MHz, plus period
- DC505—to 110 MHz, plus period

Digital Multimeters:
- DM501—4½ digit
- DM502—3½ digit

Signal Generators:
- FG501
- FG502

Power Supplies:
- PS501
- PS502
- PS503A

Mainframe Oscilloscopes:
- SC501
- SC502
- MR501

You should also select one of the regular, portable, storage oscilloscopes with a bandwidth at least to 15 MHz, plus storage capability. If a lot of digital servicing is anticipated, you might go ahead and specify one of the 50 to 100 MHz portables designed especially for that type of field service. Also select a small battery portable, such as the Tektronix *211* series, and be happy to trade off some bandwidth for totally portable operation. These oscilloscopes can easily fit into some of the briefcase tool kits typically used by field engineers. Once you have to stand on a ladder balancing a 20 pound, $3000 oscilloscope, you will surely see the wisdom of this purchase.

Chapter 16
Electrical Safety

In times past, when little in the way of electrical or electronic equipment was used in the hospital, electrical safety was not a big consideration and could be all but ignored with little consequence. Today, though, technological proliferation has made electrical safety a much larger and more important consideration. It is the job of all persons using or servicing electrically operated equipment to be on guard for certain defects and problems that could possibly forewarn of impending disaster.

ELECTRICAL SHOCK

Almost everyone with training in the practical aspects of electricity and electronics will have some familiarity with the possibility of electrical shock and the associated hazards. And most everyone of us was taught some standard do's and don'ts, with more than a little technical mythology. For example, "that 450 volt power supply isn't dangerous because it's the current that kills you." Well, ever hear of Ohm's law, fella?

One semi-official pronouncement aimed at a particular group of electronics technicians demands the following amusing, if not contradictory, rules be adhered to:

1—Never work on live equipment.
2—When working on the live equipment that you are never suppose to work on, keep your left hand in your pocket.

Both regulations appear to be the meddlesome handiwork of someone who has never had to work on any equipment. They do, however, serve nicely to illustrate the confusion existing.

Types of Electrical Shock

In medical environments we have to consider two separate categories of electrical shock, and these are designated *macroshock* and *microshock*. Macroshock is that form of electrical shock most familiar to us, but microshock can be just as fatal under the correct set of circrumstances. In this context, the use of the term *micro* is an unfortunate choice of words because it may tend to lull people into a lax attitude, allowing them to think we are merely talking about *small* shocks. Fatal electrical shocks, whether micro or macro, are hardly small to the person who was electrocuted!

The Hewlett-Packard Company, in their publication *Patient Safety* (application note AN-718), offers the following information regarding the effects of various milliampere current levels on the "average" human body, through *intact* skin.

Current Level	Effects
1 mA	Threshold of perception. Most people cannot feel currents less than this amount.
5 mA	Amount of electrical current accepted, by convention, as the maximum harmless flow through intact skin.
15 mA	Lowest current level where the victim can still let go.
50 mA	Painful electrical shock, some fainting possible. There is also a strong possibility of mechanical injury.
100–300 mA	Possibility of fatal ventricular fibrillation of the heart.

The threshold of perception will cause only a slight tingling sensation, but no real pain. At a higher current level, in excess of 5 mA, some mild pain is generally expected, and this will cause the victim to pull away sharply. Somewhere above 15 mA, the victim's muscles go into sustained contraction, and this prevents him from letting go. As current levels increase, so does the danger until, in the neighborhood of 100 to 300 mA, the victim may suffer a fatal cardiac arrhythmia, called *ventricular fibrillation*.

The point of electrical contact for most victims is the skin, and this can have a very high electrical resistance. Typical values of skin resistance vary from around one thousand to well over one million ohms. The actual resistance at any given time is dependent upon many factors, one of which is dampness. For instance, if your skin is exceptionally dry and has a resistance of one million ohms, the current flow when touching a one hundred volt electric line is:

$$I = E/R$$
$$= 10^2/10^6$$
$$= 10^{-4} \text{ A, or } 0.1 \text{ mA}$$

This value, a tenth of the so-called threshold of perception, is clearly well within the safe region under 5 mA. But suppose, in the same situation, the skin resistance had been on the order of one thousand ohms?

$$I = E/R$$
$$= 10^2/10^3$$
$$= 10^{-1} \text{ A, or } 100 \text{ mA}$$

This value comes disturbingly close to the level that is considered possibly fatal. Since such a wide variation in skin resistance can easily occur in the same person, you are prompted to avoid any accidental electrical contacts with even moderate voltages.

Microshock

But what about the hospitalized patient? Are the rules the same for him as for other people? The answer seems to be no. The levels of current believed to be dangerous are considerably less than those given above, since under conditions when the patient's skin is pierced, a path is provided for current to pass directly into the body.

Microshock occurs when a victim comes in contact with a source of electrical current through paths other than intact skin. Resistance values through internal organs vary somewhat, but figures between 50 and 500 ohms are commonly discussed. Your internal body fluids are mostly electrolytic in nature, and this is the reason for the extremely low resistances. Consequently, these fluids make it much easier to present a high-density current to the heart.

Normally, shock from small currents is not a worry because the high resistance of the patient's skin protects the heart. In medical environments, however, piercing the high resistance of the patient's skin is an everyday, necessary, and a very normal occurance. In surgery, obviously—but also IV needles, injections, cardiac catherization, and many other medical procedures.

Although no one knows for sure just what constitutes "safe" levels of microshock, standards have been developed based on research with dogs. It has been found that ventricular fibrillation can be induced in dogs with electrical currents as low as 20 *micro*amperes at 60 H ac.

One of the most insidious things about this is the fact that such low levels of current flow can easily occur from current sources that are "stray" and not normally accounted for in electronic equipment design. These are the so-called ac leakage currents. There is some amount of controversy over exactly what constitutes a maximum safe level for stray currents such as these. One of the arguments often heard is that it is impossible to extrapolate data from dogs, which have lower body weight and different physiology than man. Be well aware, though, that not all authorities accept the value taken from dog experiments and prefer a much higher value of 100 or even 140 μA.

In this book we are recommending that the most conservative standard be accepted until some authority determines that it is incorrect. This standard takes one-half the current that caused ventricular fibrillation in a dog as the maximum safe leakage current permitted to be applied to any one patient. The dog value was 20 μA, so the standard we are adopting is 10 μA, which is more or less the standard taken as the correct value adopted by hospital insurance carriers.

Now that we are aware that some frighteningly low values of 60 Hz current can be lethal, we can do something about the situation. But first, how many patients do you suppose are electrocuted in U. S. hospitals every year? One medical authority claims the correct figure to be absolutely zero, while a noted consumer advocate put the figure around 5000 cases annually. To me, both figures ring rather hollow and sound like they are based on self-interest rather than hard, scientific investigations. The real figures are probably somewhere in between these two extremes. It is also likely that the figures for recent years are lower than the figures for past years because the awareness of medical people is so much better. In recent times, equipment manufacturers, malpractice insurers, electronics people, hospital administrators, and medical personnel have all recognized that dangerous situations can and do exist, and they have taken positive steps and efforts to reduce the incidence of such hazards. Part of their safety program is the adoption and enforcement of conservative electrical standards.

MECHANICS OF MICROSHOCK

The question might fairly be asked, "just what are the sources and causes of microshock?" Well, microshock can theoretically occur whenever a potential difference great enough to cause a current flow over 10 μA is connected across the patient.

You would naturally expect that certain equipment designs, now years out of date and hopefully no longer in use, could cause such dangerous situations. But they pale into insignificance when compared with the dangerous leakage currents from equipment of modern design when operating quite normally. Consider Fig. 16-1, for example. Capacitance exists between any two electrical conductors placed in close proximity to each other. The chassis and normal power wiring in the equipment, therefore, form the elements of the

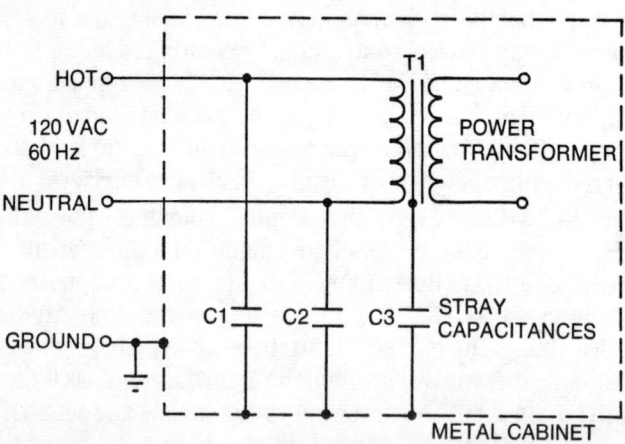

Fig. 16-1. Leakage currents from ac powerlines are caused by capacitive coupling between the power wiring and the chassis. A third wire in the power cable is used to carry these currents harmlessly to ground.

capacitors represented by C1, C2, and C3. Although these capacitances may have what seems to be very low values, they still have sufficiently low capacitive reactance at 60 Hz to allow the passage of considerable current in 120 volt circuits.

In older medical equipment, no longer permitted in hospitals, and in certain classes of consumer equipment, the power cable from the ac powerlines have only two wires (hot and neutral). In these devices, the leakage current remains on the chassis unless some path to ground is provided inadvertently. If such an appliance is used out of doors, or in a basement with a concrete floor, it can cause mild shocks in the threshold of perception. That current, though, is considerably larger than the current required to place a patient in danger from microshock.

Equipment which is approved for use in the hospital must always have a three-wire power cord. The third wire provides a safe chassis ground, and its sole purpose is to carry leakage currents off harmlessly to ground. In such equipment, then, the normal standard is less than 5 mA flowing in the third-wire ground lead and less than 10 μA escaping to ground through other paths.

Leakage current levels are measured by an ac microammeter, which is usually called a leakage tester when purchased specially for hospital use. These are covered in Chapter 15. Most testers are equipped with a probe and a ground fitting that can be inserted into the ground hole on any convenient duplex wall receptacle. The probe is then touched to equipment chassis, and the leakage current is read from the meter. Normally, the current will be less than 10 μA, but any more than this amount indicates a failure that must be diagnosed and corrected.

POTENTIALLY DANGEROUS SITUATIONS

Let us assume a situation in which a patient is connected to an ECG machine that is grounded. It is of an older design, so we find that the patient's right leg is connected directly to the same chassis ground serving the powerline. (Modern ECG machines connect the patient common through a special right-leg amplifier or isolation circuit.) The patient is also connected to some other electrical appliance, say, to an electric bed. This bed has a ground wire carrying 100 μA of leakage current to ground. Since the ECG machine is also grounded, a parallel path exists for this leakage current to flow to ground both through the ECG machine and through the ground wire of the bed. Assuming a nominal patient resistance of 500 ohms and a ground-wire resistance of 0.1 ohm, it is easy to see that most of the current would flow through the ground wire rather than the patient. In such a parallel circuit, the amount of current flowing through the patient would be:

$$I = \frac{(100 \, \mu A) \, (0.1)}{(500 + 0.1)} = 0.02 \, \mu A$$

This value, of course, is clearly within the safe limits of even the most conservative standards. However, if the ground wire on the bed should break, or if the power outlet ground should be faulty, then the full 100 μA would flow through the patient to the ground of the ECG machine. This is obviously a dangerous situation because the leakage current is ten times the maximum safe level of 10 μA.

Two-wire appliances such as lamps, radios, and television sets present a special danger in the hospital environment. A patient with an indwelling catheter, IV needle, or open wound would be in danger should a leakage current choose that path to enter his body. If another person should touch both the patient and that appliance, a possibly fatal current could flow, yet be so small as to never be felt by the person making the conductive bridge. Recall that a current as little as 10 μA is officially dangerous, yet the threshold of perception is one hundred times higher (1 mA). For this reason, most hospitals and their insurance carriers ban all two-wire appliances from patient care areas. The only way these can be considered even remotely safe is if they are operated from an approved isolation transformer that is itself grounded and fitted with a three-wire cord.

Consider the second example in Fig. 16-2 where we again have two instruments or appliances connected to the patient. These could be the ECG monitor and an electrical bed, as in the previous case, or they could be any two other instruments. For each instrument, the sum of the resistances of the electrical wiring and the ground contacts is one ohm, as measured from true ground. Assume that the first instrument has a leakage current of 4 mA and that the second instrument is passing 2 mA. The voltage drop between the two chassis is:

$$E = IR$$
$$= (0.004)(1) + (0.002)(1)$$
$$= 0.006 \text{V ac}$$

If the patient's electrical resistance is the standard nominal value of 500 ohms, the current is:

$$I = E/R$$
$$= 0.006/500$$
$$= 12 \,\mu\text{A}$$

If we accept the 10 μA standard, this is clearly an intolerable situation. But an even more dangerous situation exists if the current in one or the other ground increases to a higher value. The classic situation, most often quoted in the hospital safety literature, uses a floor-buffing machine in the next room as a frightening and seemingly occult cause of patient electrocution. The economics of construction dictate (in typical wisdom) that outlets on walls between adjoining rooms must share the same powerlines. Thus, a buffing machine plugged into the adjoining outlet in another room could seriously upset the ground potentials of any medical

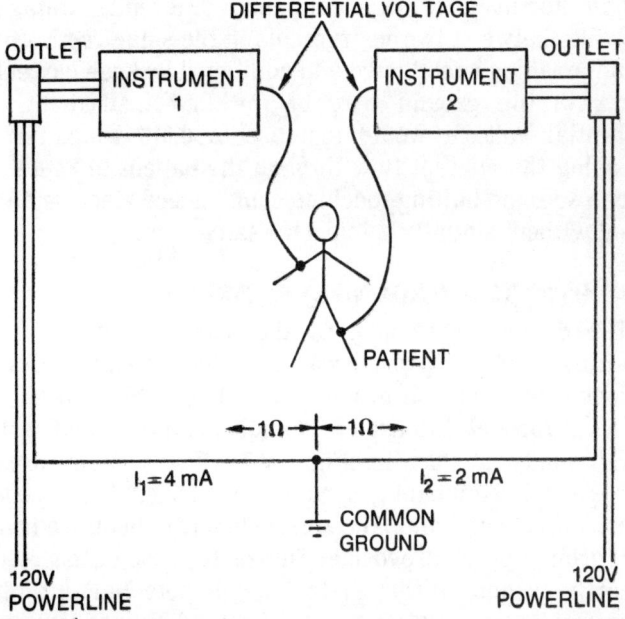

Fig. 16-2. One cause for possible electrocution due to excessive leakage currents.

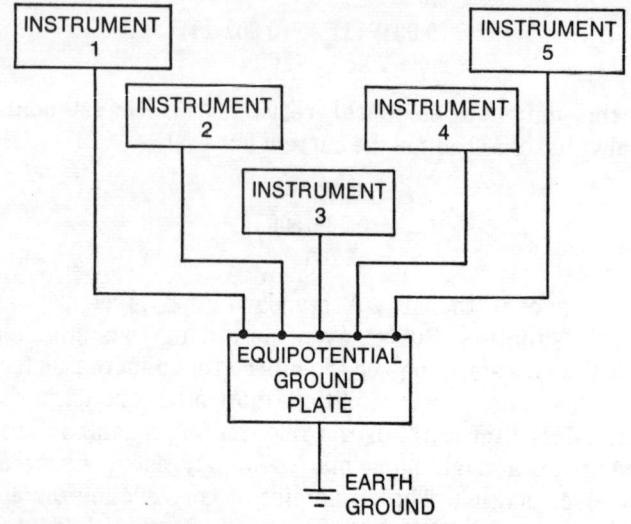

Fig. 16-3. An equipotential ground system (EGS) is used to keep differential ground potentials reduced to a value low enough to prevent a situation such as that in Fig. 16-1.

instrument sharing the same powerline. In the second example, for instance, we calculated a differential voltage of 0.006 volts between two instruments in the same room. If the buffing machine contributed and additional leakage current of 10 mA in the ground wire of the first instrument, the differential voltage would increase to 0.016 volts, further increasing the current flow through the patient to 32 μA. As you can see, the buffing machine could indeed electrocute the patient without actually being in the same room.

EQUIPOTENTIAL GROUND SYSTEMS

The dangers presented by the buffing machine in the preceding example arise because of the grounding system employed. Such unsafe ground currents can be reduced to a safe level through the use of an equipotential ground system (EGS) such as that in Fig. 16-3. This system uses a heavy-gauge, redundant ground wire to connect the chassis of all instruments and appliances close to any patient to a heavy, local, ground plate at bedside. This plate is then connected to an earth ground. Although the actual potential difference between this ground plate and true ground may be quite high due to leakage currents flowing in the resistance of the main ground wire, the differential voltage between the instruments in the room will be well below the dangerous point.

EGS systems are commonly found in coronary care units, intensive care units, dialysis units, cath labs, special procedures X-ray rooms, and other critical care areas. All equipment, instruments, and appliances in the immediate vicinity of the patient's bed must be grounded to the equipotential ground system. This includes all lighting fixtures and permanently installed metal surfaces. Portable, temporary, or occassionally used equipment must also be equipped with heavy ground wires that can be plugged into jacks on the EGS plate. Some hospital units may keep a heavy EGS ground plug, which has a 50 or 100 ampere-size alligator clip on one end, to connect rarely used equipment to the EGS ground plate.

ISOLATED ELECTRICAL SYSTEMS

Operating rooms use some heavy current-drain appliances and may also have conductive flooring. Because of this, and to guard against the buffing machine problem, most operating rooms are equipped with an *isolated* electrical system. All outlets in any one room are powered from a single 1:1 or 2:1 isolation transformer located in a panel within the room. Although a ground wire is usually supplied, this ground becomes electrically isolated due to the transformer, so there will ordinarily be no potential between it and either of the two wires coming from the secondary winding of the transformer, and power can be tapped only across these two wires. Most isolated electrical systems are equipped with a ground fault alarm that will turn on a buzzer if any appreciable current does flow from either secondary line through the ground line. And it is designed so that the alarm will also sound if the ground wire on any appliance connected to the secondary should become open.

Another aspect of the operating room electrical environment is protection against the explosion of certain types of anesthesia gases. Some of these are indeed explosive and can be easily ignited by electrical sparks. Since these gases are heavier than air, they tend to collect near the floor, so a danger zone exists between the floor and a level 5 feet above the floor. All outlets and appliances operating at a potential greater than 8 volts must be either of an approved explosion-proof design or they must be physically located more than 5 feet off the floor.

Static electricity can also ignite such gases. Therefore, to prevent the occurance of sparks due to the discharge of static electricity, operating room floors are made of a conductive material. Personnel in the operating room must wear either special conductive shoes or conductive shoe covers over regular shoes. Equipment and furniture on rollers in the operating room must be fitted with special conductive casters. All these tactics place a resistance of 25,000 to 1,000,000 ohms between the object or person and ground. This allows a value low enough to discharge the static electricity before it becomes a spark, yet it is not so low that it becomes dangerous to operating room personnel should a catastrophic equipment failure occur in which a 120 volt line touches an ungrounded chassis. Even if the floor resistance is only 25,000 ohms, the minimum value, the current flow from the worst case 120V ac accident would amount to less than 5 mA, the value assumed to be maximum harmless amount through intact skin.

POINTS INSURING SAFE SYSTEMS

Electrical safety is no mystery, even in the medical environment where the sources of possible trouble are seemingly everywhere. The basic principles of electrical safety are known and need only be applied.

One solid cornerstone of any safety program is inspection—on a regular, periodic basis. The inspection should include a leakage test using a tester such as discussed in Chapter 15. Also, test the duplex ac outlets for correct wiring and proper blade or ground-lug tension. Instrutek, Inc. of Annapolis, Md. manufactures test devices for this purpose.

Inspection can provide a valuable defense against electrical hazards. But it can also provide a false sense of security if nurses and other personnel are allowed to fall into the unfortunate belief that all is well if there is a recent date on an inspection sticker. The inspector can guarantee only that the equipment was in proper order at the time of inspection. It must be realized that dangerous faults can occur immediately after the inspector leaves.

Nursing personnel and doctors use the equipment day in and day out, so they must provide the first line of defense in keeping electrical faults to a minimum. They should be educated to recognize anomalies and faults that might otherwise escape them. They should immediately report frayed or broken cords, deviations from expected or normal operation, "tingly feelings," overt shock incidents, and any controls, knobs, or switches that don't operate or do what they used to.

All reports concerning electrical safety should be given fast response, even if you suspect that no real danger exists. Besides the fact that you might be wrong, and a real fault exists, there is the possibility that a slow or unenergetic response might lead the staff to think, "So what, if they aren't concerned about it, why should I." The "boy who cried wolf..." might apply, but still, go see if the electrical wolf is at the door. That way you will stay free from criticism.

Testing of conductive floors is also necessary, and this should be done on a regular basis. Dirt, wax, and other assorted filth conspire to raise the electrical resistance well above allowed limits. The standard test procedure is to measure the resistance between 2 metallic discs that have a 2.5 inch diameter and a weight of 5 pounds and are located 3 feet apart.

Chapter 17

X-Ray Apparatus

X-rays are well known even in ordinary experience. Almost everyone has been X-rayed at one time or another by a medical doctor, dentist, or radiologist. In fact, it was the medical applications that caused the X-ray industry to grow. Besides medical uses, however, they are also used in industry for quality control purposes, and by researchers in the scientific fields of chemistry, physics, and biology. X-rays are a means for photographing the interior structures of objects normally opaque to visible light.

It was not until November 8, 1895, however, that X-rays were even known. Even then, their discover, W.K. Roentgen, only called them *X-rays* because their nature was not known. The name has persisted even until today, despite the fact that considerably more is known about them. In honor of their discoverer, since 1925 the internationally accepted unit for X-ray quantity has been called the *Roentgen*.

PROPERTIES OF X-RAYS

Before discussing the types of diagnostic X-ray apparatus commonly found in hospitals, let's first review briefly the physics of X-rays. These "rays" are actually electromagnetic waves, much like radio signals and light. Figure 17-1 shows a spectrum chart giving the relationship of the respective frequencies in the electromagnetic spectrum. Elec-

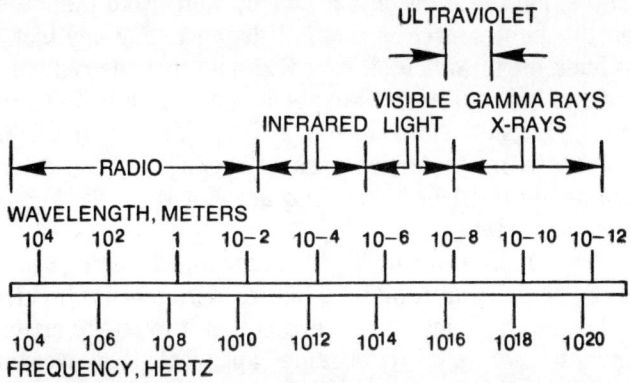

Fig. 17-1. Electromagnetic spectrum chart showing the relative wavelengths of radio, light, and X-ray waves.

tromagnetic waves are different from other types because they can travel in a vacuum and are thereby propagated even through outer space. Electromagnetic waves are said to have the following properties, some of them in common with other types of waves:

1—They obey the relationship $V = F\lambda$.
2—The relative intensity of electromagnetic waves will obey the inverse square law: their intensity is proportional to $1/D^2$.
3—They propagate rectilinearly.
4—They are not deflected by magnetic fields.
5—They produce interference and diffraction phenomena.

The first property was discussed in Chapter 13 on ultrasonic waves and is fundamental to all wave phenomena. It merely states that the velocity of wave propagation is equal to the product of frequency and wavelength. In the case of electromagnetic waves, this velocity is the speed of light, denoted by the letter c and equal to approximately 3×10^8 meters per second.

The inverse square law states that the field intensity falls off as the reciprocal of the square of the distance, $I = 1/D^2$. This simply means that doubling the distance from a point-source radiator will cause the relative intensity to diminish to a quarter of the previous intensity. This effect can be demonstrated with an ordinary flashlight. Turn the switch on and shine the light onto a nearby wall. Note the intensity when the light source is a small distance, say one foot, and then back off to four feet. You will note that the reduction in the intensity is quite a bit—to about one sixteenth. The amount of energy hasn't changed, but at a longer distance, it must illuminate a much larger area of the wall. This particular phenomenon must be taken into account when working with X-ray equipment.

It was in the study of electromagnetic phenomena, namely *black body* thermal radiation, that modern physics broke with the classical physics then prevalent. In the later part of the nineteenth century, it became apparent that Newtonian physics could not account for observed facts concerning electromagnetic phenomena. Whenever scientists find that observations in nature or in the experimental laboratory contradict a theory, then that theory must be either modified or scrapped to make room for a new all-encompassing theory.

Modern physics began in the year 1900 when a classical physicist named Max Planck proposed, in a paper presented before the German Physical Society, the notion that electromagnetic energy must be *quantized*. That is to say, it can only exist in certain discrete packages now called *photons*. According to this view, photon energy follows the relationship:

$$E = hF = hc/\lambda$$

where E = energy
F = frequency
h = Planck's constant (6.62×10^{-34} joule-sec)
c = speed of light (3×10^8 m/sec)
λ = wavelength in meters

Example. A certain electromagnetic wave has a wavelength of 6000 angstroms. What is its energy level? First, convert the units of wavelength into the appropriate MKS metric units. All terms in a problem must be in the same units of measure and we already have Planck's constant in MKS units.

$$(6000 \text{ Å}) (10^{-10} \text{ m/Å}) = 6 \times 10^{-7} \text{ m}$$

Second, set up the problem and turn the crank,

$$E = hc/\lambda = \frac{(6.62 \times 10^{-34})(3 \times 10^8)}{(6 \times 10^{-7})} = 3.31 \times 10^{-19} \text{ joules}$$

In the paragraphs to follow we shall discuss certain quantum phenomena, but only as they relate to the understanding of medical X-ray equipment. For those who wish to pursue this course of self-study, permit me to recommend some books:

1—*Relativity and Early Quantum Theory* by Robert Resnick.
2—*Thirty Years that Shook Physics* by George Gamow.
3—*Mr. Tompkins in Wonderland* by George Gamow.

The first of these is a college freshman or sophomore textbook in physics and is a little more mathematical than the other two selections. The latter titles, though, are extremely readable, popular treatments and are as humorous as physics books can be. There are surely other good books on this subject.

George Gamow, incidentally, was a participant in some of the physics research that went on in those *Thirty Years*. The *Mr. Tompkins* book is a whimsical thing in which the hero dreams of the world as it might be if Planck's constant were on the order of unity, and the speed of light was attainable, or at least approachable in ordinary conveyances.

In this book, we are going to describe five quantum phenomena: The photoelectric effect, the Compton effect, pair production, pair annihilation, and bremsstrahlung.

PHOTOELECTRIC EFFECT

Albert Einstein is perhaps best known to the general public for his theories of relativity. The first of these is called the special theory of relativity and was published in the 1905 edition of *Annalen Der Physik*. Interestingly enough, though, it was his work on the photoelectric effect that won for Einstein the Nobel prize in physics. Albert Einstein published four papers in the year 1905, all of which could have earned him a big reputation in the world of physics. Since that volume of *Annalen Der Physik* became so important to the history of modern physics, it has all but disappeared from library shelves; all copies stolen by souvenier collectors.

The photoelectric effect was first noted by Heinrich Hertz in 1887 during an experiment to confirm one of Maxwell's predictions. Photoelectric effect is the emission of electrons from a clean metallic surface when electromagnetic radiation falls onto that surface. There are at least four different phenomena which can cause electrons to be released from a metallic surface. Besides photoelectric effect there is also thermionic emission, field emission, and secondary emission.

Thermionic emission is the process that creates the electron current in vacuum tubes. The metal object is heated to incandescence, and this imparts thermal energy to the free electrons. Some of the more energetic surface electrons actually "boil off" from the surface into space.

Field emission is the attraction of electrons from the surface by a strong electric field.

Secondary emission is a problem in ordinary vacuum tubes and the mode of operation of X-ray generator vacuum tubes. This occurs when a rapidly moving electron strikes the metallic plate, imparting some of its kinetic energy to electrons in the plate. If enough energy is transferred to these electrons, they may jump off the surface, creating a secondary emission of electrons.

Figure 17-2 shows an experiment used to study the photoelectric effect. When light strikes the positive anode, electrons will be emitted. These electrons will be moving with a kinetic energy of:

$$E = \tfrac{1}{2} m_e v^2$$

where m_e = mass of an electron (9.11×10^{-31} kg)
v = velocity of the electrons in meters per second

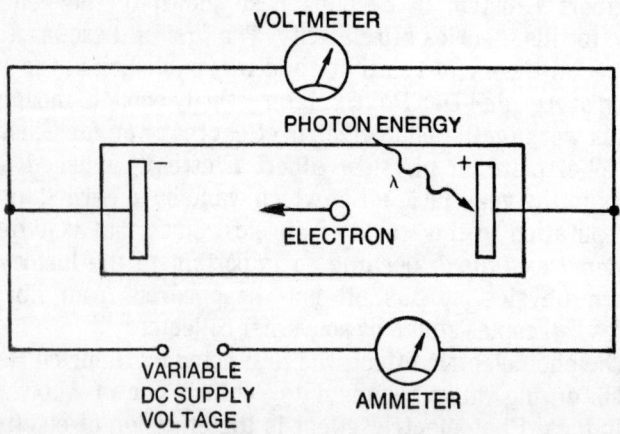

Fig. 17-2. Apparatus used to demonstrate the photoelectric effect.

The external power supply creates an electric field that opposes the electrons and creates a retarding influence on their motion. At some potential V_0 even the most energetic electrons will be retarded so that no current flows in the external circuit. The energy situation under these circumstances is:

$$eV_0 = \tfrac{1}{2} m_e v_M^2$$

where e = electron charge
V_0 = external voltage
v_M = velocity of the most energetic electrons

One interesting aspect of the photoelectric effect is that V_0 is independent of light intensity but *is* dependent upon the frequency (color) of the impinging light wave. Light photons striking the metallic surface have an energy $E = hF$ presented earlier. Each photon can only give up all of its energy to a single electron (fractions are not permitted), so we can write:

$$hF = \tfrac{1}{2} m_e v_M^2 + hF_0$$

The extra term, hF_0, is called the *work function* and is a property of the particular material comprising the metallic cathode surface. Frequency F_0 is the critical frequency that must be exceeded for the photoemission of electrons to occur. Photoemission can only occur if hF is greater than hF_0.

COMPTON EFFECT

The Compton effect is a phenomenon by which a photon can impart only a part of its energy to a charged particle such as an electron. This situation is illustrated in Fig. 17-3. In part A of the figure, an electron is at rest and lying in the path of an incident photon with energy level hF. This photon "collides" with the electron and some of its energy is imparted to the electron. This, incidentally, implies that photons carry momentum. In fact, the momentum of the photon is equal to:

$$P = E/c = hF/c = h/\lambda$$

where E = energy
F = frequency of the photon
c = speed of light
h = Planck's constant
λ = wavelength

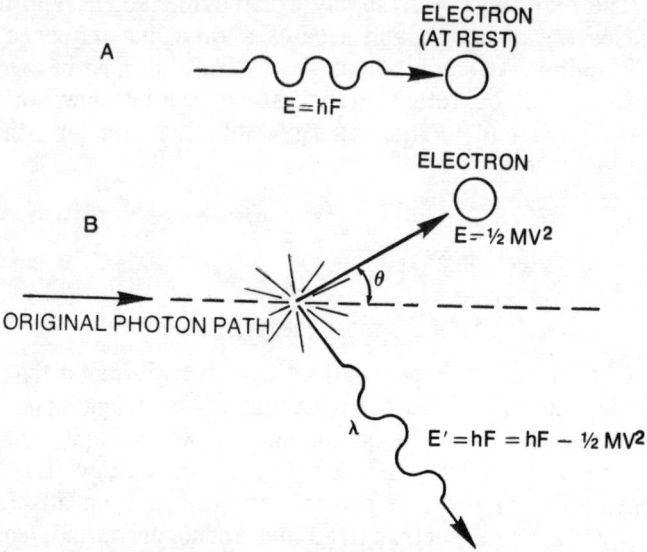

Fig. 17-3. The Compton effect is a means by which an incident photon can give up only part of its energy to a nearby electron.

The photon will still exist after the collision because it only imparts a portion of its energy to the electron. It will, however, exist at a lower frequency (longer wavelength) because of the lost energy. The energy lost to the electron will become kinetic energy, setting, the electron in motion. A particle at rest has a potential energy of $U = mc^2$, so by conservation of energy:

$$hF + U = hF' + U'$$

where U' is the potential energy of the recoiling electron, and the other terms have been previously defined.

The loss of energy means that photon hF' has a longer wavelength, λ'. The difference in wavelength, $\Delta\lambda$, is given by:

$$\Delta\lambda = 1/F - 1/F' = (h/Mc)(1 - \cos(\theta))$$

where θ is the angle of deflection shown in Fig. 17-3.

The kinetic energy of the moving electron is:

$$E = hF\left(\frac{\Delta\lambda}{\lambda + \Delta\lambda}\right)$$

BREMSSTRAHLUNG

The word *bremsstrahlung* is German for *braking radiation*. An example of bremsstrahlung is shown in Fig. 17-4. An electron with kinetic energy E_1 approaches and is deflected by the heavy nucleus of a nearby atom. After the deflection, the electron has a new level of energy, E_2. By considerations of energy conservation:

$$E_1 - E_2 = hF$$

X-rays are generated by bremsstrahlung, and they are merely photons (electromagnetic waves) with a wavelength of approximately one angstrom (10^{-10} meters).

X-RAY TUBES

Figure 17-5 shows an elementary X-ray tube. Electrons are boiled off the cathode by thermionic emission, much like as in any other form of vacuum tube. These electrons are accelerated through a potential to an energy of eV. Their kinetic energy upon striking the target anode is:

$$eV = E = \tfrac{1}{2} m_e v^2$$

Since the energy of the emitted photons is related to the kinetic energy of the impinging electrons, we can conclude that the energy level of the emitted photons is proportional to photon frequency, so the predominant frequency of emitted X-rays shifts higher as voltage across the tube is increased.

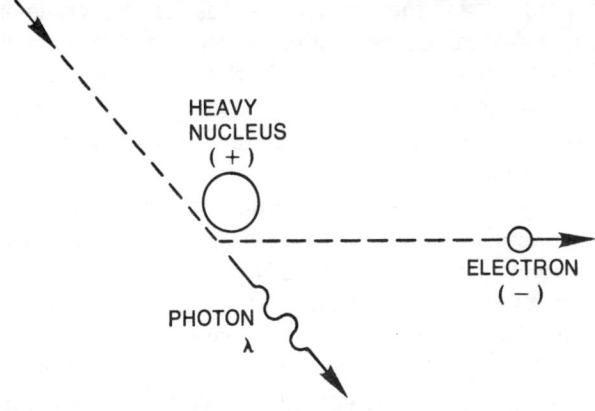

Fig. 17-4. Diagram of a bremsstrahlung collision by which X-rays are produced.

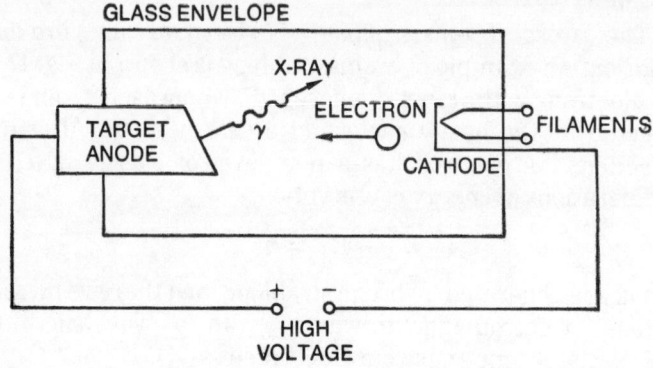

Fig. 17-5. An elementary X-ray tube.

Not all electron kinetic energy is converted to X-ray photons, however. In fact, a considerable amount is turned into thermal energy. Consequently, the target anode must withstand a large amount of heat. This problem is partially overcome through judicious construction of the target anode; tungsten targets embedded in a massive copper structure seem popular.

In all areas of engineering people speak of *trade-offs*—which actually means *compromises*, but is more palatable. This is also true in X-ray tube design with the target anode size. Maximum thermal capacity requires the largest possible target area. Best photographic resoltuion, on the other hand, requires the smallest possible target area. The target anode area, then, must be considered a trade-off in X-ray tube design. Anode geometry (see Fig. 17-6) provides a partial answer. By beveling the anode surface 15 to 19 degrees, we can reduce apparent focal size of the tube while, at the same time, keeping the true area large, as required by thermal considerations.

Heat generated by electron bombardment of the anode and electrical heating of the cathode filament causes at least one other problem. Like all electron tubes, the X-ray tube must operate in a vacuum. This requires that the cathode and anode structures be inside an evactuated glass envelope. Manufacturers of such tubes are very careful to design the glass envelope and anode-cathode structures to have similar coefficients of thermal expansion, so that the seals where wires pass through the envelope are not broken during the expansion/contraction cycles. Some tube designs use an intermediate glass shield between these structures and the overall glass shield, and this intermediate shield has a coefficient of expansion midway between the two.

X-ray tubes with anodes such as those just discussed are called *stationary anode* designs. Figure 17-7 shows a housing for such a tube. There are three requirements which must be met by the housing:

1—Electrostatic shielding of the high-voltage section.
2—Radiation shielding.
3—Heat dissipation.

The first of these is amply met by a metallic construction and adequate grounding.

The second requirement is occasioned by the fact that X-ray tubes fire radiation in many directions, not just in the direction desired. To overcome this, X-ray machine manufacturers line the insides of the housing with lead shielding.

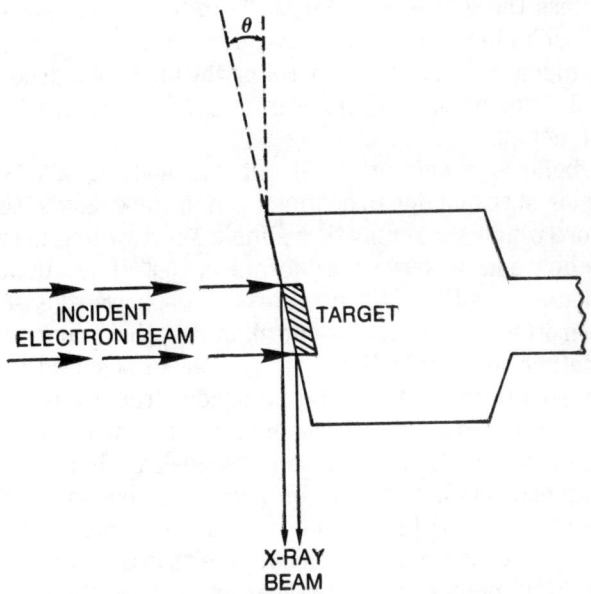

Fig. 17-6. Use of a small-area X-ray target embedded in a large copper heat sink allows proper heat dissiapation yet retains the small-size focal spot needed for resolution.

303

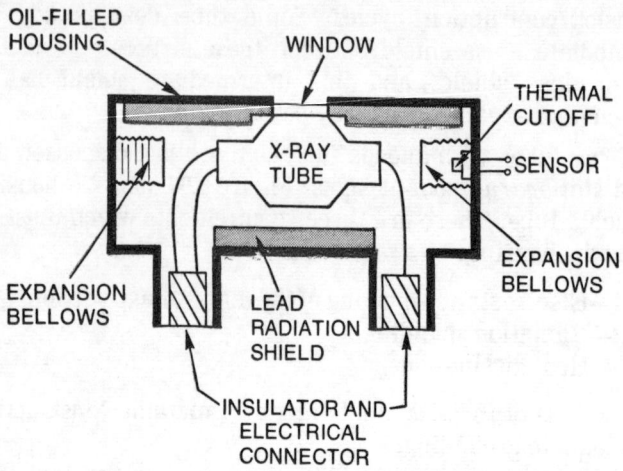

Fig. 17-7. Construction of the X-ray tube housing prevents leadage of X-rays in undesired directions and keeps personnel from contacting lethal high-voltage points.

X-ray tubes must be operated at voltages between 30 and 150 kilovolts. Such high potentials can easily arc across an air gap unless the gap is very large. Transformer oil, however, has a much higher dielectric strength, so a gap filled with oil can be much smaller. Thus, by filling the high-voltage housing with oil, the manufacturers reduce substantially their size requirements.

A bellows assembly inside of the housing allows for expansion of the oil due to heating from the tube. Some include a sensor (which needs only be a simple Microswitch) in one or both bellow ends to serve as a thermal cut out. If heat builds up an amount to sufficiently compress the bellows, this sensor will turn off the power supply and allow the tube to cool down.

Another solution to the heating problem is shown in Fig. 17-8. In this illustration a rotating anode structure is used in the X-ray tube. Instead of a spot or small rectangle of tungsten for the target, we have a tungsten disc instead. In this type of target construction, the electron gun or cathode is placed so that its electrons strike only the rim of the rotating anode disc. In this way, we gain a small focal area that is down to a few square millimeters, yet the heat is allowed to dissipate through the entire anode assembly, which could have an area well over a thousand square millimeters. In the use of a rotating anode we see:

1—Higher thermal loading for a fixed focal size.
2—Reduced number of milliampere-seconds required for a given focus.

HIGH-VOLTAGE POWER SOURCES

X-ray machines require anode potentials ranging from 30,000 volts to over 100,000 volts for proper operation. This potential is usually supplied by a large, oil-filled, high-ratio transformer energized from the ac powerlines. Permanently installed X-ray machines usually operate from a 240V ac power, but more than a few make use of the three-phase power available in almost all hospitals. In any event, these high-voltage transformers typically have turns ratios on the order of 1:400.

The X-ray tube must also have a filament transformer to heat the cathode. Since this transformer operates at very low voltages, it is usually connected to one side of the high-voltage supply (see Fig. 17-9) in order to reduce the possibility of cathode-heater arcing.

The circuit in Fig. 17-9 is a simple, self-rectified, X-ray generator in which the X-ray tube is connected across the ac secondary of the high-voltage transformer. The tube will, however, only conduct current on the half-cycle in which the anode is positive with respect to the cathode. There are several problems with this technique that severely limit its application. One of these is the fact that X-rays can only be

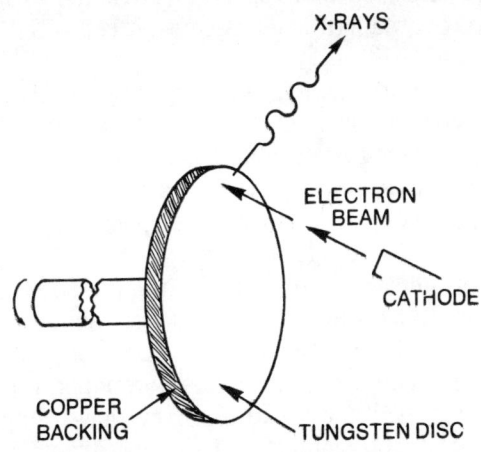

Fig. 17-8. Construction of the rotating-anode X-ray tube.

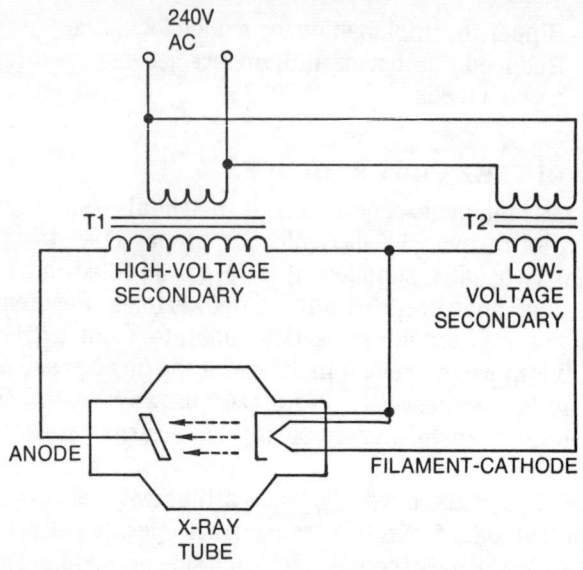

Fig. 17-9. Circuit of an obsolete, self-rectified, X-ray generator.

produced during the half-cycle when the anode is positive. Another is the fact that the X-ray tube becomes an open circuit on the negative half-cycle, which "unloads" the secondary of the high-voltage transformer and allows a very high voltage to exist across the tube. If of an appreciable amplitude, these reverse potentials can cause arcing. Yet a third limitation is that the hot anode assembly can to give off electrons by thermionic emission and these are attracted to the cathode during the reverse half-cycle because it is positive relation to the anode.

These problems can be eliminated by rectifying the high voltage. Some X-ray machines use a single-diode, half-wave arrangement where the rectifier is in series with the cathode side of the X-ray tube. Others, also half-wave, use two vacuum-tube rectifiers connected in series, one in the cathode and the other in the anode circuit.

Another solution to this problem that also eliminates the second and third limitation mentioned above is to use a low-voltage rectifier in the primary circuit of the high-voltage transformer. This method thus eliminates the need for high-cost, high-voltage rectifiers. This low-voltage diode is used to shut off the primary of the power transformer on the reverse half of each cycle. But because the current flow in the primary is in one direction, there is a tendency toward magnetizing the transformer core, unless some current is made to pass through the primary on the forbidden half-cycle. To allow this, a resistor is placed in parallel with the diode; it does not, however, have a value low enough to permit significant energization of the secondary during the unwanted half-cycles.

Classifications

X-ray machines can be classified by their power-supply configuration. Self-rectified power supplies, usually limited to portables, are called *one-pulse* machines see Fig. 17-10A) because each ac input sine wave produces but one half-wave pulse across the X-ray tube. These circuits have a 60 Hz ripple.

Full-wave rectified power supplies have a 120 Hz ripple and produce two power pulses across the X-ray tube for each ac sine wave. These, naturally enough, are called *two-pulse* machines (Fig. 17-10B). Two-pulse designs are the limit of a single-phase power system because there are only two halves of the ac sine wave.

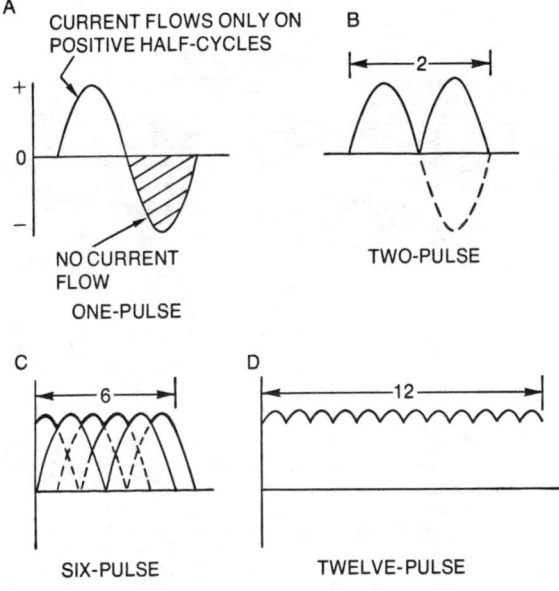

Fig. 17-10. Power supply ripple waveforms: (A) one-pulse (half wave), (B) two-pulse (Full wave), (C) six-pulse (full wave, three phase), and (D) twelve-pulse (dual, full wave, three phase).

In three-phase systems, however, there are two halves of three different sine waves, so you can make a *six-pulse* machine. A three-phase power supply will therefore produce the waveform of Fig. 17-10C across the X-ray tube.

In many three-phase systems, the primary windings are connected in the *delta* configuration while the secondary windings are connected in the *wye* manner. This has been found to be more efficient when compared with use of the same configuration on both sides of the transformer. A variation on this delta-wye theme is to use two secondaries for each phase. The X-ray tube cathode is connected so that wye-configuration secondaries feed rectifiers that produce a negative cathode potential. At the same time, the alternate secondaries are delta connected to rectifiers of a polarity that produces a positive voltage on the anode. These waveforms can be algebraically added to give the waveform shown in Fig. 17-10D, and this is the *twelve-pulse* type of system.

TYPICAL X-RAY MACHINES

Figure 17-11 shows the elements of a *simple* X-ray machine. Power is supplied by autotransformer T1. There will

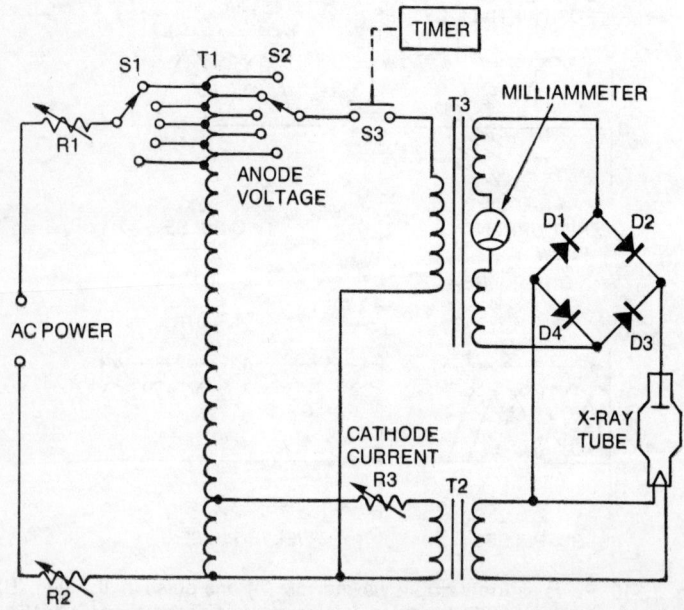

Fig. 17-11. Circuit of an elementary X-ray generator.

always be some source resistance in any power supply, and this also holds true for the ac power lines. Even though this source resistance is very small, it can still cause a great deal of trouble in high-current systems such as the X-ray room and is quite capable of causing a significant reduction in available voltage. This creates line regulation problems.

This same loading phenomenon can be demonstrated using a simple flashlight bulb and a small 1.5V battery. First, measure the open terminal voltage (no load) and then connect the lamp (or a low-value resistor) across the battery and again measure the voltage. The second voltage measurement will be significantly lower than the first, and this is due to the internal resistance of the battery. This internal resistance is added into the circuit in series with the load resistance, and that means we can use the standard voltage-divider equation to find the actual delivered load voltage.

Ballast resistors R1 and R2 in the primary circuit of the autotransformer are used to compensate for this phenomenon. The circuit is made in such a way that it operates at a voltage lower than the ac line potential. This way, variations can be accommodated by adjusting the ballast resistors (a technique not limited to medical X-ray equipment, incidentally).

The X-ray tube anode potential is set through selection of the position of front panel switch S2. This switch determines the kilovoltage applied to the tube by varying the primary voltage applied to high-voltage transformer T3. Although the full-wave bridge rectifier is shown here as being made from solid-state diodes (as well they might be in recently made equipment), they may actually be large vacuum-tube diode rectifiers.

The X-ray tube cathode current is set using a technique once familiar as the volume control circuit of early radio receivers; they vary the voltage applied to the filament. This is the function of potentiometer R3. The voltage across the filament determines the amount of current flow, which in its turn determines the amount of heat built up in the filament. The filament will boil off (thermionic emission) more electrons when it is hot than when it is cool, so this establishes the current available in the anode path.

The length of time for the allowed exposure is set by the timer circuit. In very early (and very crude) machines of low output, this was controlled by a handswitch. In all recent machines (past several decades), some sort of timer has been used. Four types of timer have become more or less standard: a clockwork mechanism, synchronous motor mechanism, impulse timer, and photo-controlled timer.

Clockwork timers are handwound spring-loaded gear trains. These are reminiscent of kitchen cooking timers, but provide a range of intervals from 0.1 to about 12 seconds. These timers are used mostly in portables and dental machines that use low-current X-ray tubes.

The synchronous-motor timer is actually something like an electric alarm clock in that it used a synchronous motor to drive a gear train. These are capable of exposure intervals from 0.05 to about 30 seconds.

The impulse type of timer uses digital electronic counters to set the exposure times. The time base of the digital clock uses the 120 Hz ripple component from a full-wave rectifier circuit. Since their circuits can easily discriminate even one pulse at these rates, it becomes possible to count from 1/120 second (0.0083 sec) up to whatever overflows the particular counter in question. This method allows the designer to set the maximum range of the timer by simply choosing a digital counter chain that is long enough.

A photo timer is an ionization chamber or photocell connected into a circuit designed to terminate the exposure when a certain amount of radiation has been delivered. This is not strictly a *timer* as such, but serves a similar function and is used in fluorography.

DESIGN VARIATIONS

Please understand that X-ray electronics is a vast field and cannot be adequately treated in one chapter of a medical electronics book. It is, in fact, a proper subject for a book of its own. This chapter presents an overview treatment and does not take into account some of the ramifications of X-ray technology and differences in philosophy between manufacturers. This treatment, therefore, has been much simplified.

Take, for example, the matter of typical X-ray machine controls. There are three basic controls: anode voltage, cathode current, and time. But they can be implemented in different ways and may well be interrelated in many cases. In many medical X-ray machines, for instance, the anode-voltage and cathode-current controls are mechanically linked in order to prevent any settings that would exceed the maximum load the tube is designed to handle. This little bit of precaution is used to protect the multikilodollar X-ray generator tube that could easily be damaged.

In some machines there is also a special potentiometer in the primary of the filament transformer to compensate for variations in current due to changes in the kilovolt control. An X-ray tube is normally operated in a saturated mode, so anode voltage changes will not affect the cathode current. That's what the theory says—but in reality some changes do occur. The compensation resistor in the filament primary is ganged to the anode-voltage control in order to overcome this problem.

There may also be a saturable transformer regulator connected in series with the primary of the filament transformer. Its function is to smooth out powerline fluctuations that could be transmitted to the X-ray tube filament and thereby intensity-modulate the X-ray beam produced by the tube.

A *falling load* generator is also sometimes used. In that type of system the X-ray tube operates at its maximum rating initially, but loading is reduced as the exposure time increases. In one system using this technique, the falling load characteristic is created by connecting the primary of the high-voltage transformer through a stepping switch that selects taps on a series-connected resistive voltage divider.

SCATTER REDUCTION

Several types of scatter shields are used on X-ray tube housings. These are designed to contain the X-rays within the smallest possible area, thereby limiting scatter. Some machines are fitted with a cone or cylinder to guide the X-ray beam. These are most common on dental machines and low-powered medical machines intended for making films of small areas of the body. Cones, cylinders, and slit masks are used for this purpose on certain small industrial X-ray machines made for quality-control inspections.

Collimators are also used in many medical X-ray systems to restrict the beam size and reduce scatter. These are lead-lined shutters covering the window on the X-ray tube housing, and these can be adjusted to the minimum size needed to perform the prescribed X-ray procedure. Each shutter has at least a three millimeters thickness of lead shielding. A light and mirror assembly, and possibly a crosshair for aiming, is used to prealign the shutters. Specifications require that the X-ray field be perfectly coincident with the light-beam field viewed through the mirror.

IMAGE INTENSIFIERS

The image intensifier is a special electron tube that uses electron acceleration to produce a brighter image than is normally possible with fluoroscopy. In fact, brightness intensification of two or three hundred times is possible.

Figure 17-12 shows a diagram of a typical image-intensifier tube. X-rays enter the glass window on the left side and strike a fluorescent screen, which is sandwiched with a photoelectric cathode. When light photons from the fluoroscreen enter the photocathode, electrons are emitted into the vacuum space where they are then subject to an electric field from an outside potential. They accelerate through this considerable potential and gain quite a bit of kinetic energy by the time they strike the aluminized phosphor screen. Consequently, when the electrons collide with the atoms of the phosphor screen, they produce a visible light emission in a manner like any cathode ray tube. This light is

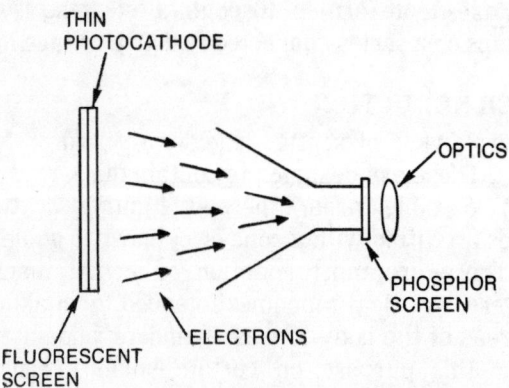

Fig. 17-12. Basic construction of an image-intensifier tube. Electrons emitted by the photocathode sandwiched to the X-ray sensitive flouroscreen are accelerated through an electrical potential before striking a phosphor screen. Kinetic energy picked up by the electron produces an image on the phosphor screen that was brighter than that on the fluoroscreen.

considerably brighter than that on the fluoroscreen because of the increased energy level imparted to the electrons.

Optics at the output focus the light beam and feed it to where it is to be viewed. In typical units, this light might go to a TV camera or to a 35 mm movie camera.

SOME X-RAY TERMS

angstrom—unit of wavelength. One angstrom equals 10^{-10} meters.

Bucky grid—A specially aligned and motor driven grid structure located between the patient and the film. It is used to reduce scatter.

collimator—shutter assembly made of lead that is used to adjust the size of the X-ray field.

curie—unit of radioactive decay equal to 3.7×10^{10} disintegrations per second. See *Elementary Modern Physics* by R.T. Weidner and R.L. Sells, alternate second edition. Allyn & Bacon, Boston, 1974 (p340).

fluorescence—ability of certain materials to emit light, or glow, when bombarded by X-rays.

fluoroscope—fluorescent screen that allows real-time examination of body parts as they are being X-rayed.

Heel effect—the intensity along any axis of the X-ray beam in the patient plane is not constant, but is maximum in the center and falls off toward the edges of the field.

penetrometer—aluminum "filter" used to check X-ray film exposure. It produces uniform gradations of shading on the film. Anomalies indicate faults.

rad—a unit of absorbed dose of ionizing radiation equal to an energy of 100 ergs per gram of irradiated tissue.

rem—a dosage of ionizing radiation that will cause the same biological effect as one roentgen of X-ray or gamma-ray dosage.

roentgen (r)—international exposure dose, which is a measure of the ability of radiation to ionize air.

stereoscopy—films of the same object but taken from slightly different angles are viewed on a special optical box to produce a stereo effect.

X-ray—electromagnetic radiation with wavelengths less than approximately one angstrom.

X-ray tube—special diode vacuum tube designed to generate X-rays.

Chapter 18
Lung, Blood Gas, and Dialysis Machines

The equipment discussed in this chapter are related, after a fashion, in that they follow the flow of gas through the lungs and into the blood stream, in which waste products accumulate through bioligical processes and must sometimes be removed through a kidney dialysis machine. Thus, we shall treat these various instruments in this order.

RESIPRATORY MEASUREMENTS

According to one definition, respriation is the exchange of gases between the external environment and the blood. In humans this exchange takes place in small sacs in the lungs called *alveoli*. These sacs are the point of exchange between the outside environment and the blood as oxygen comes into the body and carbon dioxide waste products leave it. Pulmonary function tests are used to assess the efficacy of this process. Unfortunately, though, no one single test will give all of the information that is required. In place of a comprehensive test, there is instead a collection of tests that can be considered together where appropriate.

The lungs in humans are elastic bags or sacs located in the body's thoracic cavity. The right lung has three lobes or sections while the left lung has but two since it must allow room for the heart. In the back of the throat, there is a little "trap door" called the *epiglottis*, and this prevents liquids or food from entering the respiratory system. Following this is the *trachea*, which branches into two further tubes, called the left and right *bronchi*.

Breathing is allowed by pressure dyamics and the thoracic musculature, primarily the diaphram, that allows the volume of the thoracic cavity to expand. Since this cavity is a closed system, expansion of its volume creates what is essentially a slight negative pressure. Atmospheric pressure forces air in through the mouth and the elastic lungs expand.

The ability of the lungs to expand and contract is measured by a factor called *lung compliance* and this is expressed as the derivative dV/dp, where V is the volume of the lungs and p is the intra-alveolar pressure. This pressure, incidentally, varies from a positive pressure of about three torr to a negative pressure of approximately the same magnitude over the inspiration/expiration cycle.

Pulmonary function is dependent upon many factors that include the properties of the mouth, all of the air tubes, the condition of the musculature, and the compliance of the lungs. Some of these parameters can be assessed by examination and analysis of certain volume changes during specific phases of the respiratory cycle. Figure 18-1 shows a graph of various volumes relating to respiration. Normal breathing of a resting subject is shown in the figure as the resting tidal volume (RTV). The graph shows the normal changes in lung volume due to regular resting respiration. There are several other features of this waveform that will prove of interest: expiratory reserve volume (ERV), residual volume (RV), total lung capacity (TLC), inspiratory capacity (IC), vital capacity (VC) and functional residual capacity (FRC). These can be defined as follows:

- **ERV**—this volume measurement is the amount of gas that can be expired under maximum effort after completing an inspiration/expiration cycle. This is defined as the volume change from the negative half of the tidal volume waveform and a maximum effort expiration.
- **RV**—this is the volume of the gases remaining in the lungs after a maximum effort exhalation. The patient is forced to breath out as much air as possible.
- **TLC**—this is the maximum amount of air the lungs can hold after a maximum effort inspiration. TLC is the sum of two other factors, RV and VC.

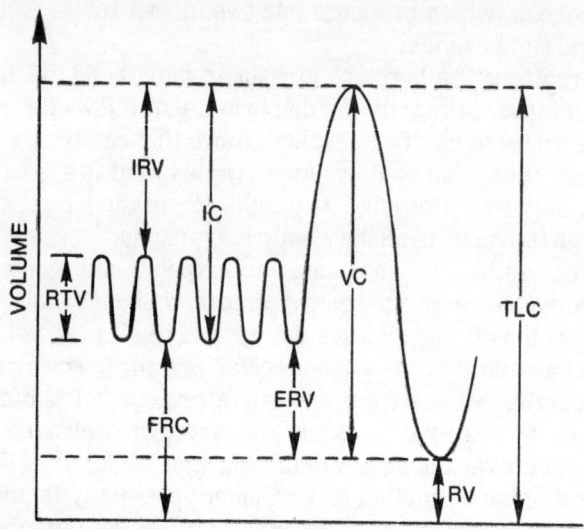

Fig. 18-1. Graph showing the various types of respiratory volume in humans.

- **IC**—the inspiratory capacity is the volume of gas that could be inhaled if a maximal inspiration effort is made. Measurement is made from the end of a normal resting respiration cycle, the low point on the tidal volume feature of the waveform in Fig. 18-1.
- **IRC**—the inspiratory reserve capacity after normal inspiration at rest.
- **VC**—vital capacity is the difference between total lung capacity and residual volume. If can be expressed as the total volume change when a maximum inspiration is followed immediately by a maximum expiration.
- **FRC**—this measurement determines the amount of air remaining in the lungs when a normal respiration expiration has occurred. It can be expressed as the total volume change between zero and the inspiratory capacity minimum point.

Another test often made in pulmonary laboratories is the *minute volume*, mentioned briefly in Chapter 14. This is the volume of air taken into the lungs during one minute of normal respiration. The minute volume can be determined on paper by multiplying together the tidal volume and the patient's respiration rate in breaths per minute. In electronic equipment this can also be found by integrating the volume flow signal.

SPIROMETERS

All lung volumes can be measured on an instrument called a *spirometer*, of which several different types are common. One of the most common of the recording spirometers is known as the *bell* or *water* spirometer (Fig. 18-2). The bell is inverted in a tank of water and counterweighted so that atmospheric pressure and the weight tending to force the bell to move up is exactly counteracted by the weight of the bell tending to force itself down.

The cable supporting the bell passes by the chart of a drum recorder, called a *kymograph*. When the spirometer is at rest, only atmospheric pressure affects the air inside of the bell, so the chart recorder pen remains at zero.

The patient is seated and the mouthpiece positioned so that he can breath into it. The patient's nose is blocked with a small clip so that air cannot escape by passing through the nostrils.

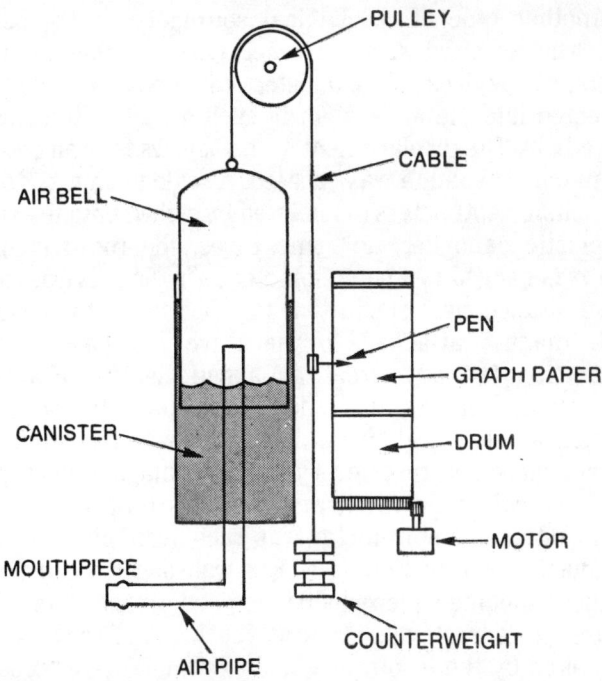

Fig. 18-2. Water-displacement or "diving bell" spirometer.

When the patient exhales air into the mouthpiece, this increases the amount of gas inside the bell. The bell then rises in order to allow the air pressure inside to be at equilibrium with the atmospheric pressure. This motion causes the pen attached to the support cable to fall, scribing a line on the chart paper. Similarly, when the patient inhales, air pressure in the bell decreases, the bell's weight forces it to fall, and this causes the pen to rise.

Two bell sizes are common, 9 and 13.5 liters, but the smaller is probably the more common of the two. The kymograph is usually a multispeed design that can move the chart at speeds of 32, 160, or 1900 millimeters per minute. Not shown but also included in the spirometer system will be a carbon dioxide absorber.

An alternate version of this instrument uses a slide-operated, linear potentiometer with its wiper terminal ganged to the support cable, in place of a pen, to generate an electrical signal that is proportional to volume. This signal can be processed, if desired, to yield several other parameters, or it can be fed directly to the chart recorder.

Another type of mechanical spirometer is the bellows type. This is often seen on respirators or other breathing assistance devices. A cannister containing a bellows is connected into the air system in such a way as to catch the expired air. The displacement of the bellows tells an observer how much air volume was exhaled. A scale in units of volume (e.g., cubic centimeters) is painted or etched onto the side of the plastic cannister. In some cases, the rod driving the bellows is ganged to a potentiometer as in the previous case to derive an electrical signal that is proportional to volume. A small magnet attached to the drive rod passes a coil concentric to the rod to create a magnetic field that changes as the patient breathes. This field interacts with the coil to generate an electrical signal that varies with the respiration. A timer circuit is reset every time the magnet generates a signal, but will sound an alarm if allowed to time out.

An ultrasonic spirometer was once available and used a transducer such as Fig. 18-3. The transducer has a pair of obliquely mounted piezoelectric crystal transducers. These are used to generate ultrasonic waves that are fired across the path taken by the inspiratory and expiratory gases breathed by the patient. One transducer is pulsed while the other acts as

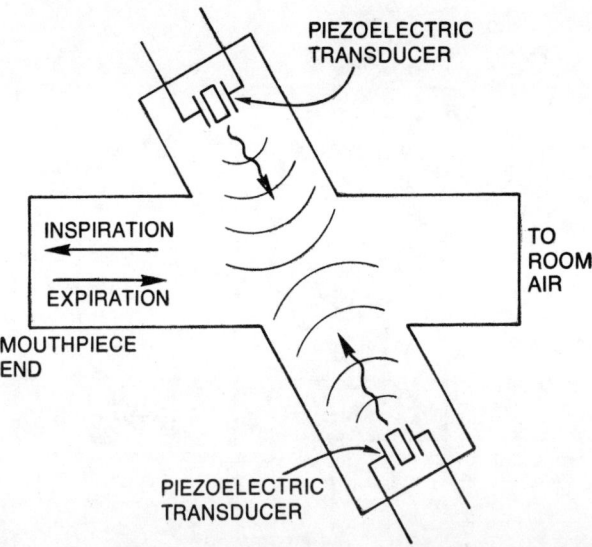

Fig. 18-3. Construction of an ultrasonic transducer for an electronic spirometer. The transducers are both used for transmit and receive in order to accurated measure the Doppler shift due to air speed.

the receiver. A determination of the time of travel in the downstream direction is thus obtained. Next, the situation is reversed, and the other transducer is pulsed so the upstream transmission time is obtained. This information is then used by the instrument to calculate the flow volume, respiration rate, etc.

GAS MEASUREMENTS

Pulmonary function laboratories can measure both pulmonary gases and blood gases. A general discussion of blood gas instrumentation was given in Chapter 12 and so will not be repeated here. We will, though, discuss the techniques used to measure the partial pressures of oxygen (O_2) and carbon dioxide (CO_2) in inhaled and expired gases.

Measurement of oxygen concentration is made easier by the fact that oxygen is among the few molecules that will respond to a magnetic field. A special transducer is constructed so that oxygen passes through two coils of nickel wire. One of these coils is in the field of a permanent magnet, but both are part of a bridge circuit. The coil in the magnetic field experiences a varying flux because of the oxygen flow, and this causes a varying bridge current to flow.

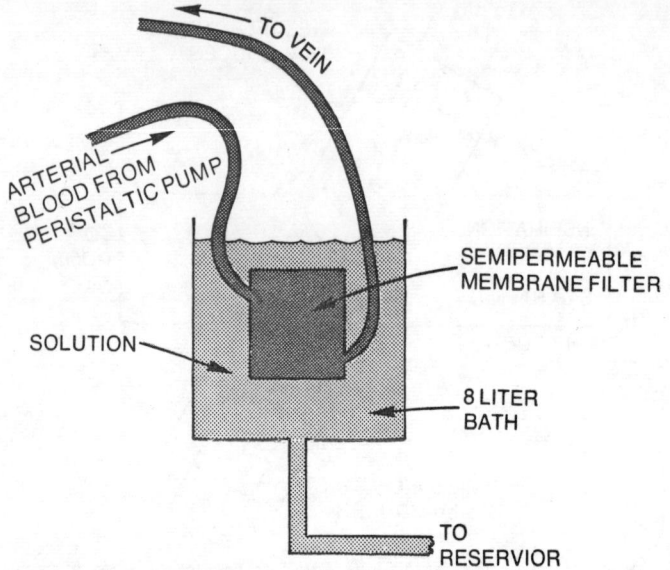

Fig. 18-4. Diagram of a renal dialysis machine.

The measurement of carbon dioxide is made easier by the fact that CO_2 has infrared absorption properties. The relative CO_2 concentration in the patient's exhaled gas can therefore be calculated by measuring the infrared properties of the gas and comparing them with those of a known calibration gas that has either zero or a calibrated amount of CO_2 present. These calibration gases can be purchased from local bottled-gas suppliers or can be made up in-house if proper facilities are at hand.

KIDNEY DIALYSIS MACHINES

Human kidneys have two principal functions. They eliminate waste products from the blood and the assist in the control of certain elements in the body. Renal failure is fatal unless artificial means of fulfilling the kidney's functions is provided.

The method currently in favor is called *dialysis*, shown in a highly simplified diagram in Fig. 18-4. The patient will have a bypass inserted between a vein and an artery of the arm (called an *A-V shunt*). This tube is kept from clotting by the passage of blood. When it is time to dialyze—on the average of two or three times a week—the bypass is removed and tubing to and from the dialysis machine is attached to the open ends.

Blood from the arterial side of the A-V shunt is passed through a peristaltic pump (see Fig. 18-5) to a disposable coil filter, which is semipermeable to H_2O and certain crystalloid substances but nonpermeable to most of the large molecules and colloids found in the blood.

This filter assembly is immersed in a bath containing elements in concentrations similar to those actually found in the blood. These are, for example, magnesium, sodium, calcium, glucose, salts, etc. The concentration of these constituents is adjusted to cause osmotic pressure to force the unwanted substances out of the blood line and into the eight-liter bath. Fluid in this bath is recirculated several times and is then replaced by fluid from a 120 liter reservoir.

Although not shown in this simplified drawing, there are also several safety features and controls that are either part of or peripherally related to the kidney machine. A pressure alarm, for example, is used to warn of a break in the lines from the patient. Such an alarm could turn off the machine as well

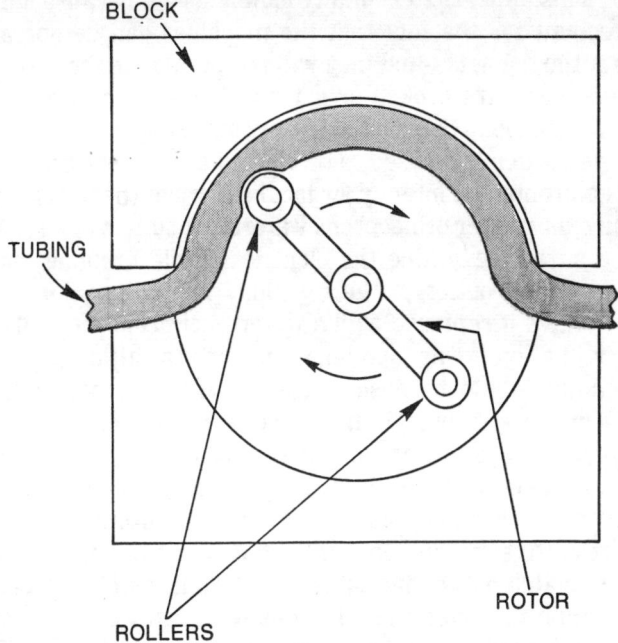

Fig. 18-5. Operation of a peristaltic pump. Fluid, such as blood, passes through the plastic tubing. The nylon rollers on the ends of the rotor arms gently push fluid forward. This is a single-rotor design, but multirotor types are also found. Speed is approximately 20 rpm.

as alert the staff of an impending catastrophy. There are also temperature regulators and controls provided.

The kidney dialysis machine is both in and of itself a "wet environment" and so must come under some rather stringent electrical safety regulations. The use of ground fault interrupters (GFI) is recommended because the dialysis fluid can get into some of the electrical circuits and create ground-line currents from the case in excess of the 5 mA "safe" level.

Many of the machines in current use may require some modification in order to bring them up to the standards met by more recent designs. It might, for example, be necessary to replace some of the regular ac power outlets and plugs of both the machine and its peripherals with rubber-covered or other waterproof types. Most older machines used regular outlets and plugs as might be found on any electronic equipment.

A bonnet over the filter bath was also used in older machines to protect against electrical shorts due to splashing water. This appears to be faulty logic, though, because it does not account for the fact that the machines can be operated without the bonnets—and they will be operated in that manner if the bonnets are broken or get misplaced. Also, it does not take into account the tendency of people to become careless with the garden hose used to fill the 120 liter reservior. Where this is a problem, contact your local electrical (not electronic) supplier for rubber or neoprene waterproof outlets.

Be sure to examine the electrical cable bringing power from the wall outlet to the machine. If it is regular black rubber, have it replaced with a waterproof neoprene cable. In one installation it was found that machines awaiting servicing or cleaning would be pushed aside with the ac power cable laying in the still full 120 liter reservoir. The electrolytes in that reservoir can impregnate the insulation of the wire and create a dangerous low-resistance situation. Replacement of the cable with a waterproof type is deemed appropriate.

Preventive maintenance is even better than educating the users to watch out for the cable because a hospital might have a very high turnover rate of personnel, requiring a constant in-service education regiem. It is also true that Murphy's law and the normal perversity of the universe tend to keep at least ten percent of the people from "getting the word." Since ten percent never get the word even if present when given, it is wise to redesign their environment to prevent their lack of awareness (or ignorance, when one doesn't care to be charitable) from causing trouble.

In normal repair operations it is wise to stock certain items. These include switches, bulbs, fuses, and other small electrical or electronic items, as appropriate. Also keep pump motors, pump impellers (water pumps), drain solenoid assemblies, and any control regulators. Where lack of service has been a problem in the locality (as it often is), you may become more than a little surprised at the mechanical dexterity and repair ability of the nurses who operate this equipment. After all, although some time may be available, repair is essential because a kidney machine is *life support* equipment and must work properly.

SOME FINAL ADVICE

Several pointers are in order for the prospective medical equipment technician. One is to be always alert to possibilities for learning. New situations come up all of the time and you will not want to be caught unaware. It is necessary that you adapt a really professional attitude toward the work. In the TV repair business or certain industrial electronics jobs, the loss from a sloppy worker is merely money and an occasional Sunday afternoon football game. In medical electronics it can be considerably more serious and can cost somebody their life. It is wise to present a positive image to the nurses, technicians, and physicians who use the equipment. If you run around in a janitor's uniform and appear to be inept, don't expect to have the confidence of the professionals you serve.

Become used to writing things down. This will take on two forms. One, carry a pocket notebook and jot down any equipment complaint that you will have to remedy later. This will not only keep your memory jogged, it will result in a high overall level of confidence from your medical and nursing customers. Also, keep extensive records of all equipment repairs, safety inspections, and examinations. Your administration will require the records for accreditation or licensure inspections and in case of a malpractice suit. Even your own efforts may be subject to such a suit, so you will want to keep the records up to date to show your competence and good faith. In this case, the records are sometimes humorously called an SYA file, and I will leave it to you to decode the meaning of the letters.

Appendices

Appendix 1

Bibliography

1. *Introduction to Medical Electronics, 2nd Edition* by Burton Klein. TAB BOOKS, Blue Ridge Summit, Pa., 1976 (cat. 830).
2. *C.E.T. License Handbook, 2nd Edition* by Joseph J. Carr. TAB BOOKS, Blue Ridge Summit Pa., 1976 (cat. 701).
3. *Biophysical Measurements* by Peter Strong. A Tektronix, Inc. Concept Series book, Beaverton, Oregon.
4. *Handbook of Biomedical Instrumentation & Measurements* by Harry E. Thomas. Reston Publishing Co., Reston, Va., 1975.
5. *Biomedical Instrumentation & Measurements* by Leslie Cromwell, et al. Prentice-Hall, Englewood Cliffs, N.J., 1973.
6. *Practical Instrumentation Transducers* by Frank J. Oliver. Hayden Book Co., New York, 1971.
7. *Diagnostic Ultrasound* by Mathew Hussey. John Wiley & Sons, New York, 1975.
8. *Elementary Biophysics—Selected Topics* by Herman T. Epstein. Addison-Wesley Publishing Co., Reading, Mass.
9. *Electronics for Scientists* by H.V. Malmstadt & C.G. Enke. W.A. Benjamin, Inc., New York, 1963.

10. *Bioelectric Phenomena* by Robert Plonsey. McGraw-Hill, New York, 1969.
11. *Physics in Medicine & Biology* by Paul Davidovits. Prentice-Hall, Englewood Cliffs, N.J., 1975.
12. *Electronic Instrumentation & Measurement Techniques.* Prentice-Hall, Englewood Cliffs, N.J., 1970.
13. *Principles of Diagnostic X-ray Apparatus.* Engineering staff of Philips Medical Systems, Ltd., London, 1973.
14. *Instrumental Methods of Chemical Analysis* by Galen W. Ewing, McGraw-Hill, New York, 1975.
15. *Radioisotope Laboratory Techniques* by R.A. Faires and B.H. Parks. London Butterworths, London, 1973.
16. *Servicing Biomedical Equipment* by Eliot Kanter. Howard W. Sams & Co., Inc.
17. *Servicing Electrocardiographs* by Eliot Kanter. Howard W. Sams & Co., Inc.
18. *Questions & Answers About Medical Electronics* by Edward Bukstein. Howard W. Sams & Co., Inc.
19. *Introduction to Biomedical Electronics* by Edward Bukstein. Howard W. Sams & Co., Inc.
20. *Microprocessor/Microprogramming Handbook* by Brice Ward. TAB BOOKS, Blue Ridge Summit, Pa. (cat. 785).
21. *Minicomputers for Engineers & Scientists* by G.A. Korn. McGraw-Hill, New York, 1973.
22. *Computer Methods for Science & Engineering* by R.L. Lafara. Hayden Book Co., Rochelle Park, N.J., 1973.
23. "Cardiac Arrest or Electrocution" by Joseph J. Carr. *O.R. TECH*, the official journal of the A.O.R.T., Littleton, Colo., Sept/Oct. 1972. (pp 6–18).
24. "A Servicer's View of Medical Electronics" by Joseph J. Carr. *Electronic Servicing*, Sept. 1972 (pp 46–53).
25. "R.F. Devices in Medical Electronics." *Electronic Servicing*, Dec. 1972 (pp 36–42).
26. "Getting Started Servicing Medical Electronics" by Joseph J. Carr. *Electronic Servicing*, Sept. 1974 (pp 32–36).
27. "Medical Electronics—A Healthy New Field for Servicers—Part I" by Joseph J. Carr. *Electronic Technician/Dealer*, May 1975 (pp 18–23, 44).

28. 'Medical Electronics—A Healthy New Field for Servicers—Part II" by Joseph J. Carr, *Electronic Technician/Dealer*, June 1975 (pp 28—33, 47).
29. "Getting Into Medical Electronics" by Joseph J. Carr. *Electronics Technician/Dealer*, Nov. 1975 (p 46, 55).
30. *Patient Safety* (AN718) Hewlett-Packard application note.
31. All Hewlett-Packard medical application notes (consult local H-P office for availability).

Appendix 2
Medical Prefixes, Suffixes, and Roots

PREFIX	MEANING
a-	absence; not
ab-	away from; off
ad-	toward
amphi-	on both sides; bilateral
an-	absence of
ante-	before; in front of
antero-	in front
anti-	against
ap-	separation
apo-	separation
bi-	two
bio-	pertaining to life
brady-	slow
cardio-	pertaining to the heart
cephalo-	head
chiro-	hand
chole-	bile
co-	together
con-	with
costo-	rib
cysto-	sac; bladder
dactylo-	digit (finger or toe)
derma-	skin
dermato-	skin

PREFIX	MEANING
di-	twice
dia-	apart; through
dys-	difficult; painful
ec-	outside of
ecto-	outside
ex-	outside
en-	within
endo-	within
ento-	within
entero-	intestines
epi-	upon
ex-	away from
exo-	outside of
extro-	outside
eu-	well, good
gastro-	stomach
hema-, hemo-	blood
hemato-	blood
hetero-	different
homo-	the same; of the same sort
hydro-	water
hypno-	sleep
hypo-	beneath; deficient, lower than
hystero-	uterus
ileo-	ileum
in-, il-, ir-	within; not; inside
infra-	beneath
inter-	between
intra-	within
iso-	equal; same
kilo-	1000
leuko-	white; clear
litho-	stone
macro-	abnormally large; large
mal-	bad
media-	middle
mega-	great size; 10^6
melano-	black
meso-	middle
meta-	more than; change; after; next
micro-	small; 10^{-6}

PREFIX	MEANING
mono-	one
morpho-	form
multi-	many
myelo-	bone marrow; pertaining to the spinal cord
myo-	muscle
neo-	new
nephro-	kidney
neuro-	nerves
ob-	in front of
odonto-	tooth
ophthalmo-	eye
ortho-	straight; normal
osteo-	bone
oto-	ear
pan-	all
para-	beside
patho-	pertaining to disease
peri-	around
pneumo-	lungs; respiration
pod-	foot
poly-	many
pre-	before
pro-	before
procto-	rectum
pseudo-	false
pyo-	pus
pyr-	fire; heat
quadra-	four
retro-	located behind; backwards
rhino-	nose
semi-	half
sphygmo-	pulse
sub-	near; moderately; under
super-	excessive; above
supra-	above
sym-	union
syn-	union
tachy-	fast; extremely fast
trans-	across
tri-	three

PREFIX	MEANING
ultra-	beyond
uni-	single

SUFFIXES	MEANING
-agogue	inducing agent
-agra	sudden acute pain
-algia	painful
-cele	tumor; swelling
-centesis	puncture into
-clasia	remedy
-ectomy	surgical excision of
-ecstasis	dilatation
-edema	swelling
-emia	blood
-graph	record
-ia	diseased condition
-iasis	a process or procedure
-itis	inflammation
-logy	study or science of
-mania	abnormally excessive preoccupation
-meter	measuring instrument
-oid	resembling
-oma	tumor
-opia	vision
-osis	fullness; excess
-pathy	morbid disease
-phobia	dread; fear
-plasty	plastic surgical repair
-rrhea	discharge or flow
-sclerosis	hardening
-scope	instrument for examining
-scopy	visual examination of
-stomy	artificial opening
-tomy	incision

ROOTS	MEANING
aden	gland
ateria	artery
arthros	joint
auris	ear
brachion	arm
cardium	heart

ROOTS	MEANING
cephalo	brain
cholecyst	gall baldder
colon	intestine
costa	rib
cranium	skull or head
derma	skin
enteron	intestine
epithelium	skin
esophagus	gullet
gaster	stomach
hema, hemo	blood
hepar	liver
hydro	water
hystera	womb
kypsis	bladder
larynx	throat
myelos	marrow
nasus	nose
nehpros	kidney
neuron	nerve cell
odons	tooth
odynia	pain
opsikas	eye
os	bone
osteon	bone
ostrium	mouth
otis	ear
pes	foot
pharynx	throat
phlebos	vein
pleura	chest
pneumones	lungs
psyche	mind
pulmones	lungs
pyelos	kidney
pyretos	fever
ren	kidney
rhin	nose
rhythmos	rhythm
spondylos	vertebra

ROOTS	MEANING
stoma	mouth
thorax	chest
trachea	windpipe
thophe	nutrition
vene	vein
vesica	bladder

Appendix 3
Medical Glossary

accretion—growth or enlargement.
aveolus—air sac or cell in the lungs.
amnion—thin membranous structure around fetus.
amniotic—pertaining to the amnion.
angstrom—unit of length, 1 angstrom = 10^{-10} meters.
anterior—situated in front of.
aorta—great artery carrying blood from the left ventricle of the heart to the rest of the body.
aortic—pertaining to the aorta.
arborizations—form resembling a tree.
arrhythmia—alteration in the rhythm.
arteriole—one of the small twigs of the artery that becomes a capillary.
artifacts—erroneous lines or marks on a graph or gram. An error in a test result.
atria—(pl.) see atrium.
atrioventricular—located between the upper and lower chambers of the heart.
atrium—upper chamber of the heart.
auricle—chamber of the heart that receives blood from the veins. See atrium.
autonomic—action that is independent of free volition.
axon—long, thin portion of a nerve cell that carries the impulse away from the main section of the cell.

bioelectric (bioelectricity)—electrical activity pertaining to a living cell.
biophysical (biophysics)—branch of science that applies the concepts of physical science to biology.
brachial—relating or pertaining to the arm.
bradycardia—slow heart rate.
bronci—(pl.) see bronchus.
bronchus—tube leading from trachea to either left or right lung.
capillaries—smallest blood vessels in the body.
cardiac—pertaining to the heart.
cardiology—study of the heart and its diseases.
cardiovascular—relating to the circulatory system.
catheter—small tube that is inserted into the body to permit injection of medications, to allow the vessel or passage open, or to permit withdrawal of fluids.
cell—smallest object capable of life.
cephalic—pertaining to the head or skull.
cerebellum—large dorsal brain structure.
cerebrum—anterior portion of the brain.
cornea—transparent covering of the center portion of the eye.
cortex—outer layer of tissue on an organ.
cortical—pertaining to the cortex.
cranium—portion of the skull containing the brain.
curare—drug that produces muscular relaxation.
cytoplasm—the matter inside a cell, except for the nucleus.
defibrillator—an electrical device used to deliver a shock to stop fibrillation of the heart.
dendrite—portion of the nerve cell that conducts impulses toward the cell.
depolarized—state of being partially or totally nonpolar.
diastole—expansion of the chambers of the heart so that they may fill with blood.
diastolic—pertaining to diastole.
dicrotic—double humped waveform.
dorsal—situated near or toward the back.
ECG—(abbr.) electrocardiograph.
ectopic—located in other than normal position.
EEG—(abbr.) electroencephalogram.

EKG—(German abbr.) used in place of ECG.

electrocardiogram—tracing of the electrical signals produced by the heart.

electrocardiograph—machine for making electrocardiogram.

electrode—conductor used to make electrical contact between a wire and a conductive surface, such as human skin.

electrodermograph—recorder for measuring galvanic skin resistance.

electroencephalogram—recording of electrical signals produced by the brain.

electroencephalograph—machine for making electroencephalograms.

electrogastrogram—recording of simultaneous electrical and physical activity of the stomach.

electrolyte—a solution in which electrical current is due to ionic mobility.

electromyogram—recording of electrical activity of skeletal muscles.

electromyograph—machine for making electromyograms.

embolus—abnormal solid or gaseous particle in the blood stream.

embryo—undeveloped stage of fetus.

EMG—(abbr.) electromyograph; electromyogram.

extracellular—outside of the cells.

extracorporeal—outside of the body.

fibula—smaller of the two bones of the leg.

galvanic—that which produces a direct current.

hemisphere—half of a spherical object.

homogeneity—all of the same sort; state of.

homogeneous—of the same sort.

infarct—area of necrotic tissue due to loss of blood perfusion.

inhomogeneity—not homogeneous.

intracellular—inside of the cell.

ion—atom or molecule that carries an electrical charge, either positive or negative.

iris—colored portion of the eye behind the cornea.

isoelectric—having the same electric charge so cannot produce an electrical current.

isothermal—a body with the same temperature in all portions.
isotropic—having the same properties in all directions.
latency—apparent inactivity.
lobe—rounded portion of an organ.
lumen—the hollow portion of a tubular organ.
manometer—device used to determine gas pressures.
membrane—a thin layer of tissue.
metabolism—the total of all processes required for an organis to live.
micron—unit of length, 10^{-6} meters.
mitochondria—small granules or rods.
mitral stenosis—narrowing of the oriface between left atria and ventricle.
myocardium—a muscle layer of the heart.
myograph—instrument for measurement of muscular contraction.
necrosis—death of tissue or cells.
neuron—nerve cell.
nuclei—(pl.) see nucleus.
nucleus—central structure (as in cells and atoms).
occipital—relating or pertaining to the rear portion of the head.
organ—group of specialized cells that perform a specific task or function.
orthogonal—at right angles or normal to.
parietal—pertaining to the upper rear portion of the head.
permeable—ability to pass through pores.
peroneal—pertaining to the outer side of the lower leg.
piezoelectric—electrical activity due to flexure of a crystal.
plethysmography—recording of volume changes due to blood flow.
pneumatic—pertaining to or operated by gases, especially air.
pneumograph—measuring instrument for recording volume changes in the thorax due to respiration.
pneumotachygraph—instrument to measure respiration rate.
posterior—pertaining to the rear.
protoplasm—substance of water, inorganic, and proteinaceous material making up the parts of the cell.

psychogalvanic—electrical activity produced by mental stress.

pulmonary—pertaining to the lungs.

pupil—variable-size aperture in the center of the eye.

radical—group of atoms that can be replaced by a single atom.

radioisotope—artificially produced radioactive element.

retina—light-sensitive membrane in the eye.

rheobase—smallest electrical current that will produce stimulation.

sagittal—pertaining to or parallel to the midline of the body.

scalp—skin of the head covered by hair.

semipermeable—permeable to certain substances.

sinoatrial node— (SA node) collection of heart cells that functions as the natural pacemaker.

sinus—irregular cavity.

sphygmomanometer—blood pressure measurement apparatus.

spirometer—measuring instrument for determining respiratory air volume.

stereotaxic—precision positioning.

synapse—junction where impulse transmits from one nerve cell to another.

systemic—affecting the entire body.

systole—period during which the heart contracts.

tachycardia—excessively fast heart rate.

thermistor—electrical component that exhibits resistance changes due to temperature changes.

thermocouple—device that creates a voltage proportional to temperature.

thoracic—pertaining to the thorax.

thorax—section of the body between abdomen and neck.

thrombus—clot of blood remaining at its site of origin.

tibia—large, innermost bone of the leg.

tissue—collection of similar cells that perform a specific function or take a similar form.

torso—trunk of the body.

trachea—main tube passing air from outside world to the lungs.

transducer—device that converts energy from one form to another for purposes of measurement or control. In this context, the energy converted to is usually electrical.

ulnar—pertaining to the larger bone of the human forearm.

utero—Latin dative for uterus.

uterus—organ in the female for protection and nourishment of the embryo.

vasoconstrictors—agents that narrow the blood vessels.

vasomotor—agent affecting the size of a blood vessel.

ventricle—lower chambers of the heart.

venule—small vein connected to the capillaries.

viable—able to live.

Index

A

Absolute-value amplifier	102
Acceleration	46
Action potential	13
ADC	86
Advice	323
Air flow transducer	259
Air pressure	49
Alarm,	
balloon pump	252
limit	105
module	119
monitor	91
Alpha particles	219
Alveoli	314
Ampere-hour capacity	113
Amplifier,	
absolute value	102
bandpass	60
blood pressure	48, 52
carrier	57
common mode	99
differential	16, 31
four-channel	75
gating	75
isolation	99
operational	104
pH meter	213
right leg	31, 99
summing	77
vertical	74
Analog-to-digital converter	86
Analyzer, blood gas	216
Anomoly, ECG	22
Aorta	48
Arm, ECG	17
Arterial pressure	48, 115
Artifact	109, 186
blood pressure	51
ECG	22
muscle	24
Attenuator, balancing	27
Augmented leads	17
aVF	15, 17
VL	15, 17
aVR	15, 17
A-V shunt	320

B

Balancing attenuator	27
Balloon pump	245
Bandpass amplifier	60
Battery,	
biological	11
charging	113
deep cycling	114
ni-cad	113
pack	111
Bedside monitor	90, 116
Bell spirometer	317
Beta particles	219
Bioelectronic potential	34
Bipolar limb leads	17

Blanking	68
Blood gases	319
analyzer	216
machine	314
monitor	115
Blood pressure	115
cuff	49
direct measurement	50
frequency response	51
monitors	93
processors	62
transducer	39
Blood pressure amplifier	48
calibration	60
checking	65
circuitry	55
Bovie	165
Breathing	315
Bremsstrahlung	301
Bronchi	315

C

Cable, patient	16
Calibration	
blood pressure amplifier	60
ECG	27
medical instrumentation	278
pressure transducer	45
Cardiac output computer	189, 191
Cardiac radio telemetry	196
telemetry, FM terms	201
Cardiac telemetry, servicing	207
Cardiographic lab equipment	180
Cardiomemory	245, 261
servicing	263
Cardiotachometer	91, 102
Cardioverter,	
spares and repairs	162
special equipment	272
synchronization	158
testing	160, 161
types	156
Carrier amplifier	57
Catheter	51, 190
Catheterization lab equipment	180
Cathode ray tube	67, 82
Cauterization	169
Cell,	
membrane	11
stimulus	13
Central monitor	115
computerized	123
servicing	127
Chicken heart	269
Chart recorder (see strip chart recorder)	

Chart, strip	19
Chopper	75
pH meter	213
Clark gas electrode	216
Coagulator, spark gap	171
Code, color, ECG leads	18
Color code, ECG leads	18
Common mode	18, 24
amplifier	99
rejection ratio	31
Comparator	105
Compton effect	299
Computer, cardiac output	189
Computerized central monitor	123
Computerized lab equipment	187
Concentration, photometer	225
Converter	
analog to digital	86
digital to analog	86
Coronary care unit (CCU) monitor	115
Counter	
Geiger	222
scintillation	220
Crystal	
piezoelectric	230
transducer	46
Current, leakage	274
Cut current	169
Cut oscillator	170

D

DAC	86
Damping, stylus	143
Dark resistance	105
Dead zone	135
Deep cycling	114
Defibrillator	95, 101
circuits	151
control circuits	155
ECG protection	32
energy	149
portable	149
protection circuit	32
spares and repairs	162
special equipment	272
stationary	151
testing	160, 161
types	148
Deflection	
horizontal	68
magnetic	69
vertical	68
yoke	68
Demodulator	60
cardiomemory	262

Densitometer	225
Depolarized	13
Detector	
Doppler	237
fetal heart	239
radiation	217, 222
synchronous	60
Deviation, FM telemetry	202
Dialysis machine	314, 320
Diastole	48, 93
Diathermy	228
Differential	
amplifier	16, 31
voltage	24, 57
Digital-to-analog converter	86
Digital voltmeter, ratio	194
Digitization	86
Dilution technique	189
Display	
central monitor	119
circuits	84
format	83
non-fade	69, 82
phonocardiograph	184
Distance	232
Doppler	
equipment, servicing	240
flow detector	237
flow meter	50
shift	235
Drive roller, strip chart	20
DRT	67, 82
Dye dilution	190

E

ECG	11, 95
exercise equipment	186
telemetry transmitters	203
Echoencephalograph	243
Einthoven Triangle leads	17
EKG	11
Electrical	
isolation	291
safety	282
shocks	179, 282
dangerous situations	287
Electrical wiring, test facilities	267
Electrocardiograph	11, 95
artifacts	22
calibration	27
defibrillator protection	32
electrodes	24, 34
electronics	30
exercise equipment	186
filter	24
frequency response	30
leads	14, 15
monitor-diagnostic	24
operation	19
paste	24
performance	26
power-line interference	25
preamplifier	24, 30, 98
telemetry	196
waveform simulator	269
Electrode	
Clark gas electrode	216
ECG	24, 99
electrosurgical	169
medical	34
patient	16
Electroencephalography, electrodes	34
Electromyography, electrodes	34
Electron	
beam	68
gun	67
Electrosurgical generator	165
maintenance	176
rf power	177
special equipment	270
Energy	
defibrillator	149
rf power	177
Equipotential ground system	290
Exercise ECG lab equipment	186

F

Facilities, test	266
Fatal heart detector	239
Fibrillation, ventricular	148
Filter	
and flame photometer	225
ECG	24
Flame photometer	225
Flow detector, Doppler	237
Flow meter, Doppler	50
FM	
narrow band	202
receiver	206
recording	119
telemetry	201
transmitter	203
Free-running sweep	73
Frequency response	
blood pressure	51
chart recorders	133
ECG	16, 30
oscilloscope	69
stylus	143
vertical amplifier	74

G

Galvanometer, PMMC	17, 133, 134
Gas	
blood	216, 319
measurements	319
pulmonary	319
Gating amplifier	75
Geiger counter	219, 222
Generator	
electrosurgical	165
square wave	75
Ground	
equipotential	290
reference	17
fault interrupter (GFI)	277
Guard shield	99

H

Heart	
phonocardiograph	184
pressure	48
rate	91
voltage	11
Heart detector, fetal	239
Hemostasis	169
High-voltage power supplies	305
Holter monitor	189
Horizontal deflection	68
Hot tip stylus	133

I

Idler roller, strip chart	21
Image intensifier	312
Impedance pneumograph	261
Ink stylus	21, 132
high velocity	132
Instrument	
recording	118
scientific	210
test	266
ultrasonic	228
Instrumentation, calibration	278
Intensifer, image	312
Intensity modulation	68
Intensive care unit (ICU) monitor	115
Interference, power line	25
Intra-aortic balloon pump	245
Ion	13
Ionization chamber	219
Isolated electrical system	291
Isolation amplifier	99

J

Joule	149

K

Kidney dialysis machine	320
Korotkoff sounds	49
Kymograph	317

L

Lab equipment	
cardiograph	180
catheterization	180
computerized	187
exercise ECG	186
Holter monitors	189
phonocardiograph	184
Lamp, trigger	105
Lapping pens	132
Lead	
augmented	17
bipolar limb	17
Einthoven Triangle	17
electrocardiograph	14, 15
unipolar limb	17
V	18
Leakage current	274
Leg, ECG	17
Limit alarm	105
Linear voltage differential transformer	43
Lissajous figure	68
Lown waveform	154
Lung machine	314

M

Magnetic deflection	69
Maintenance	
central monitors	127
preventive	109
strip chart recorder	139, 142
Manuals, service	268
Marker stylus	136
Medical	
instrumentation calibration	278
oscilloscope	67
Megohmmeter	274
Membrane, cell	11
Memory	
ECG recorder	261
recirculating	86
scratch pad	86
shift register	86

Meter, pH	210, 213
Microammeter	274
Microphonics	240
Microshock	284, 286
Minute volume	316
Modulation	
FM	202
frequency	202
intensity	68
Modulator, cardiomemory	262
Monitor	
alarm	91, 119
bedside	90, 116
blood gases	115
blood pressure	62, 93
CCU	115
central	115
computerized	123
display systems	119
Holter	189
ICU	115
multibed	115
OR	115
oscilloscope	84
portable	90
recording instruments	118
systems	95
temperature	115
diagnostic, ECG	24
Multibed monitor	115
Multichannel oscilloscope	75

N

Narrow-band FM	202
Ni-cad battery	113
Non-fade display	69, 82

O

Operating room (OR) monitor	115
Operational amplifier	104
Oscillator	
cut	170
sweep	72
voltage controlled	119
Oscillography	67
Oscilloscope	
free-running	73
frequency response	69
medical	67
monitor	84
multichannel	75
non-fade display	82
recurrent sweep	73
sweep circuits	69
testing	88

P

Pacemaker	91
Paddle, patient	153
Paper	
brake	136
drive	136
ECG	19
loading	142
strip chart	20
Paste, electrode	24
Patient	
cable	16
electrodes	16
paddle	153
Peak-holding circuit	64
Pen	
hollow	132
ink	132
lapping	132
maintenance	139
protection	144
strip chart	20
Period, repolarization	13
Phonocardiographs	184
pH meter	210, 213
Phosphorous	67
Photocell, trigger	105
Photoelectric effect	297
Photometer	225
Photomultiplier tube	220
Photon	220
Photoplethysmograph	38
Photoresistor	38
trigger	105
Piezoelectric transducer	230
Plethysmograph transducer	37
PMMC galvanometer	17, 133, 134
Pneumograph, impedance	261
Pneumotachometer	245, 256, 260
Portable	
defibrillator	149
monitor	90, 111
Potassium	11
Potential	
action	13
bioelectronic	34
resting	13
skin	11
Power-line, interference	25
Preamplifier	
ECG	24, 98
vertical	74

Pressure
- air — 49
- arterial — 48, 115
- blood — 115
- diastolic — 48
- swan-ganz — 115
- systolic — 48
- transducer, calibration — 45
- venous — 115

Preventive maintenance — 109
Pulmonary gases — 319
Push-pull — 16
P wave — 15

Q

QRS complex — 15

R

Radiation detector — 217, 222
Radio telemetry, cardiac — 196
Raster — 69
Ratio digital voltmeter — 194
Receiver, cardiac telemetry — 206
Recirculating memory — 86
Recorder
- cardiomemory — 262
- drum type — 131
- dual trace — 131
- electronics — 139
- servorecorder — 145
- strip chart — 19, 95, 118, 128
- X-Y recorder — 145

Recording instruments — 118
Records, service — 268
Rectal temperature probe — 37
Recurrent sweep — 73
Reference, ground — 17
Reflected wave — 233
Refracted wave — 234
Repolarization period — 13
Resistance, dark — 105
Respiratory measurements — 314
Resting potential — 13
Right leg amplifier — 99
Roller, strip chart — 20
R wave — 15, 74, 91
- detection — 158

S

Safety
- electrical — 282
- inspections — 274

Sanborn configuration — 29

Scatter reduction — 311
Scientific instruments — 210
Scintillation counter — 220
Scratch-pad memory — 86
Screen — 67
Service
- manuals — 268
- records — 268

Servorecorder — 145
Shield, guard — 99
Shift-register memory — 86
Shock
- dangerous situations — 287
- electrical — 179, 282
- microshock — 284, 286

Skin, potential — 11
Snell's law — 234
Sodium — 11
Sonic wave — 228
Sound wave — 231
Spark gap coagulator — 171
Sphygmomanometer — 49
Spirometer — 317
Square-wave generator — 75
Stationary defibrillator — 151
Stethoscope — 49
Stimulus, cell — 13
Strain guage transducer — 39
Strip chart
- drive roller — 20
- idler roller — 21
- paper — 20
- stylus — 20

Strip chart recorder — 19, 95, 118, 128
- drum type — 131
- dual trace — 131
- electronics — 139
- frequency response — 133
- maintenance — 139, 142
- paper drive — 137
- servorecorder — 145

Stroke volume — 189
Stylus
- damping — 143
- hollow pen — 132
- hot tip — 133
- ink — 21
- maintenance — 139
- marker — 136
- protection — 144
- thermal — 21, 133

Summing amplifier — 77
Surgery, electrosurgical generator — 165
Swan-ganz pressure — 115
Sweep circuit, oscilloscope — 69

Sweep	
free-running	73
oscillator	72
recurrent	73
triggered	73
Synchronization, cardioverter	158
Synchronous detector	60
Systole	48, 93

T

Telemetry	
cardiac	196
FM	201
Temperature	
monitor	115
rectal probe	37
transducer	36
Terms, X-ray	313
Test equipment, special	269
Test instruments	266
Thermal stylus	21, 33
Thermistor	36, 190, 257
Thermocouple	36
Thermodilution	190
Thyratron	174
Time	232
Trachea	315
Transducer	
air flow	259
blood pressure	39
calibration	45
crystal	46
extending usefulness	46
LVDT	43
medical	34
piezoelectric	230
plethysmograph	37
spirometer	318
strain guage	39
temperature	36
thermistor	257
ultrasonic	229
ultrasonic, testing	242
Transformer, LVDT	43
Transmitter, cardiac telemetry	202, 203
Trigger, lamp/photocell	105
Triggered sweep	73
Tube	
cathode ray	67
photomultiplier	220
X-ray	301
T wave	156

U

Ultrasonic	
instruments	228
transducers	229
Instruments	
Doppler flow detector	237
echoencephalographs	243
fetal heart detector	239
servicing	240
testing transducers	242
Ultrasound	228
Unipolar electrIsurgery	167
Unipolar limb leads	17

V

Vector pattern	68
Velocity	46
Venous pressure	115
Ventricle	48
Ventricular fibrillation	148
Vertical amplifier	74
Vertical deflection	68
V leads	18
Voltage	
common mode	24
differential	24, 57
heart	11
skin	11
X-ray supplies	305
Voltage-controlled oscillator	119
Voltmeter, ratio digital	194
Volume, minute	316

W

Wall, cell	11
Water spirometer	317
Watt-second	149
Wave	
reflected	233
refracted	234
sonic	228
Waveform	
ECG	101
Lown	154
parade	84
Wide-band FM	202
Work, memory	84
Workbenches	267

X

X-ray	219
apparatus	294, 308
classification	307
image intensifiers	312
properties	294
scatter reduction	311
terms	313
tubes	301
X-Y recorder	145

Y

Yoke, deflection	68